AMERICAN MEDICINE AS CULTURE

AMERICAN MEDICINE AS CULTURE

HOWARD F. STEIN

WITH THE EDITORIAL ASSISTANCE
OF MARGARET A. STEIN

Routledge
Taylor & Francis Group
LONDON AND NEW YORK

First published 1990 by Westview Press

Published 2018 by Routledge
52 Vanderbilt Avenue, New York, NY 10017
2 Park Square, Milton Park, Abingdon, Oxon OX14 4RN

Routledge is an imprint of the Taylor & Francis Group, an informa business

Library of Congress Cataloging-in-Publication Data
Stein, Howard F.
American medicine as culture/Howard F. Stein; with the editorial assistance of Margaret A. Stein.
p. cm.
Includes bibliographical references.
ISBN 0-8133-0737-6
1. Social medicine—United States. 2. Medicine—United States—Philosophy. I. Stein, Margaret A. II. Title.
[DNLM: 1. Anthropology, Cultural. 2. Medicine-United States. W 21 S819a]
RA418.3.U6S74 1990
306.4′61′093—dc20 89-22711
CIP

ISBN 13: 978-0-367-00319-7 (hbk)

ISBN 13: 978-0-367-15306-9 (pbk)

Dedicated to

Lawrence W. Patzkowsky, M.D., Director,
Donald C. Karns, M.D.,
Kurt S. Frantz, M.D.,
and
John W. Ronck, M.D.,
Faculty Physicians,
Enid Family Medicine Clinic, Enid, Oklahoma

with gratitude and friendship.

Man's most desperate problem is to know his fears and not be so ruled by them that they destroy his creative resources, making it impossible for him to anticipate the ramifying consequences of his actions. Socrates said, "Know thyself"; and this must naturally include, "Know thy fear."

—Jules Henry, *Culture Against Man*

Contents

Tables and Figures

Tables

Figures

PREFACE

THIS BOOK SITUATES BIOMEDICINE within American culture and argues that the very organization and practice of medicine are themselves cultural. It offers answers to the questions, What is cultural about American biomedicine? What is the nature of the fit between the culture of medicine and the wider society and historic epoch it serves and represents? What is the nature of the links among individual development of the future practitioner, medical career choice, professional socialization, institutional organization, and practitioner role in the larger society? This work is thus simultaneously about medicine and an inquiry into what medicine is about.

More broadly, this book addresses additional questions beyond the definitionally clinical realm. What is culture? How is culture organized? What needs and purposes does culture serve? In addition to being a study of American medicine as a cultural system (that is, as an ethnomedicine), this book is a meditation on the nature of culture as well.

Physicians, other medical practitioners, the popular media, and lay public alike often designate biomedicine as "medical science." Ronald Munson (1981), however, shows that although science and scientific research are tools of medical practice, the equation of medicine with science is spurious. Official, formal, scientific models are part of the picture in medicine, but they are by no means all of it. They are not the focus of this book; they are addressed in literally thousands of medical textbooks and journal articles. Moreover, the appeal to the ideology of science is analyzed as part of the complex cultural texture of biomedicine. Medicine uses science in highly symbolic, metaphoric ways. In this work, I demonstrate the symbolic construction of clinical reality within American biomedicine, a construction that utilizes but is not reducible to the discoveries of the chemists and bacteriologists of the late nineteenth and early twentieth centuries and their contemporary successors.

If biomedicine is not culturally monolithic and homogeneous (see Hahn and Gaines 1985), neither is it so heterogeneous and idiosyncratic as to be random. In this work, subtle patternings and themes that organize, underlie, and pervade biomedicine's diversity are identified (compare Payer 1988). By the time the reader finishes the book's final pages, this portrait of what is distinctively, culturally American as well as universal about biomedicine should be easily recognizable.

The focus of this book is the implicit or informal, largely unconscious models that influence medicine. These consist of a subject matter that, although acted upon and admonished in medical training, is rarely formalized in the doctrinal literature of medicine. American medicine is a cultural system, not simply a congeries of physicians and nurses, medical specialties, and institutions. It has an internal coherence based on a system of core values, metaphors, beliefs, attitudes, and themes that in turn are influenced by a deeper, largely unconscious core. The cultural value orientations of activity, mastery over nature, individualism, and future orientation (Kluckhohn and Strodtbeck 1961; Spiegel 1971); the worldview in which the human body, mind, and, most recently, the family are seen as machine-like and therefore "fixable" by clinical technologies; the philosophies of pragmatism and utilitarianism according to which functioning itself is the highest goal and human and clinical problems are simplifiable to dysfunctions—these, together with their internal, shared meanings in official medical culture and in the wider American folk or popular culture, crop up as the implicit cultural medical model.

Following Robert Hahn and Atwood Gaines, I approach biomedicine as "a cultural artifact, a complex human product shaped from human and nonhuman resources, constantly responding to historical circumstances which are in turn human transformations of themselves and their environments" (1985: 5). An ethnographic discourse on biomedicine reveals how the ***biological body is culturalized***—that is, how the body, knowledge about it, and clinical ways of dealing with it are themselves cultural artifacts that are then projected onto and into the body, thereby becoming the very nature of human biology and of that applied human biology called medicine. As Margaret Lock notes, "The body is socially and culturally produced and historically situated: it is both a part of nature and society but, at the same time, a representation of the way that nature and society are conceived" (1987: 8). Biomedicine is amenable to the same type of cultural, ethnographically based interpretation as are other ethnomedical systems. The contradictions and ambivalences within medical culture play out and embody themes that pervade the wider American culture that biomedicine serves, preserves, represents, and is employed to heal. When young physicians during their apprenticeship (intern and residency) years start a day with the exhortation, "Let's hit the wards and stamp out some disease," they are doing far more than translating dispassionate scientific investigation into clinical work. They are engaging in cultural roles and enacting largely unexamined cultural mandates for immediate and aggressive action in response to any circumstance. This book attempts to make explicit the often unofficial cultural agendas of medical work and training.

The official and officially taught medical worldview consists of (1) the "basic sciences": anatomy, physiology, biochemistry, microbiology, pathology; (2) the belief that medical science is and should be based upon rational, scientific, dispassionate, objective, professional judgment; (3) the belief that disease and its attendant suffering are ultimately to be understood in terms of pathological entities, organic in nature, and that treatment optimally consists of a technological procedure or intervention that results in a cure; (4) the belief that medical knowledge and skills are best organized by creating specialties around "organ systems." This official ethos is only the surface or manifest part of a complex cultural picture. I argue that for practitioners and teachers, the biomedical ethos often functions less as scientific reality testing than as an intricate personal, group, institutional, and cultural defense against the experience of vulnerability, fragility, infirmity, aggression, sexual desire, passivity, and death—in short, abhorred qualities or characteristics associated with patienthood. One goal of this book is to understand the dynamics and meaning of that form of contextualization—one that anthropologists are wont to call decontextualization—labeled as "biological reductionism."

In discussing Roland Littlewood and Maurice Lipsedge's (1986) analysis of the relation among culture, psychopathology, and biomedicine in the dominant culture, Joel Paris writes that "whereas the ideology which binds symptoms to culture in traditional societies tends to be religious, in the West contemporary science and biomedicine provide an analogous framework" (1988: 107). If medical science and technology possess a magico-religious aura, biomedicine's disavowed subjectivity can be equally seen in the day-to-day encounter of practitioner with others' vulnerabilities and infirmities. In addition to serving the patient, medical practice serves for the practitioner as a formidable bulwark against recognizing the common bond with the patient, that is, the human condition.

Throughout this book I state what I have recognized as a fundamental, implicit, organizing theme, if not axiom, in biomedicine: "A doctor (or practitioner) is not a patient." Howard Brody eloquently writes that

> just as to be sick is to sense an unpleasant disruption of the self-body unity ("ontological assault") . . . to perceive sickness or disability in others is to be reminded of one's own vulnerability and mortality in an equally unpleasant and threatening way. Thus much reaction to sickness that superficially appears to be solely outward-directed (that is, toward meeting the needs of the sick person) is in reality also inner-directed as an attempt to remove, resolve, or transcend this inner threat to integrity (1987: 110).

This study shall show how biomedicine—from medical practice to medical symbolism to medical education—never leaves the realm of the personal, even as the process of professionalization inculcates the sought-after belief that subjectivity has been left behind if not abolished.

In a *Family Systems Medicine* editorial on maintaining complexity, Donald A. Bloch, M.D., addresses the issue of "modulating the *total volume* of information and its organized complexity" in health care (1987a: 147). He later writes that in medical practice

> not noticing, indeed forgetting, as well as constructing simplifications is as essential to functional integrity as including all necessary information. Much of what passes for standard instrumental practice should be understood as information management. Who among us has not palpably experienced the confusion that goes with "knowing more about that than I want to"? Medical procedures are often organized to protect against unwanted information—information about despair; mutilation; about the jaws of the traps of life that bite into us all; and even about good news, sometimes more upsetting than bad (1987a: 148).

This book examines the cultural context in which certain kinds of medical complexity are welcomed as challenges and other kinds of medical complexity are ignored, discounted, or disdained; the context in which simplification into small, discrete, isolated, disembodied, and thereby manageable visceral parts performs a largely protective function against the despair, mutilation, and bad news/good news traps to which Bloch refers.

Inseparable from Bloch's issue of the "total volume" of information is the type of information accepted (sought) or rejected. Physicians eagerly, aggressively (to use a frequently and zestfully uttered physician term) seek larger and larger quantities of certain kinds of information and tend to feel less overwhelmed by it than they are intimidated by psychosocial data. From sixteen years' work with physicians as their teacher, clinical behavioral science supervisor, and participant observer, I have learned to ask of myself and of them, "What don't I/they want to know (about the patient, about the disease, about oneself), and why?" What Bloch calls "functional integrity" is, in part at least, one's defensive organization, the way one regulates self-esteem and assaults upon it, the way one maintains a sense of cohesiveness—often at the expense of the patient and patient care. For to know too much is to be vulnerable to hurting too much oneself.

The classical notion of the physician as "wounded healer" is anathema to the need for this type of social distance between doctor and patient. Despite the official ideology of patient care, for many practitioners the treatment of disease and of people who are ill is more a means than an end. For many, an unstated purpose of patient care is to reassure the physician (and medical staff/colleagues) via treatment and conquest of disease. Bloch's meditation about complexity and simplification in American biomedicine opens a rich trove of cultural issues that constitutes the subject matter of this book. This volume studies American medicine as a whole culture, not in the sense of including everything (the illusion of completeness) but rather in the sense of describing and interpreting key themes, patterns, and symbols that pervade and organize medicine and that link it with currents in American society. Beneath the bewildering diversity of individuals, ideologies, institutions, and specialty cultures is a unifying texture of meaning large enough to be called a system of meaning.

An abundance of books approach American medicine from sociological, economic, or historical points of view. This book, which offers a depth psychology-informed anthropological account, is meant less to supplant these others than to supplement them. Anthropological accounts are typically written by anthropological fieldworkers who spend at least a year doing participant observation and open-ended interviews among some group not of the fieldworker's own culture. Further, the resulting written and published accounts (scholarly presentations, journal articles, and books) are for the most part read by and written for audiences consisting of the scholar's or fieldworker's behavioral science colleagues. This book and its author depart considerably from a standard anthropological rule (if not taboo) that one should not—even cannot—study one's own "tribe." As an American and as a faculty member and clinical teacher in medical departments since 1972, I have long been deeply involved in the culture that I am about to describe and interpret. Yet, it is only within the past five or six years that I have begun to conduct a systematic, self-conscious study of my own work environment.

Permit me briefly to explain this evolution. As a graduate student in medical and psychological anthropology from 1967 to 1972, and early in my professional career as clinical teacher, I expected—and was expected by anthropological and medical colleagues alike—to train medical students, physician residents, and other health professionals how to take into account patients' cultural belief and behavioral systems, to teach them how to work with patients from cultures different from those of the student or practitioner, and to prepare them to be careful and compassionate listeners with their patients. Anthropological training at that time closely resembled medical training in that the observer's, researcher's, and clinician's subjectivity was supposed to be held in check. Professional training was expected to be a guarantor of objectivity. In those days, "reflexivity" in anthropology and "subjectivity" in medicine were fearsome and arcane matters discussed by only a few. Nonetheless, early in my work as clinical teacher and supervisor, I began to notice that many problems that interns or residents would present to me as patient problems bore the weight of the physicians' own characters, unconscious conflicts, and issues in their own families or cultures of origin, all of which contributed to the distortion of the clinical relationship and to the diminution of the quality of care. From this was born my interest in clinical relationships—indeed all varieties of relationships in medicine, including those between professionals—and in unconscious aspects of those relationships (Stein 1985g; Stein and Apprey 1985, 1987, 1990).

No sooner had I begun to focus upon countertransference in clinical dyads than I began to realize that I needed (depending on one's preferred metaphor) to cast a wider net or use a wide angle telescope. Having long participated in various types of clinical groups (in academic and community practice settings alike), I began to notice and hear a wide variety of clinical attitudes and beliefs voiced by clinicians and to observe treatment and doctor-patient interaction practices, discrepant with the official biomedical model. These occurred in a wide variety of settings—clinical decisionmaking conferences, case conferences, formal medical seminars and grand rounds, informal hallway consultations between practitioners and staff, and so forth. I soon came to realize that although in earlier work I had briefly mentioned and illustrated small and large group dynamics, and although I had always framed clinical relationships against the background of some vague notion of medical and American culture, it was now time for me to expand this picture of "the subjective in medicine" to encompass group, institutional, and larger cultural processes.

A cornerstone of American medicine, the doctor-patient relationship is enshrouded by an aura and by values of privacy, confidentiality, and exclusivity. A widely taught, and publicly expected, medical ideal is that the physician works in behalf of the best interest of each individual patient and leaves group and societal matters outside that sacred space. One of the main tasks of this book is to demonstrate how truly crowded—with people, their mental representations, group agendas and rules—a patient encounter in an examination or hospital room can be and the consequences of this for clinical thinking and practice. Just as I learned that teaching a medical student or resident how to listen to or talk with a patient is always mediated by that individual student or resident's individual conscious and unconscious forces (together with my own), I have likewise learned that teaching the subject of clinical behavioral science is always mediated by the ***group processes***, ***institutional structure***, and ***professional cultures*** through which the ultimate subject of medicine—the patient "out there"—is refracted. As I hope to demonstrate throughout this book, "individual" and "group," "personality" and "culture" are not two distinct entities or processes but are aspects of dynamics that permeate medicine and all of human life.

The organization of this book is as follows. The Introduction orients the reader to the ethnographic study and anthropological interpretation of American biomedicine as a cultural system. Chapter 1 explores the core values by which medicine is organized. Chapter 2 identifies and interprets key metaphors and symbols that undergird the identity system of medicine. Chapter 3 discusses the moralistic role played by medicine in and in behalf of society and demonstrates how the function of social control lies beneath the more explicit functions of beneficence and the naturalistic search for disease etiology. Although a widespread image of the physician (and other health care workers as well) is that of the solitary individualist, Chapter 4 describes the profound influence group dynamics has upon medical thinking and practice. In turn, Chapter 5 considers the deep split within biomedical culture between care-giving and the pursuit of financial self-interest, a split made all the more ironic and paradoxical by the proliferation of corporate medicine in the early 1980s.

Chapters 6 and 7 turn attention from professional thinking and practice to the process by which one becomes and wishes to become a biomedical practitioner. Chapter 6 describes the professional socialization process of medical school, internship, and residency by which a layperson is transformed into a member of the medical guild. Through a series of life-history vignettes, Chapter 7 establishes linkage among individual physicians' family-of-origin experiences, unconscious structure, and the choice and meaning of medical practice as at least in part a solution to developmental issues. Beginning at the macrolevel of culture, the book culminates at the microlevel of individual personality and thus offers an interpretation, for American culture and elsewhere, of how individual psychodynamic structure and group culture are not distinct entities but facets of a unitary dynamic process. The brief Conclusion advocates the wider usage of the ethnographic approach in future research into the culture of medicine, in medical teaching and supervision, and in the formulation of medically related social policy.

As a discourse on the culture of medicine, this work is addressed to a wide audience inclusive of behavioral scientists of various disciplines (medical anthropologists, medical sociologists, clinical psychologists, social workers, psychoanalysts, pastoral counselors, family therapists, family social scientists) teaching and/or conducting research in medical settings; physicians of primary care (family medicine, internal medicine, ambulatory pediatrics), psychiatric, and other medical specialties teaching in medical settings or working in community practices; clinicians or professionals of any field who are interested in better understanding and fostering health-related change in their own institutional and professional cultures; and members of the lay public interested in better understanding the complexities of clinical culture and their place within it.

It is my contention that we can only begin to solve medical and social problems if we identify them correctly in the first place and understand the stake we often have in their misdefinition. It is not enough for health professionals to direct their clinical gaze outward toward patients' and families' life situations and worldviews in order to intervene (or recognize the constraints on intervention). We in the health and health-related professions must take at least as seriously the cultural world of medicine and identify those broader issues in American culture that underlie the often acrimonious debate about public policy. The present volume is a step in that direction.

Howard F. Stein
Oklahoma City, Oklahoma

ACKNOWLEDGMENTS

IF I MAY PARAPHRASE John Donne, no author, no book, is an island. The stimulation, encouragement, and tenacity of many people helped make this book possible. When I first arrived at the University of Oklahoma Health Sciences Center in 1978, then chair of family medicine, Norman Haug, M.D., took me aside and said somewhat as follows: "I know that you've done a lot of research and writing on ethnicity. In no way do I want to discourage you from continuing that line of development. However, I'd like you to give some thought to looking around in medicine. You might find something interesting to write about." Dr. Haug, having long departed academe for private practice, remains a "guardian spirit" of this project.

I have been blessed with many mentors (now friends), inside and outside of biomedicine, who have steadfastly encouraged my use of depth psychology as a tool in the study of biomedical culture and its history: Lloyd deMause, George De Vos, Ph.D., Henry Ebel, Ph.D., Warren Gadpaille, M.D., Weston La Barre, Ph.D., Jeanne Spurlock, M.D., G. Gayle Stephens, M.D., and Vamık D. Volkan, M.D.

Soul-searching and culture-searching discussions (and correspondence) with the following colleagues have influenced the ideas developed in this volume: Maurice Apprey, Ph.D., Lisa C. Baker, Ph.D., Alvah Cass, M.D., Roger Elliott, P.A., M.P.H., Robert F. Hill, Ph.D., Thomas Johnson, Ph.D., James W. Mold, M.D., Charles Nuckolls, Ph.D., Lorna Amarasingham Rhodes, Ph.D., Johanna Shapiro, Ph.D., and Jeffrey R. Steinbauer, M.D.

Three reference librarians at the University of Oklahoma Health Sciences Center Library have generously conducted countless bibliographic odysseys on my behalf: Virgil Jones, Joy Summers, and Ilse von Brauchitsch.

Without the diligent and creative editing by Margaret A. Stein, M.A., this book would likely not exist. Ms. LaVonne Wolfe assisted in the word processing of this book.

To Dean Birkenkamp, executive editor, Westview Press, goes my deep gratitude for making possible the fruition of a project that is both interdisciplinary and ambitious—what some colleagues have politely termed "neither fish nor fowl."

From my father, Charles D. Stein, I learned to listen to a symphony and to read an orchestral score as a whole, not just as melody here, harmony there, counterpoint, orchestration elsewhere. From him I have learned to discern the music of a group, the texture of a culture. When I was a child, I attended Pittsburgh Symphony concerts with him and often thought him to doze off amid glorious music. I was wrong. From him I also learned that sometimes in order truly to hear, one must close one's eyes to avoid being distracted by sight.

H.F.S.

INTRODUCTION

An Anthropological Interpretation of American Biomedical Culture

People live in groups, which are variously called bands, tribes, chiefdoms, ethnic groups, nation-states, communities, empires, religions, neighborhoods, organizations, institutions, corporations, and so forth. Into some of these (for instance, multi-generational ethnic groups or tribes) people are born and learn future adult roles and identities. Into others (for instance, corporations or professions) people are recruited as adults from the larger society and are socialized (trained) for membership in that group. In either case, people feel that they belong to, and identify with, these groups. Culture, as I use it in this book, refers to a shared and constantly renegotiated sense of definition and affiliation with a particular group or groups and the action that derives from and validates this self-definition. People often say, "I *am* a Baptist, black, Hungarian, Jew, mill worker, lawyer, physician, nurse. . . ." The sense of shared identity, of overlapping meanings and their associated symbols and rituals, becomes expressed in the fantasy of "we-ness." "I am" becomes "we are," and vice versa. Further, what "we do" follows from what "we are."

For many influential late nineteenth and early twentieth century social theorists—Emile Durkheim, Edmund Spencer, Arthur R. Radcliffe-Brown, Alfred Kroeber, Franz Boas, Ruth Benedict—society and culture could not and should not be described and analyzed as the product of persons. For some theorists, each society or social group had its distinctive culture; for others, the culture itself was regarded as the social unit. However, common to these writers was the belief that cultures or societies were things unto themselves with forces distinctly their own. According to this view of society-as-organism, people were more "products" of their culture than active fashioners of it. Through the socialization or enculturation experience of being a child and growing up within a group, one internalized that culture and eventually bore its stamp. Cultures, ethoses, institutions all felt palpably "real" to those who invested their very selves in them and who incorporated these values and ideals into their own psychic structures. Organizations and societies all felt "larger than life," something to which people belonged that gave them a sense of place and purpose. Entire anthropological theories, notably the "superorganic" models of culture advanced by Alfred Kroeber (1948) and Leslie White (1949), supported this virtually universal lay or folk perception: that culture was somehow there, immortal, beyond the mere existence of the individual.

Yet, reifications notwithstanding, organizations and societies truly exist only as a result of what individuals in groups believe and do. In *The Social Construction of Reality*, sociologists Peter Berger and Thomas Luckmann write that

> the objectivity of the institutional world, however massive it may appear to the individual, is a humanly produced, constructed objectivity. The process by which the externalized products of human activity attain the character of objectivity is objectivation. The institutional world is objectivated human activity, and so is every single institution. In other words, despite the objectivity that marks the social world in human experience, it does not thereby acquire an ontological status apart from the human activity that produced it (1966: 60–61).

Berger and Luckmann then note "the paradox that man is capable of producing a world that he then experiences as something other than a human product" (1966: 61).

It seems to me that we cannot, even if we try, stray from human biology. Human relationships, language, symbolism, and culture itself are all expressions of species-specific biology and efforts to cope with biological inheritance. The experience of being a child and of being a familial animal constitutes much of the substance from which culture is built (La Barre 1951, 1954, 1972). Through culture we tend to respond to, if not continually recreate, society and nature as though they were our bodies, our early mother-infant symbioses, our families, and the contents of our primitive psyches.

Contrary to what many social scientists have thought for nearly a century, the family is not the agent and executor of the internalization of (impersonal, external) culture. Instead, culture is largely a result of the externalization and recreation of family (La Barre 1954). Culture is created and sustained by the outward proliferation of largely out-of-awareness family contexts. As Edward Hall (1977) notes, people experience and respond to others, society, and the environment as though these were "extensions" of self. This phenomenon is at the heart of what psychoanalysts and psychiatrists (see for example, Devereux 1967; Kernberg 1965) call ***transference*** and ***countertransference***. As I shall use these terms, transference refers to the patient's unconscious reaction to the practitioner, and countertransference refers to the clinician's unconscious response to the patient. Their distinction thus lies in the "who" rather than the "what" of the subjective reaction. Both terms refer to perceiving, feeling, and acting toward current persons as though one were reliving the tribulations and passions of one's formative, childhood experiences. These unwitting processes serve deep, out-of-awareness purposes for the management of anxiety, which is one of the main functions of culture (Róheim 1943).

A complex network of thinking (perception, cognition), feeling (affect), and behavior (roles) organizes the group into a cultural system. This network includes values, attitudes, beliefs, rules, roles, statuses, together with underlying, mostly unconscious, fantasies, anxieties, conflicts, and feelings that are expressed indirectly through symbols or directly through action. This latter, often termed *acting out* in psychiatric literature, refers to deeds that, although rationalized by those who are performing them, are done in order to avoid remembering and feeling painful and forbidden things. Many anthropologists in recent years prefer to limit the definition of culture to cognitive, symbolic elements and to distinguish them from behavior. As this book explains, I find it useful to see them as part of a single system, but, in contrast to many anthropologists, especially those of the 1930s and 1940s, I do not see this system as static, consistent, or necessarily harmonious. Cultural wholes are ridden by conflict, ambivalence, contradiction; nevertheless, their participants or inhabitants may consciously—but for deeply unconscious reasons—perceive and experience cultures as far more smooth sailing than they are.

The approach I take to medical culture and to universal cultural process is that people are constantly creating, negotiating, revising, internalizing, and externalizing their culture and that culture is always a process and never a thing—even when a group's inhabitants (and social scientist apologists!) perceive and experience their group as something beyond them of which they are a part. I show that even in institutional and large group-psychology, the individual is never merely a passive product or conduit of culture.

Now, I do not imply that the early theorists' organismic cultural monolith was without fissures. Ruth Benedict was a passionate poet striving to have her individual voice heard, and Alfred Kroeber's magisterial volume *Anthropology* (1948) concluded with the clarion call that anthropology's foundation—like that of culture itself—should be the individual:

> While psychosomatic individuals do and must precede societies of individuals and the cultures of human societies—must precede them conceptually and evolutionistically—and while psychology is therefore in one sense a science that underlies both sociology and anthropology, nevertheless, in this mid-twentieth century, we have the curious situation that sociologists and anthropologists perhaps explain their proper phenomena less often in terms of the underlying psychic factors than psychologists are cognizant of the overlying sociocultural ones (1948: 848).

As American society's dominant clinical ideology and institution, ***biomedicine*** is organized according to the "medical model," which is its philosophical and methodological foundation, and which now serves both allopathic (M.D.) and osteopathic (D.O.) medicine. Kroeber's words bring me to the central question of this study (and to what deserves to be the guiding question behind any cultural inquiry): What is the culture of American biomedicine for? (What is culture for?) That is, what meanings, purposes, fantasies, and motives does it serve for those who participate in it? How do its participants use, create, revise, invest in, and repudiate it? This book explores the cultural production of medical knowledge and practice, *and* inquires into the processes that produce culture as biomedicine's context. Although in this book I at times discuss medical roles and values as abstractions, I do so because they are nodal points in a shared mental world—never because I believe they somehow exist apart from those who breathe significance into them.

Culture is not relative only to itself. We must continue to ask what people use culture *for*. If, as Richard Koenigsberg writes, "cultural ideas, beliefs and values may be viewed . . . as an institutionalization and social embodiment of primal human phantasies" (1975: viii; also see Devereux 1980a; La Barre 1954,

1972, 1984; Spiro 1982a; Stein and Hill 1977; Muensterberger 1970; deMause 1974b, 1982; Stierlin 1976; Binion 1976, 1981; Gonen 1975; and Erikson 1958, 1963a, 1974), how do we go about understanding the process by which such institutionalization and embodiment take place?

The Nature of Ethnographic Fieldwork

To answer the preceding question, I employ a psychoanalytically sensitive ethnographic method. The goal of this method is a descriptive and interpretive account of a group's way of life, so as to evoke and offer insight into what it is like to be a member of that group. Such a narrative is based on many months if not years of observation, participant observation, open-ended as well as directed interviews, examination of documentary materials, and other data-gathering methods—the whole of which is called "fieldwork." Whatever culture is relative to, it is also relative to the self of the observer and interpreter. In his analysis of Balinese cockfighting, Clifford Geertz writes that

> the culture of a people is an ensemble of texts, themselves ensembles, which the anthropologist strains to read over the shoulders of those to whom they properly belong. . . . As in more familiar exercises in close reading, one can start anywhere in a culture's repertoire of forms and end up anywhere else. . . . Societies, like lives, contain their own interpretations. One has only to learn how to gain access to them (1972: 29).

In this statement, Geertz crystallizes the anthropological approach, which aspires to comprehend a culture from its members' point of view. Any narrative—like any narrator—can go on endlessly. One goal of ethnography is to discern nodal points or themes that are played out in the multitude of variations (narratives). Moreover, an astute listener and observer (and clinically, an interpreter who helps the informant/patient to better understand himself or herself or the group to understand itself) can help the informant or patient to uncover texts and meanings that neither realized heretofore existed. In this book, my goal is to trace the articulation of contemporary medicine with wider cultural currents and to interpret the nature of the fit among individual practitioner, medicine, and culture. In the inquisitive spirit of Geertz's book, *The Interpretation of Cultures* (1973), my approach is to look over the shoulders of medical practitioners, practices, ideologies—themselves all "cultural texts"—to compose a "thick description" of various cultural texts from the natives' own viewpoints, and to demonstrate the utility and validity of a psychoanalytic approach to the interpretation of culture. The ethnographic method that gives the lead and direction to the informant(s) finds themes, motifs, and preoccupations in the informant's leading. The ethnographer of modern medicine can talk not only with people to elicit these central organizing ideas, feelings, and fantasies (also see Nurnberg and Shapiro 1983) but can approach the medical literature itself as a cultural text that will reveal medicine's central concerns at any given time.

Ethnography refers in part to the detailed description and interpretation of a group's way of life, beliefs, values, expectations, rules, conscious and unconscious levels of meaning, attitudes, roles, and the consequences of these for behavior. One strives to learn how the members of the group see, feel, experience, cognitively construct their world—that is, to comprehend the native or indigenous viewpoint (for example, the peasant who plows Mother Earth versus the farmer who plows a fall acreage or financial investment). This cultural construction of reality often differs markedly from the external observer's viewpoint (for example, the medical epidemiologist who might approach the incidence and prevalence of a disease through official United States Census tract units or through the boundaries of community mental centers' "catchment areas" rather than in terms of the indigenous ethnic, religious, or rural community's definition of its own boundaries). In terms borrowed from linguistics, these two frameworks correspond to the ***emic*** and ***etic*** constructions, respectively. One goal of ethnographic work is to help build a corpus of rich, intensive emic studies that further permit one to develop a comprehensive cross-cultural ethnological etic theory, not only about the individual group one studied but about commonalities and variations in being human. Ideally, these methods and models help us to know what is culture or era specific and what is species specific, that is, universal.

The ethnographic method—which can be dated from the anthropological fieldwork of Bronislaw Malinowski in the Trobriand Islands, off northern Papua New Guinea during World War I—consists of systematically eliciting knowledge of what it is like to live as a member of a particular group. Methods or techniques commonly used in ethnographic research include naturalistic and participant observation; open-ended or nondirective interview; long-term, intimate familiarity with the group achieved by working closely, if not living, with the group, often for years; and the selection of a number of key "informants," people knowledgeable of the group's meanings and history, who help one navigate, expand one's network, and avoid getting into too much trouble (for example, violating taboo).

Ethnographic research moves from the theoretical to the applied when the observer's goal is to ***help the studied group to do something*** (for example, solve some problem, achieve some task or goal; see Morley 1988) rather than simply to use knowledge derived from the study to build theory (and careers in more academic anthropology departments). For example, as a behavioral scientist who teaches and supervises in medical training settings, I study physician-patient relationships, family dynamics of patients and doctors, and the cultures of clinics and hospitals in order to teach more effectively and to help practitioners be better healers. Along the way, as a theoretical anthropologist, I use emic materials to construct etic theory about the nature of culture.

In ***Pragmatics of Human Communication***, Paul Watzlawick, Janet Beavin, and Don Jackson write that "a phenomenon remains unexplainable as long as the range of observations is not wide enough to include the context in which the phenomenon occurs" (1967: 20–21). Although this elegant formulation is true, to be even truer one must add to the ***range*** or ***breadth*** of observations their ***depth*** as well. Observational and clinical contexts are composed not only of assorted personnel and social units—individuals, families, institutions, communities, cultures—in various relationships; these units and relationships can be unconsciously linked by out-of-awareness feelings, meanings, fantasies, and wishes. In clinical teaching and theoretical work, I have been striving to build what might be called a psychoanalytic systems theory (Stein 1982d, 1985a, 1985g; Stein and Apprey 1985, 1987)—a phrase that to some might be a heresy and to others an oxymoron! This book continues that effort.

There is a common misperception in the United States that psychoanalytic therapy is "talk therapy," and likewise that psychoanalytic theory is simply a theory about words, their associations with other words, and their cognitive or symbolic (verbal) meanings. Although many psychoanalysts are not immune to the isolation of idea from affect, such a misapprehension of psychoanalytic thinking misses the whole point, and radical innovation, that psychoanalysis introduces: namely, the reintegration of feeling with thinking. Heinz Kohut writes that "Affects are at the heart of psychoanalytic knowledge. Words by themselves do not constitute the primary data of psychoanalysis. . . . What endows words and other symbolic structures with significance is the communication of affects" (1984: 172). I would add that what Kohut writes of "psychoanalytic knowledge" is equally true for ethnographic knowledge: that sentiment is an intrinsic part of all cultural structures, and of the observer's understanding of those structures, a point to which I shall return repeatedly in this study of American medicine.

Documentary research complements naturalistic and participant observation, open-ended and focused interviewing, and other direct, interpersonal field techniques. A careful perusal of the following documentary sources within the culture(s) of biomedicine has helped me to formulate, test, and corroborate impressions of patterns and meanings within biomedical culture and in the wider American culture: *The Journal of the American Medical Association, Family Medicine, The Journal of Family Practice, The New England Journal of Medicine, Modern Health Care, Family Systems Medicine, Medical Economics, The Society of Teachers of Family Medicine Newsletter, Family Practice News, American Medical News* (American Medical Association), *Continuing Education for the Family Physician*, and the academic programs and other promotional brochures from academic and professional medical societies.

As if this contextual complexity were not overwhelming enough for teacher and resident alike, I have discovered through sixteen years of clinical teaching and supervision that unconscious factors in teacher, intern, resident, and staff constantly affect all that we see and do, setting limits upon our clinical capacities and judgment (R. Smith 1984, 1986; R. Smith and Stein 1987). Physicians and social scientists are for the most part trained nowadays to pay virtually exclusive attention to "context," which is defined as the world "out there" of the patient and family. Yet, if we have learned anything from the near century of contributions from psychoanalysts and others influenced by psychoanalytic insights (Freud 1910: 144–145; Balint 1957; Binion 1981; deMause 1982; Devereux 1967; Katz 1984a; La Barre 1978; Stein 1985h; Stein and Apprey 1985, 1987), we know that we participate in the context we observe. By systematically understanding the process, dynamics, meaning of observation, inference, and intervention, we become more aware of where we stand and why and thereby liberate ourselves from inner compulsions to take exclusive theoretical and clinical stands.

Author's Experience as Data Base

This book is based on sixteen years' experience as clinical teacher, supervisor, and ethnographer in medical education settings. From 1972 to 1978, I taught in the Department of Psychiatry and Community Mental Health Center at Meharry Medical College in Nashville, Tennessee, working with medical students and with psychiatry and family medicine residents on the psychiatry service. Employed since 1978 in the Department of Family Medicine and the Physician's Associates (PAs) Program at the University of Oklahoma Health Sciences Center in Oklahoma City, Oklahoma, I have also coordinated the teaching of behavioral sciences in the rural, community-based residency programs in Enid and Shawnee, Oklahoma. In that time I have logged some 85,000 miles by car to the Enid and Shawnee sites alone.

Formally, I have been officially designated as a behavioral science teacher/supervisor of graduate PAs, interns, and residents and a consultant to the residency training programs proper rather than to the wider clinic settings. On "paper," in my formal job description, I teach medical students, physicians, and PAs. I have nonetheless negotiated a wider informal job description—with the encouragement of administrative and medical support staff alike—so that in effect the "net" of my interest and activity encompasses the entire training context. For instance, in the past I have coordinated monthly joint conferences between family practice residents and interns in pastoral counseling. I have offered supportive counseling for staff members as well as residents. I have been asked to contact and bring in speakers from the community for monthly clinic meetings attended by all employees and residents. I have arranged with a local county health department for a bimonthly conference offered by its director on family medicine and community medicine. Awareness of the clinic network, ideology, and conflicts positions me to have a sense of the whole that transcends any member or unit who brings to me the perspective of a part. Another way of putting this is that various clinical employers have come to value my role as internal ethnographer of their clinical, academic, and quasi-corporate cultures.

A further source of insight and vignettes for this book derives from my work as co-facilitator of intern, resident, and postresidency community practitioner Balint groups in the Department of Family Medicine, University of Oklahoma Health Sciences Center, Oklahoma City. These groups were inaugurated in the Oklahoma City residency program in 1984, where I now serve as Balint coordinator. The groups have consisted of three to sixteen intern or resident members (depending on a variety of scheduling constraints) plus two to five faculty members (physician and behavioral scientist) per group. These groups meet twice monthly for an hour or slightly more each. ***Balint groups***, as developed by psychoanalyst/psychiatrist Michael Balint among general practitioners in the United Kingdom (Balint 1957), consist of research-cum-training seminars in which participants present and discuss cases involving personally difficult physician-patient, physician-physician, and physician-staff relationships.

Balint groups, which have historically been more established and accepted in the United Kingdom than in the United States, are designed to complement formal, scientific, biomedical conferences. Ideally, Balint seminars are a safe place in which physicians can ventilate and better understand, for instance, cases about which they have intense, often disturbing feelings; cases in which they feel "stuck" in their interactions, in which their use of the same clinical problem-solving techniques fail to work; and cases in which the physician harbors an unrealistic expectation of the relationship with the patient or of medical procedures. In Balint, participants have the opportunity to slow down the harried pace of practice, to think over issues, and to show feelings that they do not permit themselves to show during patient care.

Although not intended to be therapy sessions, Balint seminar discussions are indirectly therapeutic in that they help presenter and other participants to understand emotional factors in the physician (and others in the case) that contribute to the vexing, nagging nature of the clinical or professional interaction (Scheingold 1988). By coming to understand one's personal reactions to a patient, a patient's family member(s), medical colleagues, and the like, one can thereby improve patient care and team morale. In such a safe, supportive, trusting, and compassionately confrontive atmosphere, physicians (teachers, interns, residents) and behavioral scientists "wrestle with the bear." Such struggles have less to do with adjusting medications than with coming to terms with the experience of medicine and medical education. The vignettes presented throughout this book, many of which derive from Balint groups (and from individual counseling prompted by the Balint process), are considerably altered and disguised to preserve confidentiality.

Since 1980, I have also offered an ethnographically-oriented course on behavioral science in occupational medicine for graduate PA students in a masters of public health program and for resident physicians in the occupational medicine residency program. These varied teaching activities, together with a considerable amount of time spent in individual resident consultation, supervision, and "shadowing" (in clinic and hospital examination rooms); participation in regular clinical case conferences, mortality and morbidity conferences about the inpatient service, and grand rounds; and numerous individual counseling/therapy sessions with residents and faculty have offered me the opportunity to conduct sixteen years of ethnography and to formulate and test hypotheses about the cultural organization of American medicine. I have found that in working with family physicians, my ethnographic orientation is taken seriously only as I immerse myself in their intensely practical, time-consuming, hands-on world.

MEDICINE AND CULTURE

Clinical categories and their meanings can take us to the heart of a society (Stein 1979b, 1982e). In all cultures, including scientific or biomedical methodology, problem definition constrains problem solution. Questions prefigure answers. The two are inextricably linked by the usually unexamined premises they share. The social construction of problems is a key to group preoccupations.

Currently within the American culture, a social process has occurred whereby a wide gamut of problems are redefined and managed as more narrowly biomedical issues. As a result of this transmuting, matters rich in personal meaning and embedded in social significance are denuded of their larger context. This *medi-*

calization of problems in the West is an example of the way groups define problems and formulate their solutions in keeping with the cultural *ethos*, that is, with the distinguishing characteristics and shared assumptions that pervade a group and its constituent institutions. When premises are sacred and therefore must not be questioned, the range of solutions must be narrowed, even as some solutions must be doggedly pursued. Sadly, as with Ptolemaic astronomy, by adding yet another "corrective" epicycle to earlier failed solutions, the next solution removes us even further from the capacity to reformulate the problem itself. In this respect, biomedicine has much in common with sacred doctrine and ritual practice.

A given society may comprise multiple subdivisions, each with its distinctive clinical realm. For instance, in a widely cited work, Arthur Kleinman, Leon Eisenberg, and Byron Good offer the following distinctions among "professional, folk and popular" constructions of clinical reality.

> Studies of the social context of health care disclose three structural domains of health care in society: professional; popular (family, social network, community); and folk (nonprofessional healers) (Kleinman 1973). The great majority of health care takes place in the popular domain: 70% to 90% (Zola 1972; Hulka, Kupper and Cassel 1972). Most illness episodes never enter the professional or folk domains (Hulka, Kupper and Cassel 1972). When they do, decisions about where and when to seek care, how long to remain in care, and how to evaluate treatment also occur in the popular domain, most commonly in the context of the family (Zola 1972; Litman 1974; Freidson 1970b). Each domain possesses its own explanatory systems, social roles, interaction settings, and institutions (Kleinman 1975). For example, a sufferer is a sick family member or friend in the popular domain, a specific type of patient in the professional domain, and a client of one sort or another in the folk domain. These roles can be quite distinct. . . . Clinical realities are thus culturally constituted and vary cross-culturally and across the domains of health care in the same society (1978: 254).

These useful distinctions are also quite fluid. What is included in and excluded from biomedical culture changes; likewise, various groups vie for possession of the coveted title "professional." Similarly, the relationship between traditional ethnic medical beliefs and practices and mainstream, acculturated beliefs and practices—that is, between "folk" and "popular" domains, respectively—can sometimes be viewed in terms of a clear-cut distinction, and at other times in terms of a continuum or even a bridge between cultural worlds. Many members of ethnic cultures augment if not supersede their original medical cultural repertory with beliefs and practices common to national American society—for example, the high value on medical technology and purchase of over-the-counter drugs at pharmacies. Acupuncture, regarded by the biomedical establishment in the early 1980s as an exotic folk practice of China, has by now been partially absorbed into biomedical professional culture and has become an alternative (popular) treatment modality. Biofeedback has even more successfully been incorporated into biomedical practice, having originated in an amalgam of behaviorist psychology and 1960s counter-culture.

How a society feels about and acts toward its practitioners can also reveal much about the dynamics of that group. Non-Western societies as diverse as the North

Alaskan Eskimo, the Yokuts and Western Mono of aboriginal California, the Navaho and Apache, and a Mayan village in Chiapas ambivalently if not dichotomously view their native healers (Foster and Anderson 1978: 114–115). Those who can heal can also hurt, if not kill, via witchcraft. George Foster and Barbara Anderson propose that

> in societies in which most illness is attributed to witchcraft, it is not unreasonable for people to believe that the specialist who can control and fight sorcery also has the requisite power to practice it himself when it suits his needs. And, by the same token, it is reasonable to assume that when disease is believed to be the result of natural causes, the role of the curer is seen as more nearly benevolent (1978: 115).

Social mistrust of biomedical practitioners during the past two decades in the United States calls into question their latter assumption. Malpractice litigation is the functional equivalent of the witchcraft accusations made in small-scale, non-Western societies. Subjective factors among patients and among the general population can override naturalistic models of disease etiology and can lead to egregiously personalistic interpretations of physicians' competence. "Mal-practice" is ultimately the psychological heir to deep as well as ancient fears of "mal-evolence."

Yet another vital issue in the ethnographic study of clinical systems is the relationship between clinical thought and action. Universally, clinical conceptualization and choice of treatment modality are part of a single, if not formally articulated, system of thought and action. How a problem is treated is an extension of how that problem is understood. Eisenberg, for instance, writes, "Working models of the disease process determine the data that physicians gather, inform the ways in which facts are integrated into a diagnosis, and circumscribe the boundaries of interventions designated as therapeutic" (1977: 10, also see 1988). Different treatment procedures derive from different kinds of assumptions and explanations. In an elegant study of the American cultural construction of pain, Thomas Johnson writes that

> much of the public believes—indeed, has been led to believe—that physicians should be able to eliminate their pain. In society today, medicine has come to be seen as very powerful, and the primary functions of the physician have come to be pain relief and prevention of death. The amazing successes of the anesthesia revolution of the 19th century and the antimicrobial revolution of the 20th century have led patients and physicians alike to see pain as a scourge to be eliminated or treated and death as an enemy to be conquered. . . .
>
> Physicians are professionally enculturated to eliminate pain, to see pain as something to be defined, measured, fixed. Millions of dollars and research hours have been spent trying to objectify and quantify pain (1989: 43).

On the basis of much ethnographic work, anthropology holds that the medical component or ethnomedical system of a culture is embedded in the ethos of that culture, which pervades all institutions. For instance, in writing of Morita therapy in Japan, Christie Kiefer observes that

> Morita Therapy is . . . a kind of cultural institution, subject to the same influences that shape other institutions in this society. One sees characteristic Japanese patterns. . . . One begins at once also to see the fit between Morita Therapy and the prevailing social attitudes of the Japanese. . . . Even the types of neurotic disorder for which the technique is most often used . . . are the sort which one would expect to flourish in the Japanese social atmosphere. In short, the study of a treatment modality tells us a surprising amount about the society in which it is practiced (1976: 11).

Problems, medical ones included, are often unconsciously designed so that they cannot be solved except at the partial, symbolic level. People often formulate and address certain problems in order to avert others. To put it this way requires, I believe, that we investigate what an individual or group wishes to know and not to know about itself and the world. This perspective aids us in understanding why some problems are intractable to solution. The persistent character of the problems discussed in this chapter points to issues that transcend contemporary American scientific medicine and that concern the functions of human culture (see La Barre 1972; Róheim 1943; Devereux 1980a; Stein 1980a, 1980b, 1983d).

Rather than reifying, say, the medical institution appointed by the larger society, I shall explore the interplay between institution and society, the nature of the boundary between them, the cogwheeling between small organizational and larger cultures, and finally the process by which the larger cultural ethos or configuration integrates various subsidiary units such as biomedicine. As Ruth Benedict writes, "The significant sociological unit is not the institution but the cultural configuration" (1934b: 244) that pervades a wide assortment of social institutions. More recently, in her introduction to a cultural study of health and medical care in Japan, Margaret Lock remarks that "medically related conceptions are embedded in a mesh of cultural concepts, what Peter Worsley (1982) has called a 'metamedical' framework. Isolation and study of components such as a 'medical system' or 'tradition,' a hospital, a clinic, or a healing session, are artificially bounded units superimposed by the social scientist who undertakes the analysis" (1987: 2–3).

Moreover, although in American culture physicians, social workers, and other official diagnosticians label categories of persons as sick, deviant, diseased, criminal, and the like, this book argues that the cultural configuration, its ethos, and interlacing themes are quite often shared by those who are labeled as well as by those who label. This book identifies the cultural dynamics that link these two ostensibly different groups and in the process it will force us to rethink the boundary between culturally defined pathology and normalcy. I show how cultural deviants and cultural exemplars are consciously and explicitly opposite poles of a common, underlying, unconscious structure. In the present study, the categories of patients, clients, and deviants represent the officially labeled abnormals; the category of biomedical clinicians occupies the role of Benedict's "abnormals of extreme fulfillment of the cultural type" (1934a: 64).

Many naturalistic, ethnographic studies by medical sociologists and medical anthropologists have contributed to our understanding of mainstream medical culture through the analysis of deviance: for example, Robert Edgerton's (1967) study of mental retardation and his cross-cultural study of deviance (1976); Sue

Estroff's (1981) study of chronic mental illness; Howard Becker's (1963) sociological study of deviance; Michael Agar's (1973) and Robert S. Weppner's (1973) studies of the life-ways of street addicts; John Schwartzman's (1975; see also Schwartzman and Bokos 1979) studies of the family and wider social network of heroin addicts; James Spradley's (1970) study of urban drunks; and my own studies of alcoholism and drug abuse (Stein 1982d, 1985a). Such studies as these vividly portray cultural norms through the examination of (those categories of) persons who are classified as *violating* them. The present work describes and interprets that group of people who view themselves and are socially defined as ***articulators and enforcers of the norm*** and investigates the relationship between that delegated group and the wider society. Thus, this book explores the nature and meaning of "social control" (an implicit function of "patient care") and the fear of loss of control in American medicine and society.

In an early use of the term *group fantasy* (which Lloyd deMause [1982] designates the cornerstone of his theory of culture and history), Weston La Barre draws attention to the group dynamics that constitute a culture's process. These dynamics often function unconsciously to draw attention to specific categories of "bad" people in order to avoid examining those sacred premises and beliefs that act as widely shared defense mechanisms:

> It is true that group fantasy confines and delimits our private psychoses, but if the culture of the group comes to resemble a psychosis itself, by a kind of *folie à deux* to the nth degree, then the group is worse off than when it started. In this unconscious and unwitting way, all social groups are in the long run either therapeutic, that is adaptive to a real world, or anti-adaptive. Man is like an existentialist spider who spreads out a moral net of symbolism over the void out of his own substance—and then walks upon it. But the final safety of the net depends always on the integrity and the soundness of the postulated points of reference to a real physical world (1962: 67).

In describing and explaining biomedicine's "moral net of symbolism," I try to understand the process of clinical thinking and clinical work, to portray the inner "substance" out of which such thinking and work are constructed, and to identify the dimly perceived medical group fantasies that influence a physician's attempts to diagnose, assess, label, and treat *others*.

Group fantasies refer to the conscious and unconscious experience of what it is like to be a member of a particular group at some era in its history. Now, in our society especially, which prides itself on its rationality, realism, and objectivity, a view that shared fantasies influence our behavior is a bitter pill to swallow. Psychohistorian Gerhard Bliersbach recognizes the irony inherent in "the fact that one should be in the grips of collectively shared fantasies—unconsciously, no less!—at the same time that one is habituated to taking the category of *fantasy* very lightly" (1987: 338). The widespread resistance to recognizing the degree to which all human behavior is affected by unconscious process is reflected by the fact that "in colloquial speech, the term 'fantasies' has a pejorative connotation" (1987: 338). I hope to demonstrate the defensive, homeostatic, and adaptive functions of the group fantasy of objectivity and rationality in medicine and in the wider culture from which biomedicine derives its role and status.

MULTIPLE MODELS IN BIOMEDICINE

In biomedical environments, "facts" are the most highly valued category of information. What constitutes a fact is frequently illustrated by allusion to the 1950s television detective series "Dragnet." A few years ago, I inquired of a physician colleague whether he might include in a medical school course titled "The Basis of Medical Practice" reading materials on culture and the physician-patient relationship. He replied, "The course is so short and is packed with facts they've got to have. My rule about what to include or not include is what Sgt. Joe Friday said: 'Give me the facts, just the facts, ma'am.'"

From the first day of medical school through the final day of residency, one is warned of all the facts that one must amass, have at one's command. One is further taught how these facts are rightly and wrongly organized and what constitutes useful and not-so-useful facts. I have often found it ironic that while medical students, interns, and residents are willing and eager to learn thousands of anatomical, biochemical, and microbiological terms that are Latin and Greek in etymology, they often dismiss and balk at learning even a small list of psychoanalytic, family therapy, or anthropological terms, many of which are rooted in the same linguistic traditions. Clearly, not all "facts" are equal. As much of this book shows, dominant biomedical values, metaphors, personal and group dynamics, and the process of training itself determine the contexts that qualify or disqualify ideas as sufficiently biomedical "facts."

The value and metaphor of factuality notwithstanding, biomedical decisionmaking and patient care are not altogether based on rational, scientific, objective factors. Consider for example, the *medical model*, American society's dominant clinical framework for conceptualizing and treating issues that are subsumed under the rubric of disease. According to this model, the physical body and its constituent parts are the units of clinical discourse. To interpret the preeminent role of the medical model in American medicine, we must distinguish between two of its separate yet interrelated dimensions: (1) the medical model as part of the imperfect, culture-transcendent history of science, (theories, methods, and discoveries that heighten knowledge about reality); and (2) the medical model as folk or ethnoscience that adopts and conforms the scientific method to cultural (group-shared) premises, meanings, and fantasies. Stated differently, *as science*, the medical model is capable of generating new knowledge about living systems. As *culture*, the medical model constantly bends novelty to cultural expectation and tradition.

This is not to deny the genuine advances and progress in reality testing that have occurred within the medical model. The discovery by Antoine Lavoisier of the role of oxygen in combustion was a genuine advance over the preeminent phlogiston theory. The microbial theory of Louis Pasteur and his successors was superior in reality testing to the theory of spontaneous generation that it superseded. No shibboleth of cultural pluralism or relativism could have impugned the improvement in truth value that the oxygen and microbial theories represented.

But when these theories are advanced as the whole story about human suffering, when they become ideology rather than disciplined play, then the medical model as a theory of disease and a form of treatment has coopted science for culture. That is, when researchers or clinicians, and the group whom they serve, draw premature closure around the conceptual boundary of the problem—and further link it with such cultural elements as therapeutic activism, the dread of death, and the search for control—then science is in fact abandoned even as it is invoked as a methodology. Of the psychohistorical roots of biomedicine Henry Ebel writes that

> like all religions, it began as an *anti*-religion. Never again would unhygienic "holy men" and "holy women" do nothing for their patients because death was to be welcomed.
>
> Death, the new religion proclaimed, is the worst thing that can happen to you because you are all chemistry and physics, so there is no "soul."
>
> Since this philosophical position claimed to be founded on the proclamations of an oracle known as Objective Truth, fully measurable and replicable, most everybody bought into it (1988: 5–6).

As I hope this book demonstrates, a scientifically and culturally precise discourse on American medicine must distinguish between two systems of meaning of the very word *biology* (as in biomedicine, the biomedical model, or biopsychosocial). One system comprises the subject of open-ended, naturalistic inquiry into human origins, human nature, and human affliction. The other contains a powerful American cultural metaphor that absorbs and condenses into an overarching ideological framework many disparate and changing cultural elements, including biology in the first sense.

No society is without its core tensions, rifts, cultural contradictions. As Matthew Arnold wrote in 1869, and Weston La Barre wrote a century later in 1972, the history of Western civilization can profitably be explored as a struggle between Hebraism and Hellenism, between two interlocking and inseparable conceptions of human nature. (Correspondence with Henry Ebel in the summer and fall of 1988 persuaded me that these polarities are essential to an understanding of the deification of medical science and technology in the twentieth century United States.) From the Jews come abject humility in the face of the Almighty; the sense of one's smallness in the universe; submission to God's will; the majesty of God the Father; the sense of awe in the halting gaze at reality; the lively if sometimes oppressive sense of sin and with it a belief in human fallibility and imperfectability; preoccupation with and hatred of one's evil; and the recognition that we distort things even as we try to understand them. From the Greeks comes a far sunnier, more optimistic view of human nature and accomplishment. Hellenism is characterized by its faith in reason, its confidence, its elegance, and its simple beauty; the belief that humankind's limits are boundless, as is the knowledge that we can attain on our own; the belief that human will and agency are our true fate; the belief in objectivity, in human control over the future, in perfectability; the prerogatives of the son (contemporary feminists would surely add "daughter"); and the elevation of the self above group and gods alike. On its sinuous historical odyssey, this struggle has at present solidly come out on the side of the Hellenists, in biomedicine as elsewhere.

Of the countless critiques of biomedicine that have been voiced since the mid-1970s, that of George Engel (1977) most closely resembles the approach I take in this book. If I read Engel correctly, he is not strictly aligned with either *cultural relativism* (the belief that all concepts or ideas are so completely embedded in a cultural or historical context that any attempt to derive universal application is misguided and futile) or *essentialism* (the doctrine that thoughts or ideas necessarily correspond to forms or entities in nature). Thus in formulating the need for a biopsychosocial model to complement the biomedical model, he believes an enterprise called "science" is still possible (also see Bronowski 1956). According to Engel, all models do not have identical truth value with respect to the real world; some are better than others. It is not enough to approach comparative ethnomedical (or ethnophilosophical) systems from linguistic and relativist viewpoints alone. Ptolemaic epicycles and Galilean orbits, phlogiston and oxygen, supernatural voice and superego, are not simply functional equivalents in different explanatory systems (see La Barre 1974). Engel courageously argues that

> not all models are scientific. Indeed, broadly defined, a model is nothing more than a belief system utilized to explain natural phenomena, to make sense out of what is puzzling or disturbing. The more socially disruptive or individually upsetting the phenomenon, the more pressing the need of humans to devise explanatory systems. . . . Such culturally derived belief systems about disease also constitute models. These may be referred to as popular or folk models. As efforts at social adaptation, they contrast with scientific models, which are primarily designed to promote scientific investigation. The historic fact we have to face is that in modern Western society biomedicine not only has provided the basis for the scientific study of disease, it has also become our own culturally specific perspective about disease, that is, our folk model (1977: 130).

In this passage, Engel reveals the Janus-headed character of biomedicine: One aspect points to science, while another aspect points to culture. Because of the virtually sacred status of science and technology in our culture, however, it is easy to confuse the practice of medicine as science with the appropriation of science by culture (for example, the recent tendency to label virtually any social "problem" as a medical one, replete with diagnosis, treatment, prognosis, and outcome). The naturalism and aestheticism of Leonardo daVinci as he strives to be a cartographer of the human body differ radically from, say, the aggressiveness and dominance of the warrior-physician who wants to "get in there and obliterate disease with a blast of steroids" and for whom the patient represents a refractory obstacle to that form of military conquest known as cure. The prohibition against dissecting the human body and against directly observing its interior, a ban that dominated the Middle Ages, has given way to our current biomedical prescription that visualization is virtually the only trustworthy means of gaining scientific knowledge of disease.

Although many investigators and critics argue that biomedicine *is the American ethnomedicine* (that is, our cultural medical subsystem of health-related beliefs, definitions, diagnoses, customs, and symbols), the actual professional socialization and practice of American medicine are far more complex. To borrow Audrey Richards's distinction between a person's "expressed" and "deduced" purposes (1956), the biomedical model may be the most expressed view of medicine by its practitioners and educators. But it is not the only one that can be deduced by the observer as affecting teaching and patient care. The biomedical model may reign as the ideal, yet it is far from a complete description of real medical training and practice; or, said another way, biomedicine functions as medicine's official, or formal, worldview, yet it interacts in actual clinical supervision and decisionmaking with countless unofficial, or informal, worldviews that are intrinsic and extrinsic to medicine. The medical model, which occupies the manifest, conscious level, contends with models at latent, unconscious levels.

The biomedical model is socially normative in the sense that it prescribes the physician's behavior; when physicians teach medical students and resident physicians, this is the model they most often invoke and believe they are using. Yet it is far less than normative in the descriptive and statistical sense of what physicians actually think and do. If we are to understand the world of American medicine, we must accept a mélange of doctrines, authorities, and practices as the cultural "actuality" (Erikson 1964: 164) that cannot be reduced without distortion to something simpler. American medicine includes the biomedical model but cannot be wholly explained by it. Any cultural analysis, social criticism, or policy planning that only considers the medical model mistakes a part for the (admittedly elusive) whole.

Since the mid-1970s, numerous paradigms have been advanced to complement if not supplant the biomedical model, among them the "ethnomedical model" proposed by Horacio Fabrega (1975); the "explanatory models" approach advanced by Arthur Kleinman (1980); the "disease/illness" distinction formulated by Leon Eisenberg (1977) and elaborated by Arthur Kleinman (1980) and Robert Hahn (1984), among others; the "biopsychosocial model" propounded by George Engel (1977); the "semantic illness networks" approach offered by Byron Good (1977); and most recently the "critical medical anthropology" model offered by Nancy Scheper-Hughes and Margaret Lock (1987) (for an overview and critique of these models in clinically applied anthropology, see Phillips 1985). In *Social Context of Health, Illness, and Patient Care*, Elliot Mishler (1981) offers an analysis and critique of the biomedical model. He discusses four tacit assumptions that underlie biomedical knowledge and practice: That disease is commensurable and explainable biologically; that the doctrine of specific etiology accounts for pathology; that diseases are universal in their morphology and process; and that biomedical physicians consider themselves biomedical scientists who are governed by such values and attitudes as rationality, objectivity, and neutrality (value-free science). By placing biomedicine in historical and sociocultural contexts, Mishler reveals the extent to which supposedly culture-free medicine is in fact culture-laden and that health, sickness, and treatment are social, as well as biological, processes.

All the foregoing writers decry the reductionism and mechanistic quality of the biomedical model and its avowed interest only in the disease-entity. Likewise, all argue for a more comprehensive, humane, systems view of the treatment process that includes patient, family, community, and cultural perspectives. A point not developed in these critiques, however, is that biomedicine is in its own culturally distinctive way a systems or a biopsychosocial model, albeit not one that Engel or the other authors would endorse. The view of what humans and diseases are; what the clinical relationship ought to be like; the significance of such concepts as placebo, compliance, and control in medical culture; the value orientations that underlie medical practice; the plausibility of including biofeedback and family therapy within medical theory and procedures (while excluding modalities such as chiropractic, for instance); the diffidence with which physicians approach patients about remuneration; the difficulty with which most physicians approach the emotionality of death and dying, preferring instead to pare it down to a technical issue—these are decidedly biopsychosocial aspects of medicine that deserve systematic analysis as well as social criticism.

In practice, there is considerable overlap and vacillation between the formal scientific model and the congeries of folk or lay models. Kleinman's distinction between "disease" and "illness" (1980, 1983a) directs our attention to the fact that practitioners and patients (and families) often bring widely disparate constructions of clinical reality (that is, understandings of what the problem is, how it should be treated, what its expected outcome is) to the encounter. Following Eisenberg (1977), Kleinman initially identified "disease" as the physician's model and "illness" as the patient's model. These understandings and expectations often fail to overlap. Moreover, Kleinman also regarded "disease" as a condition that precipitates patients' subjective responses, called "illness," to diseases (1980, 1983a). On the one hand, reflecting a kind of semantic relativism, disease and illness were to be considered differing explanatory frameworks between doctor and patient. On the other hand—and appearing to contradict this first approach—disease was also conceptualized as a palpable reality that prompted "illness" responses and explanatory accounts by the patient, the patient's family, and the wider lay social networks. This view gives a nod to the common dichotomy made by physicians: that although their own thinking is objective, that of patients and family members is subjective.

In subsequent formulations, Kleinman (1983b) broadened the concept of disease to denote the model of any (not only biomedical) practitioner. He concluded that illness is not only a consequence of disease, but its negotiation and definition actually precedes any consultation with a practitioner. Kleinman's wider concept of "disease" now seems to denote an official practitioner model. The possibility, however, that physicians might turn to multiple models, or might employ biomedical disease/diagnosis and intervention as a subjective defense against identification with the patient's suffering, is not considered in Kleinman's more formalistic, although admittedly elegant, dichotomy.

This dichotomy overlooks and omits many nuances of clinical decisionmaking that are germane to this book. As a term, ***disease*** subsumes multiple interrelated, but often scarcely articulated, ways a physician or other practitioner thinks and acts. In one sense, it is a model of scientific, naturalistic inquiry; in another sense, it is a metaphoric, highly variable way of thinking about and acting toward someone labeled (diagnosed) as having a disease or toward the disease itself. In my experience, the model(s) that physicians use to make clinical decisions is not reducible to

Kleinman's category. Indeed, because the practice of medicine is influenced by the physician's own subjectivity (Stein 1982h, 1983b, 1985g; Stein and Apprey 1985), the physician's own conscious and unconscious response to the patient's condition often becomes incorporated into the diagnosis, treatment plan, prognosis, and outcome.

Ensuing chapters illustrate how multiple models come into play, concurrently or sequentially, in medical practice. American medicine is *syncretic*, as are all cultural belief systems (although members of all societies protest their group's individuality, uniqueness, distinctiveness from others). Biomedicine is more diversified, contradictory, pluralistic, and situational than its official doctrine and self-image would suggest. It has selectively incorporated beliefs, values, attitudes, and practices from diverse sources. Thus, for instance, although Foster's (1976) concept of "naturalistic" and "personalistic" medical models makes the scientifically welcome distinction between objective, reality factors in illness and self-referential, often animistic views of illness, it considers Western biomedical practice far more uniformly and consistently naturalistic than it actually is.

A careful study of the language and process of decisionmaking in American medicine reveals a "both/and" adoption of these two models. For example, a practitioner may use naturalistic medical diagnosis for personalistic, subjective ends. Close to the surface of the microbiological model of disease often lurks a patently demonological conception of disease. Fantasies enshrouding acquired immune deficiency syndrome (AIDS) and notions of "good" versus "bad" cholesterol number among the most current American examples. The physician is variously scientist, detective, sleuth, hunter, and exterminator of evil invaders that have overrun and possessed the body. Likewise, a young physician's clinical decisionmaking is often more influenced by the practice and authority of a particular physician with whom the younger doctor worked during medical school or during residency training than by a strictly impersonal, scientific judgment.

Such practices do not disprove the existence of the naturalistic model. Nor do they say that physicians are really subjective in their approach to diagnosis and treatment. Rather they commend our closer attention to the interplay of models, of ways of thinking and feeling, in actual medical decisionmaking and to a comprehension of those situations that find one or another model emphasized. Further, a strictly cognitive approach to medical models and their use does not suffice to account for physicians' behavior. Which model(s) they use on a given occasion is closely tied to how they *feel* about the patient, disease, situation, colleagues, cost containment, and so on. Medical models are affect-laden cognitive structures.

Numerous situationally invoked alternative treatment models surface alongside the official scientific model. For instance, often-hospitalized or clinic patients are carefully watched or perhaps treated, and they improve without a final medical diagnosis having been established. Physicians may then formulate a humorous diagnosis of "Looked sick, got better" to give themselves some sense of explanation and closure. A second example is the cost-containment-inspired "Treat 'em and street 'em" approach. Once a patient is admitted to the hospital, clinical and administrative "wheels" move quickly to complete the course of inpatient treatment, to "move 'em in and move 'em out" (idiomatic of cattle drives). This model of care is discrepant with the official scientific model (and with the quasi-official model of compassionate care). A third situational conception of treatment was articulated by a physician at the conclusion of a case presentation on management of migraine headache. Having reviewed the various etiological theories of migraine and after discussing a variety of medical and psychosocial management approaches, he sarcastically added:

> What's the correct ER [emergency room] management of headache? [He was referring specifically to the issue of moonlighting, whereby resident physicians work in various emergency rooms to gain additional medical experience and income.] It depends on what you want. If you want to get the patient out fast—because of the patient load, or because your turn is up soon—think Demerol [a pain medicine]. That'll usually make them happy, and you're out of the woods.

From my experience working with practicing faculty and resident physicians, I am persuaded that any conceptual framework that distinguishes too sharply between the practitioner's purportedly coherent, systematic, and immutable framework and the patient's supposedly loosely associated, highly flexible, and changeable framework misses the point that practitioners and patients are epistemologically in the same boat. They both must constantly try to make sense of their world and act in accordance with that process of comprehension. Kleinman, for instance, writes that "vagueness, multiplicity of meanings, frequent changes, and lack of sharp boundaries between ideas and experiences are characteristic of lay EMs [*explanatory models*]" (1980: 107). The same is true of physician EMs at the operational (as opposed to the ideal) level.

Just as lay belief systems and EMs are not fully thought through, formally integrated, and fixed (except occasionally in the form of a delusion), medical practitioner, resident, and medical educator belief systems and EMs are more rigorously systematic in doctrine than in practice. Dan Blumhagen's cautionary note about the systematicity of lay models obtains, I believe, for practitioner models as well:

> When we speak of individual belief systems, particularly as these are applied to laymen, there is a danger that we will be seduced by the term "system." Systematicity, coherence and interdependence are aspects of *professional* belief systems. It is an unusual individual (or, indeed, practitioner) who has worked out *all* the interconnections of his belief system so that it has become an integrated whole (Berger and Luckmann 1966). It is more likely that a person will have a *set* of beliefs about illness which are only loosely interconnected, if at all. The connections between the isolated beliefs may be supplied to meet the need to explain a particular situation. In addition, in a particular situation, both the interconnections and the items of individual beliefs appear to be continuously reworked (in part through the construction of a series of explanatory models) to provide a framework for dealing with a particular illness (Blumhagen 1980: 199–200).

What is true at the microlevel of individual health-related decisions obtains at the macrolevel as well. Neither biomedical culture nor the wider American culture is static. Biomedical culture participates in and represents powerful societal currents. In the culturally experimental and ecumenical, if not radical, 1960s and early 1970s, biomedicine's boundaries were more expansive, inclusive, and permeable. This was the halcyon era of the behavioral sciences in biomedical education. For at least a generation, numerous behavioral and social scientists had been working within academic and community medical environments. Many clinical and community psychiatrists sought to redefine their professional identity and their work away from the traditional, bounded medical model and toward inclusion of psychodynamic, familial, community, and cultural aspects of disease and treatment. Many psychiatrists at that time labeled themselves behavioral scientists and then claimed that psychiatry was in fact a behavioral science.

Since the latter part of the 1970s, the national retreat to fundamentalist ideologies and practices in religion and politics has been paralleled in biomedicine by a resurgence of the medical model and a narrowing of the boundaries of clinical interest. In the context of a back-to-basics cultural and clinical fundamentalism, mainstream psychiatry has embraced the search for a more biochemical and genetic etiology of mental illness and for more pharmacological treatments.[1] Many behavioral scientists teaching and practicing in medical settings now find it advantageous to call themselves specialists in "behavioral medicine." This exemplifies the current acculturation of the behavioral sciences to the dominant biomedical model (which many nonphysician behavioral scientists consciously disavow) and to the prevailing medical power structure. Practitioners of behavioral medicine offer clients, patients, and biomedical colleagues (via referral and consultation) those kinds of treatments that make most cultural sense to physicians and other biomedical practitioners. For instance, behavioral medicine colleagues often offer to help physicians get noncompliant patients to be more compliant with prescribed medication regimens, diet, exercise, stress reduction, and lifestyle change (as with diabetics, hypertensives, cigarette smokers, poststroke and post–acute care rehabilitation).

Offering brief, focused, procedure-oriented, largely impersonal interventions, behavioral medicine practitioners dispense a new "product" (to use a contemporary marketing/corporate metaphor). This approach is congruent with the biomedical ethos and with the traditional doctor-patient relationship (which is largely authoritarian, cognitive, restricted in scope to symptom removal). Like mainstream biomedical practitioners, specialists in behavioral medicine often have little interest in the subjectivity of their patients (or themselves) and tend not to inquire deeply into the meaning and significance of the patient's symptoms and illness experience. Although practitioners of behavioral medicine are drawn from such diverse fields and training programs as family therapy, clinical psychology, social work, and educational psychology, it is the common implicit cultural rubric they share with biomedicine that renders their service valuable.

Issues addressed by behavioral medicine consist of those that physicians have difficulty solving themselves within the biomedical model (such as persuading patients to take their medications and on schedule). Behavioral medicine personnel are akin to military "reinforcements." They perform their role according to clinical language, relationships, and interventions that conform to medical culture. Stated differently, although the new cultural content might be different, in its underlying form and assumptions behavioral medicine poses no threat to biomedicine. Hence, it qualifies as yet another "allied" health service. Behavioral medicine has been relatively successful (adaptive) within biomedicine because it offers change that does not undermine the emotional and assumptive framework of medicine (see Gregory Bateson's discussion of "first order" [behavioral, doctrinal] change without "second order" [underlying assumptions] change, 1972).

In short, within biomedicine, numerous professional cultures and academic disciplines are interacting. Multiple models of clinical reality are in use. At the same time, as the remainder of this book will establish, a core culture can nonetheless be recognized.

The American Medical System and the Larger Culture

This book demonstrates how profoundly biomedicine is affected by the cultural continuities and changes it shares with other institutions of American society. It shows how profoundly nonmedical are many of those features we often take to be distinctive features of biomedicine. Sickness and healer roles, together with the very definition of what qualifies as legitimate illness, are inseparably bound up with shared notions about the self and its boundaries. This collective self-image, together with the range of deviation allowed within the cultural category of normal, is not only a social fact but an important value. In the United States, for instance, disease conceptualization and treatment are embedded in the value system of self-reliance, rugged individualism, independence, pragmatism, empiricism, atomism, privatism, emotional minimalism, and a mechanistic conception of the body and its "repair" (de Tocqueville 1944; Kluckhohn and Strodtbeck 1961; Ohnuki-Tierney 1984). The horror of dependency is a powerful fuel that keeps the biomedical conceptual, diagnostic and treatment system going. B. Hocking writes that "because the sick are dependent, sickness is seen as deviant behavior, undesirable, and only to be legitimated on certain terms ([Talcott] Parsons' sick role concept). Legitimation of sickness has become the prerogative of the medical profession which uses the biomedical concept of disease as its yardstick" (1987: 526).

The biomedical conceptualization and treatment of disease have been welcomed and have successfully "diffused" (in the sense of being widely incorporated into the host society) in American culture precisely because they fit so well with the image of the self as a physical object that can be broken and fixed. This book explores the ramifications of this image for all aspects of medical practice and training.

In this anthropological view, "disease, health, and illness are seen as culturally defined conditions expressing cultural codes and social circumstances as well as organic conditions" (Estroff 1981: 206). Cultural beliefs, values, attitudes, roles, images, and the like govern the definition, experience, expectations of treatment, and outcome of illness episodes *for practitioner and patient alike*. Now, although American society has long been characterized as multiethnic, multicultural, and pluralistic (see Stein and Hill 1977) and thus contains a multiplicity of cultural health belief and action systems, I demonstrate that an overarching American medical cultural system nevertheless exists. I establish that the psychocultural system of biomedicine is relative to American society in the sense that it draws heavily from the core values, symbols, meanings, and themes that pervade American society. Moreover, I also establish that the issues with which biomedicine grapples and the way the grappling is expressed are likewise relative to the human condition and are thus local expressions of universal issues.

For instance, American medicine's obsession with activity and procedural prowess is a contemporary version of males' fear of identification with females and their need to overcompensate by emphasizing the virtues of "doing." Although the term *care* occupies center stage in the polemics and official self-image of contemporary biomedicine (many health care clinicians call themselves providers), the nurturant, succorant, affective role associated with care rank it far beneath the active, virile, masterful virtues associated with cure. Further, the means to the "conquest" of disease is control. On the eve of the era of corporate for-profit medicine, Estroff, for instance, wrote that "modern western societies, especially contemporary U.S. society, have constructed layer upon layer of protection from seeing or dealing with those who are differently able and who suffer. . . . We seem most intent, especially recently, on regulating and controlling, not alleviating, the dependence, anger, and pain of those who suffer—physically, mentally, and socially" (1984: 369).

In a work on clinical supervision of the treatment of borderline personality patients, James Masterson writes that

> to the degree to which you have not resolved your own depression (not necessarily an abandonment depression), you will have great difficulty tolerating your patient's depression, because it stimulates your own. It resonates with a lot of the things which you experienced as a child which you have repressed, and it stimulates them and starts tugging on them; they start pushing up, trying to get release (1983: 188).

Masterson's point applies as much to biomedical physicians as to psychotherapists. Any clinician's (physician and nonphysician alike) emotional response to the patient (from authoritarian overdirectiveness and control, to rescue fantasy–derived overinvolvement, to subtle rejection and abandonment) interferes with and directs the treatment process itself. The process and structure of assessment, diagnosis, and treatment can be heavily contaminated by acting out—albeit rationalized by individual physicians as well as their medical colleagues. Such countertransference to the case and to patients can represent practitioners' struggle to sustain their own repression.

Numerous writers (Davidson 1986; Masterson 1983; Katz 1984a; Stein 1985g; Stein and Apprey 1987; Balint 1957) analyzed countertransference as an *individual* therapist or physician response to the patient or family. In this book I focus on *group* and even wider *cultural* dynamics that in effect institutionalize the physician's avoidance of emotional and cultural issues by paradoxically acting out emotion-driven responses to patients. The further cultural paradox of biomedicine is that it insists that it is beyond culture and that the patient's culture is for the most part inconsequential to diagnosis and treatment. Medical education, from premedical to the basic sciences (anatomy, physiology, biochemistry, microbiology, pathology) and finally to clinical training during internship and residency direct the medical student and resident away from (and hence largely deprive them of) access to unconscious and cultural issues in themselves and in their patients. While on the surface, biomedical values of professionalism, objectivity, and therapeutic distance allow the physician to harbor a scientific demeanor toward the patient, beneath this idealistic attitude lies an effort to protect the physician from the frailties and fears that patients evoke in doctors.

Beginning in the late nineteenth century, the pseudobiological doctrine of *Social Darwinism* argued that individuals and groups should and do compete with each other, unprotected, for survival. Only the (supposedly) biologically superior survive the struggle. Its empathy denuded ethic contends that "If you can't make it on your own, you don't deserve to live." One must "make it" unaided on one's own, "like a rolling stone."

At local and national medical conferences in the 1980s, one hears less about the quality of the clinical relationship and more about "the bottom line," the "packaging" of health care, medical care as "product" or "commodity," patients as "consumers," "managed care," and family physicians as "gatekeepers." Here a societywide shift in values, a profound culturewide diminution in compassion, and a flaunting of social Darwinist sink-or-swim ideology are culturally displaced onto medicine as if medical cost containment were the entire issue. In many respects physicians are placed (and many accept the role) in the position of policing and executing draconian social policy. In a phrase, medicine acts as the delegate or agent of the wider ethos, while medicine and the wider culture collude in defining the problem as a singularly medical one. Michael L. Glenn, M.D., writes that

> today the biomedical model has made a dramatic comeback. Several fields of medicine have edged closer to it; and this rapprochement has not been accompanied by any pronouncement about retaining the psychosocial insights of the past 30 years. Rather, accompanied by head shaking, excuses (economy, pragmatism), and appeals to what the public "really wants" from its physicians, the primary care fields, family medicine included, have set off for "safe" terrain once again (1988: 324–325).

What composer and conductor Gunther Schuller observed of the predicament of classical music in the United States of 1985 describes the state of medicine as well. Schuller spoke of

> "the disaster in America's public schools. . . . So instead of being concerned with the lack of musical literacy, what do the symphony orchestras do? Educate? A little: a few outreach programs—good efforts but drops on a hot stone. No, they plan better marketing techniques; they increasingly adopt the not-always-scrupulous methods of the big corporations—as if their only obligation were to survive and be solvent. Basically, they are opting not for audience education, venturesome programming and artistic integrity—I mean, the symphony orchestra exists to transmit the highest achievements of mankind!—but for better merchandising. . . .
>
> This Nielsen-rating mentality is unfortunately also behind the hiring of most of our music directors. The orchestra boards—most of them lay people—rarely know who is a good conductor, let alone a great one. They have to look it up in *Time*

> magazine. Mostly they're influenced by the latest marketplace hype and 'superstar' press clippings. So they usually get some exotic type, frequently non-American, who's got a smart, well-connected agent." . . .
>
> As the process of deterioration continues—the product becoming more "synthetic and homogenized"—the enlightened audiences of former years, he says, are not there anymore (quoted in Tassel 1985: 26).

It requires little more than the transposition of this passage from the language of music to the language of medicine to recognize a familiar clinical tone. "The industrialization of medicine" (Kormos 1984; Stephens 1984a, 1984c) or the "McDonaldization" of medicine (Ritzer and Walczak 1986) has redefined quality of care in terms of meeting the bottom line of cost effectiveness. Questions of who shall be served and how much they should receive are reduced to the patently social Darwinist dynamics of the "marketplace." In medicine as in music, the deeper truths we might discover about ourselves and human existence are set aside as a trivial pursuit under the cozening spell of a kind of cultural kitsch. Brief, mechanistic, "tough" individual and family therapies are designed to convince therapist and patient(s) alike that it is literally worthless to delve deeply or broadly into human afflictions. Minimalism in music and art is thus one with its counterpart in the once hallowed doctor-patient relationship, now relabeled a "therapeutic contract" or an agreement between the "consumer" of medical care and the "provider" or "product line manager."

In his book, *The Physician's Covenant: Images of the Healer in Medical Ethics*, William F. May notes the antipaternalist trend in modern biomedicine and the problematic shift toward greater patient responsibility in the physician's view of the relationship:

> [Antipaternalism] deals only with sins of excess, not of defect. Patients marked by liberty alone, without moral responsibility, can expect only technical services from professionals, no more. Radical antipaternalists today rail exclusively against the overbearing professional, but professionals are increasingly "underbearing" rather than overbearing. In the commercial world of today, antipaternalism often combines with libertarian assumptions to produce a callous, minimalist ethic (1983: 52).

Minimalism extends far beyond biomedicine. It is a powerful trend in what is often called "serious" contemporary music. It is the attitudinal hallmark of a rage-ridden and nuclear war–dreading age that has withdrawn from intimacy, commitment, and I-Thou relation and has replaced these with contractual, carefully circumscribed, limited laissez-faire relationships in which accountability is king. Partners to the relationship vigilantly watch the counterplayer—with the accounting book always in close range—for one false move, ready to accuse the other of having the worst intentions. Empathy and insight are difficult to attain if practitioners strive to make themselves immune to the very kind of data that would increase these qualities.

If in the depiction of the world of medicine the reader discerns a portrait of the age as well, the reader will recognize that the institution of medicine is one canvas upon which our society portrays itself. Healer, healing institution, and culture are always—although always with imperfect fit—made for each other, for they presuppose and complete one another. In the portrait of medicine lies a self-portrait of the society that medicine serves and embodies. Chapter 1 begins the canvas with a sketch of the role values play in American medicine.

Notes

1. Wayne Katon and Arthur Kleinman, for example, write that the "professional ideological basis of clinical practice is well illustrated in psychiatry by the call to return to a narrow medical model to resolve psychiatry's 'identity crisis' (Ludwig and Othmer 1977)" (1981: 256). Ironically, 1977 was also the year that saw the publication of Engel's landmark paper in *Science* calling for a "biopsychosocial" model—a way of thinking that had been adumbrated by the "radical" era from which the mainstream American society was now in full retreat.

ONE

Medicine, Value Orientations, and Their Meanings

This chapter identifies core values in biomedicine and explores the roles they play in healing relationships. The very identification of who and what should be treated, selection of admissible clinical data, choice of therapeutic modality, and expectation of outcome are themselves based upon value-laden assumptions. The considerable literature on the "health belief model" (see Jette et al. 1981) suggests that patient perception of susceptibility to a disease condition, severity of the consequences of that condition, and efficacy of recommended health action directly influence actual health-related behavior. Likewise, medical anthropologists have long contended that how a person or family diagnoses, defines, and explains the condition of illness determines "what are to him self-evident or necessary treatment pathways" (von Mering 1961: 52; Kleinman 1980). Values not only propel the behavior of patient and family; they likewise direct the action of the medical clinician. In this chapter I explore how values affect clinical thinking, judgment, decisionmaking, and action.

Writers on the subject have repeatedly noted that persistence in treatment, compliance with a clinician's treatment plan, improvement, satisfaction, and so forth have more to do with the patient's (or family's) perception of effectiveness (that one's expectations of therapy are being fulfilled) and with quality of the healer-client relationship than with the healer's theoretical model or specific skills (Ford 1978; Kleinman 1980; Phares 1979; Strupp and Bergin 1969). Yet clinicians highly value those theories, authorities, and techniques that they use to achieve their goals, to organize their inner and interpersonal worlds, and to minimize their anxieties. Patients and families may ascribe the favorable or unfavorable outcome of treatment to the personality of the clinician(s), to their relationship with the clinician, or to the degree of congruence between the clinician's beliefs and theirs. At the same time the clinician may attribute success to his or her paradigm or armory of "tricks" and may explain clinical failure by blaming the patient (or the patient's family, social class, or culture). Thus, there may be considerable congruence or disparity between the clinically related values of patient and practitioner. The values of the family, of the medical practitioner, and of the medical specialty to which the practitioner belongs play a vital, if also silent, role in the clinical assessment that takes place reciprocally among clinician, patient, and family. To locate the place of values in medicine, we must identify what values are, which turns out to be inseparable from identifying what they are for in human affairs.

Values: Basic Premises and Clinical Implications

Values are standards according to which people aspire to live, "measuring rods" by which they assess where and who they are in relation to who they feel they ought to be. Psychologically, values occupy the superego in the dual sense of serving as ideals and as sources of often severe judgment when one fails to live up to them. They prescribe and proscribe behavior. Values are among the criteria we all hold before (and above) ourselves to determine whether we are "good" or "bad." Values likewise play a vital role in delineating boundaries between self and other, between "us" and "them"; these identity boundaries often come to haunt patient care in biomedicine. John Spiegel defines three tasks that values perform:

> [Values] have an evaluative component—that is, they serve as principles for making preferred selections between alternative courses of action; an existential component, which means that the value orientations help to define the nature of reality for those who hold the given values; and finally, they have an affective component, which means that people not only prefer and believe in their own values, but are also ready to bleed and die for them. For this reason, values, once formed, can be changed only with the greatest difficulty (1971: 190).

Florence Kluckhohn (1953) posits four overarching problem areas of human life—relationships between people, our relationship to nature, our relationship to time, and our relationship to activity—each containing three distinct value orientations that are in turn hierarchically ranked. The "relational" value orientation consists of individualism, collaterality, and lineality. In relationships governed by individualism, the family or group prizes the distinctiveness of each person. In decisionmaking each person voices his or her opinion, and the group decides by majority vote. Collateral relationships place the family or group above the individual; indeed, the individual may be said not to exist. Decisionmaking is by consensus so that a sense of harmonious oneness will prevail. Lineal relationships are ruled vertically in a system of authoritarianism and loyalty, nurturance and dependency, dominance and submission. Stability is preserved as each individual maintains his or her sense of place.

The "human-nature" value orientation proposes that we can relate to nature in three distinct ways: mastery over nature, subjugation to nature, and harmony with nature. We can likewise orient ourselves to "time" by preferring the future, the past, or the present. We can prefer three different orientations to "activity": doing (which emphasizes success, achievement, mastery, improvement), being (which emphasizes spontaneity, the expression of feeling, impulsiveness), and being-in-becoming (which focuses upon personal development, integration, individuation). (See Table 1.1, categories 1 to 4, for an interpretation of these value orientations within American biomedicine.)

TABLE 1.1
DOMINANT VALUE ORIENTATIONS IN AMERICAN BIOMEDICINE

Category		Value (1st order)	Value (2nd order)	Value (3rd order)
1.	Relation to People[a]	Individual	Lineal	Collateral
2.	Relation to nature[a]	Mastery over nature	Subjugation to nature	Harmony with nature
3.	Time[a]	Future	Past	Present
4.	Activity[a]	Doing	Being	Becoming
5.	Locus of control	Inside (self)	Outside (other)	Between (interactive)

[a]Based on Kluckhohn and Strodtbeck (1961) and Spiegel (1971).

Dominant values live in uneasy truce with those that are subordinate (Devereux 1967: 209–213). In fact, they are often in conflict with one another in unconscious structure, family relations, and cultural roles. What I am (at the group level, what we are) is intimately connected to what I am not (what we disavow) but am tempted or afraid to be. De Vos writes that "individuals 'freeze up' when asked to learn something that might threaten an incompetence that is a protective part of one's identity, be it sexually or socially defined. For example, many boys and men 'cannot cook.' Just as many women and scholars 'cannot learn' to fix a leaky faucet" (1980: 114; see also De Vos 1975a). Values and value orientations are thus far more subtle and dynamic matters than one might at first consider them to be. As a defense against ambivalence, and as a hedge against mortality and fallibility, humans tend to reify values into invariant "they." One might speak of "serving" values, as though they had a life apart from oneself.

In the context of this discussion of values, consider the quandary voiced by a family medicine intern in dealing with patients whom he found personally, rather than medically, difficult. He was at an impasse about whether to assign dominance to the medical value of caring (personal) or to that of curing (biomedical) as a basis for self-esteem.

> When I go to family medicine clinic, it's my most dreaded day of the week. I don't mind *medically* difficult patients. It's difficult to be direct with patients we don't like. But there's little choice here who you see. How do you get rid of patients? Refer? Limit the time of the visit or schedule regular visits? You need a strategy to make them less dependent on you. Am I really doing them any good? Is it the best option they have? Should the physician be satisfied with no change in the patient's condition? I'm costing someone money. Is it all I can do? Am I an incompetent physician? I'm not satisfied with the patient's progress. . . . It's frustration when you don't *know* what's wrong with the patient.

For healers, intervention often seems less an opportunity to help than a compulsion to change others. It is as though they must prove to themselves through their patients that they are able to heal. In this way the patients become an extension of the healers' fantasied omnipotence. Paradoxically, the value of healing or change can itself interfere with the treatment process. The "need to heal" or "need to change" can become a source of clinical distortion as well as accomplishment (Stein 1982h). A family physician who especially enjoys obstetrics and surgery explained to me:

> I like to do a lot of OB [obstetrics]. There's an end point, and you know you're done. The woman is pregnant, I deliver her baby, and that's a cure. You can see the results of your work, a finished product. I know they say now that pregnancy isn't a disease, but you know what I mean. I get the same feeling doing surgery, and I know that's the reason people go into surgery and OB. They want results. They want something to show for it when they're done. Surgeons like to cut it [the diseased organ or tissue] and be finished. They go in, take out the appendix, and there's no question they've made a cure. A generation ago the patient would have died because they didn't have surgery and they couldn't do a cure. It's so different treating chronic illnesses. You do your goal setting, but end up feeling like a failure because the patient isn't cured.

This rich, poignant remark clearly establishes the value and personal significance of activity and doing; it also identifies those prized types of biomedical practice (specialties, some of which roles are incorporated into family medicine) through which those cherished values can be realized. Further, it illustrates the image of the physician-as-technician as many physicians' often elusive highest aspiration.

Doing is not a self-evident activity devoid of context or meaning. If I may oversimplify to make a point, doing means something very different to a peasant fatalist than it does to a boundlessly optimistic capitalist (see Stein 1983c). What is sorely needed in clinical ethnography, assessment, and treatment is careful attention to contending value orientations within medicine. The distinction between an active and passive orientation to problem-solving helps one to understand how individuals or groups experience problems (such as independence-dependence, or initiative-helplessness). Manipulation of the environment (alloplasticity) or manipulation of the self (autoplasticity) can be valued solutions to problems. Such distinctions as act-upon/acted-upon and initiator-of-action/recipient-of-another's-action are likewise useful in assessing a valued locus of control (Schwartzman 1982). (See Table 1.1, category 5.)

The dichotomy between active and passive underlies the dominant physician images of doer, fighter, and technician and the value orientations of individualism, mastery over nature, future orientation, and internal locus of control. Although this polarity is a value distinction, it is also a deeper, or "meta," organizing value. The wish and ability to "take charge"—over another person, over a situation, over a procedure—contrast with the feeling of being at the mercy of another, paralyzed into inaction, unable to do anything in the face of death. The quest to dominate medical situations expresses this search for ways to be active, to keep the upper hand, to enlist others (patients, their families, medical consultants, one's clinical staff) to work at one's behest. One young resident explained:

We want to give service, but we sure don't want to feel used, manipulated in return. I don't know what's worse, to get sued by a patient or to feel burned, a sucker, for doing what you thought was right. So then what do we do? We start to practice defensive medicine, assuming that everybody's out to get us, to try to talk us out of meds or into unnecessary surgery. You always try to keep one up on your patients. That's no good, for you get just as bad as the patients you mistrust. I guess I've just got to be more careful so that the manipulators don't take advantage of me. . . . Some patients *dare* you to try to take their disease away. They really drive you crazy if you try to cure them. Take away one symptom, they come back at you with another one, as if they're trying to beat you at some game. I like the kind of patient who wants to get better. They're good compliers, and you don't have to worry about what tricks you've got left up your sleeve to outsmart them. Why can't we dissect every medical problem like we did in anatomy?

The distinction between active and passive is less clear-cut than might be expected. Lurking behind the dread and conscious renunciation of the passive position (clinical manifestations of which are listening, waiting, "going along with nature," doing nothing) is a deeper wish for the forbidden pleasures of passivity (fulfilling dependency wishes, being taken care of). Because of its strength, this second wish must be disavowed all the more ardently. A foundation block underlying the doer identity of the biomedical physician is, if I might put it in a formula, "A doctor is not a patient." A doctor is one who, in taking care of others and their ailments, manages the patienthood of others and resists the lures and dangers of passivity. The avowed role obligation of patients is to use the socially acceptable transitional state of patienthood in order to become again an active member of society.

Physicians often make value compromises, tempering some professional values and standards in order to enhance others. A family physician in the Great Plains contrasted his practice style with that of academic physicians in the university hospital:

At the university hospital, they're purists when it comes to treating kids who come in with congestion, flulike symptoms, no fever, but whose moms insist on antibiotics. For the purists, the rule of thumb is, "No antibiotics without ear involvement [infection]." If the ear isn't red, the kid isn't going to get antibiotics no matter what the mom says. She might say, "My regular doctor's always given us antibiotics when Johnny's got like this" or "My mother always got antibiotics for me when I had the flu." But the purists don't budge. I've seen people leave mad, not getting what they came in for.

I'm more liberal with antibiotics. As a doctor, I'm offering a service to people. We're selling a service by being doctors. You wouldn't think of going back to a clothing store where you went to buy something and they wouldn't sell it to you. "I'll get it somewhere else then," that's what you'd say. It's the same with patients; they'll continue going to another physician until they get what they're after. If what I give them isn't going to harm them, why shouldn't I give it to them? Some other time, they'll be back for something I can treat them more scientifically for.

Here, "pure" (biomedical orthodoxy, or officially correct way to think) contrasts with an implicit "impure" (compromise), which the physician illustrates to mean offering the patient a "service" that assures patient satisfaction and, as importantly, the return of the patient for later service. This pragmatic, patient-pleasing intervention is distinct from the equally pragmatic but empirical decisionmaking and action discussed in the Introduction. In the radical empirical model of decisionmaking, the physician acts prophylactically as if a specific biomedical process were occurring and could be remedied by the course of action he or she prescribes to the patient (or patient's family). The physician, however, omits the step of awaiting diagnostic confirmation before commencing treatment. In either case, the value of doing is carried out.

There are also admixtures of the placebo and biomedical form of treatment. Many family physicians prefer to have patients who do not routinely request antibiotics. Nevertheless, they will offer a compromise to those patients who request them. One physician explained:

> I'll ask them [adults], "What do you usually take for these symptoms?" If I am sure the symptoms are viral, and the patient says he takes antibiotics for them, I'll suggest that he take aspirin and Tylenol and fluids, but that if he isn't feeling better in three days, then he can fill the prescription for antibiotics that I hand him. A lot of patients never fill the prescription. I know of one doctor who postdates the prescription three days after the clinic visit. Either way, if the patient really believes he needs antibiotics to feel better, he's got them.

This physician explains the biomedical model to the patient, who counters with, "I really need antibiotics" (or "a shot" of antibiotics). The physician compromises by offering his or her own scientific clinical judgment, asking the patient to act first on it (to "buy some time"), but expressing a willingness to work within the patient's model if the patient does not feel better within a stated time period. The physician might not call the antibiotic a placebo in this case, but the physician makes it clear that he or she is prescribing it because the patient requested it, not because the patient's model coincides with the physician's ideal model.

This physician's reasoning illustrates how complex, situational, and often strategic values can be in patient care. Several additional distinctions are useful in understanding clinicians' meanings and uses of values. One can speak of ***explicit*** and ***implicit*** values (C. Kluckhohn 1951) or ***manifest*** and ***latent*** values. These pairs, in turn, may or may not correspond to the distinction between values held ***consciously*** and those held ***unconsciously***. Moreover, just as values can be classified according to their content, they can also be categorized by the context to which they refer. Some values are held idiosyncratically, some are shared only within the family or professional discipline, and still others extend beyond the group to society. Some values are uniformly adhered to and are thus (or appear to be) context free, whereas others come into play only in certain contexts or situations. One can likewise distinguish between those values that in fact underlie behavior (***operant*** values) and those values by which a person claims to be guided (***expressed*** values) (see Richards 1956: 118–119).

For example, as a basis for action the clinical ideal of definitive, scientific diagnosis and rationality in clinical decisionmaking may not match the reality of radical empiricism and pragmatism (what works). In one instance, a forty-seven-year-old male went to his family doctor complaining of occasional chest pains.

He had a normal electrocardiogram (EKG) during his stress test but an abnormal reading at rest—an unusual reversal of the "typical" picture. His family physician prescribed a calcium blocker (Cardizem), saying that "it works with a lot of people for a lot of cardiac symptoms. But we don't know why it works. But if it doesn't help, it also doesn't hurt. I want you to give it a try to see if it helps."

These distinctions are far from academic. They have consequences for patients and practitioners alike. For example, it is important to wonder what frame of reference to assign the value assertion by a father in his initial visit to the clinic: "In our family, the children's health always comes first." Is it a family fiction that flies in the face of observed fact? Is it a value rigidly adhered to regardless of the situation? Is it a proclaimed ideal that he "somehow" contrives to subvert?

The core constellation of American values—which includes self-reliance or inner-directedness, autonomy, independence, mobility, privacy, individuality, and future orientation—is systematically counterposed with such values as other-directedness, hierarchical authority, dependency, fixity, community, consensus or conformity, and past orientation (Devereux 1967). Americans pride themselves on their freedom but are fascinated with foreign tyranny and the pomp of British royalty. American parades, football homecoming games, and beauty contests all have their kings and queens.

For many, official core American values represent immigrant forebears' shared attempts to distance themselves from more underlying and enduring historical values. Mobility can be a flight from dependency, from being tied down to place or relationship (Stein 1974a, 1980c). Self-reliance can be a vehicle for pulling oneself away from domination by hierarchical authority. One flees into the future in order to escape from the past. A profound melancholy underlies cheerful optimism. Americans believe that they can master anything yet dread being mastered by anyone or anything ("Better dead than Red"). This holds not only for "old Americans" (Yankees) or long-acculturated ethnics but for each successive wave of immigrants or for internal immigrants (blacks, Hispanics) eager to trade old lives for new.

Moreover, the very words used to express American values can be confusing if not misleading to the observer. For instance, "individualism" is often wrongly assumed to mean individuation, whereas the former is a panicky retreat from relationship and the latter is the growing awareness of personal distinctiveness. Likewise, "mobility" refers to the wish-become-need to keep on the move, to avoid settling down too permanently, whereas "motility" denotes the capacity of the growing baby to feel and explore his or her environment with (optimally) a minimum of anxiety and a maximum of autonomy. In short, a person can consciously avow that a value has certain life-shaping meanings, but observation of that person's actual behavior, expression of feelings, and use of words can make the case for the presence of other, powerful, and out-of-awareness values.

The Sick Role and Its Associated Values

According to biomedical culture, there exists an ideal, defined as health, from which disease can be identified as a deviation. Diseases each have (ideally) discretely identifiable (objective) signs and (subjective) symptoms that biomedical practitioners can observe and treat. Even before the formulation of the problem-oriented medical record in the 1970s and diagnostic-related groups (DRGs: diagnosis-based medical reimbursement for hospitalized patients) in the 1980s, biomedical assessment, diagnosis, and treatment were conceptualized as problem-solving. With the patient's cooperation and compliance, the physician would search for the correct name of the medical problem and would prescribe to the patient its solution, which would lead to the restoration of health (defined as the absence or resolution of the presenting problem).

As I have stated earlier in this chapter, one of the principal motivations and implicit functions of the biomedical-problem model is to widen the social distance between physician (or other practitioner) and patient. Through the activism of diagnosis and the metaphor of physician as applied biological scientist, practitioners can and do persuade and reassure themselves that the patient, not the clinician, has the "problem" (disease) in need of "fixing," that the practitioner can muster the forces of knowledge and procedure to repair the "problem," that problems and vulnerabilities are conditions from which patients, not practitioners, suffer (Devereux 1980a: 260–261). To be sanctioned to "repair" another (active) is to remove oneself from an intolerable condition of patienthood (passive). (This paragraph benefited from my discussions with James Mold, M.D., during 1987 and 1988.)

Spiegel refers to "the way cultural values are built into the personality as a mechanism for the control of anxiety" (1971: 316). Fred Sander (1979) similarly maintains that value orientations are heir to ***primitive splitting***, itself a means of managing anxiety. In primitive splitting, which occurs early in human psychological development, the infant constructs bipolar sets of mental representations. Pleasurable experiences of the self and of others (usually mothering figures) evolve into an "all good" set of images. These are split off from frustrating and painful images of the self and others, which evolve into an "all bad" set (Volkan 1976).

> The world and self in the infant's blurry eyes are either good *or* bad and thus hopefully within the sphere of the infant's omnipotent control. . . . This "splitting" tendency of seeing human nature as good or evil, the environment as beneficent or menacing, of man as master of, the slave of, or in harmony with nature, are matters of "basic value orientations." F. Kluckhohn (1953) first systematically studied how all cultures express and reflect such generalized views, giving its members a sense of their relationship to the world (Sander 1979: 123).

Numerous studies argue that the relationship between health and illness, normal and abnormal, is one of degree instead of kind (Barrabee and von Mering 1953; von Mering 1970; Mead 1947; Zborowski 1969; Opler 1957; Bakan 1968; Grinker 1973; F. Alexander 1948, 1950; Freud 1901, 1927, 1930; Devereux 1956; La Barre 1972). For example, Roy Grinker writes that "health and illness vary only in degree of smoothness of transactional operations, in nearness to equilibrium or disintegration, and degree of de-differentiation in response to stress, signaled by anxiety" (1973: 194). By placing the individual against the cultural base, one can place in context the ordinary and the extraordinary. One must study the "well" in order to understand the "sick" and study the "ill" in order to understand what is hidden and obscured in the "healthy" because what is explicit in illness is implicit in health. Deviation from the norm is a guide to the norm through its distortion, exaggeration, or florid expression.

Nevertheless, if health and illness are usually dichotomized into opposites, then we have a right to wonder why the compartmentalization is so important to those who insist on it. George De Vos (1975b) argues that one must not accept cultural cognitive categories or taxonomies at face value but must look beneath them to determine the extent and kind of emotional investment they contain. Whereas some categorizations are matters of simple utility and convention, others are so heavily overdetermined that they are imbued with elements of stigma or contamination. Consider, for example, the categories of "chronic illness," "disability," and "rehabilitation" in American culture and medicine.

In American culture, those who are afflicted with chronic illness or disability and are in need of long-term care or rehabilitation are often regarded as different in kind, not degree, from those who are only temporarily, acutely ill. This categorical distinction between the able bodied or healthy and the disabled or chronically sick is a cue to the swift cultural current of anxiety among those who ardently wish to perceive themselves, and to be seen by others, as well. The rigidity of the boundary, and the tenacity with which it is maintained, gives form to the fear of pollution or contamination from the other side. The categorizing of health-related differences serves as a culture-wide defense mechanism for the well who are terrified at the prospect that they might indeed be sick. Ernest Jones cogently argues that "the only tenable definition of an insane person is a person who threatens to unmask the unconscious (i.e. insane) mentality which the community finds intolerable" (1948: 204). Because what the statistically normal community finds intolerable is actually part of itself, it must remask itself as clearly distinguishable from those it labels deviant. There does indeed exist a continuum, a connection, between health and illness, between temporary illness and chronic illness, but this recognition—that acute could be chronic, that decay and death are the lot of us all—must often be denied.

In the model of the "sick role" offered by Talcott Parsons (1951), one that has held up remarkably well during the years, illness is a form of deviance, both statistically and functionally, from the normal. Treatment is a rite of social control which purpose is to restore to functional normalcy the disequilibrium in relationships of all concerned, although a designated patient may be the focus of the ritual process. The patient is permitted by family, medical professionals, and society at large to enter the sick role and temporarily abdicate normal role obligations. The understanding remains, however, that the patient will participate diligently in the treatment process, respond to medical efforts in his or her behalf, and recover and reassume his or her conventional social roles (spouse, parent, worker).

Douglas Uzzell proposes that illness is a "strategic role," a form of "legitimate deviance," and that "withdrawal from interaction becomes a mechanism for maintaining interaction" (1974: 374). The negotiation not only of the sick role but of the entire social rite of illness is a complementary mirroring process between patient and society. Social roles, including clinical ones, do not exist independently of the motivations that infuse them. Donald Tuzin notes that "acknowledging the subjective component enables us to consider the mechanisms of symbolic attachment as they are grounded in the motivations of individuals" (1977: 199; also see Koenigsberg 1975). Otto von Mering reminds us that we must attend to illness as a form of "internal and external problem solving" (1970: 277) that includes "the value which illness may have in an individual's life task and way of life" (1970: 279).

In light of these perspectives on the sick role, it becomes apparent that in American culture chronic illness and disability create an insuperable problem: They defy the very normative basis of American culture. How this anomaly is dealt with reveals to us core cultural conflicts and defenses against them. The topic and practice of rehabilitation and rehabilitation medicine occupy a rather marginal status in medicine, just as the chronically ill and disabled are marginal in the wider society. The chronically diseased patient, the patient in need of long-term rehabilitation, the patient whose disease cannot be cured but only controlled or maintained—these are stigmatized along the continuum from the individual caregiver to national federal funding priorities. Likewise, within health care, disability medicine has tended to be regarded as a medical pariah.

An explanation of this outcasting can readily be understood if one recognizes the fit, or congruence, between dominant American cultural values and numerous official medical and popular medical slogans (see Kaufman 1988; Kaufman and Becker 1986). Among the core American values are freedom, (upward) mobility, courage, success, achievement, productivity, future orientation, active agency in one's life, independence, change, mastery, will, aggressiveness in the pursuit of one's goals, physical attractiveness (youth and beauty), and the like. Social status, standing, standing on one's own, and stature all are associated with erect posture and the ability to move oneself ("motivation!") and keep personal control of one's movement.

Official professional scientific medicine, and the popular lay "health culture" (Weidman and Egeland 1973) that shares with it a common cultural system of meanings, gives voice to these selfsame values and orientations. This is readily evident in the following list of ubiquitous slogans and phrases: "emergency" medicine; "intensive," "acute," and "critical" care; "heroic" and "extreme" measures; "wonder" and "miracle" drugs; "radical" surgery; "dramatic" recovery; the "new lease on life" that surgery provides; "quick-action" medication; aspirin that brings "fast, fast, fast relief"; and so forth. A vital strand in the Judeo-Hellenic-Christian tradition and literature is the overcoming of disability or handicap by personal strength of will or faith (Hill 1978; Trautmann and Pollard 1975). When religious faith does not suffice, then—as Faust's "bargain" with the devil attests—the willful renunciation of faith often becomes the path for attaining one's ambitions. The clinician often has considerable difficulty admitting that nothing can be done, because that would require that he or she question the activity-mastery premise of medicine.

As an agent of restoration to social productivity (work, functioning), the giver of health care becomes seriously impaired in relation to the disabled. How the clinician reacts to feelings evoked by the disabled patient influences how he or she treats and responds to the needs of the patient—in fact, what he or she perceives those needs to be. The disabled or chronically ill person not only reminds the care-giver of current anxieties but rekindles memory of childhood—what one never received or received only temporarily, later repudiated, yet what at an even deeper level one yearns for and must reject all the more vehemently. In American culture, one liberates oneself from and divests oneself of the past in order to pursue the future. Chronically ill or disabled people symbolize the foreclosure of the future and the reimprisonment by an even more terrifying past that gives "history" its negative valence—the childhood dependency and infantilized vulnerability of patient and care-giver alike.

From the dying leukemic patient to the listless depressive to the demanding hypochondriac with ever-new symptoms, those who have given up on or are angry with life, who insist that there is little to live for, or who are indeed ready to let go of life and die often elicit not compassion but barely disguised rage and contempt from those who treat them. Often they will be referred from clinician to clinician, or from institution to institution, as each in turn tries to be of help, feels a sense of failure, displaces responsibility on the patient for failure, and "transfers" the case to another (a process called "turfing," or "dumping"). If one can imagine in modern biomedicine the magically curative, alchemic function of medicine transmuted into the attempted conquest of death itself, then one can understand how medicine stands dumbfounded and stupefied at the prospect of treating a condition that can be neither conquered nor cured nor reversed.

This is not to deny that the identified patient has limitations, to overlook the problems inherent in chronic illness or disablement, or to assert that the problem is located entirely within the clinician or the mainstream culture. Clinicians are confronted with difficult, real-world choices regarding the allocation of medical resources. Rather, it is to emphasize that cultural attitudes and values, which represent patterned defenses, superimpose and inject problems where others already exist (such as paralysis) and create them before they are even present (such as dread of aging). Further, there are chronically ill and disabled patients who seek gratification of dependency wishes or economic gain through their illness and who stand to lose these if they improve. The sufferer's increasing self-isolation and ostracism by the social environment often become a vicious spiral. Otto Fenichel remarks that "the symptoms may acquire secondarily the significance of a demonstration of one's own helplessness in order to secure external help such as was available in childhood" (1945: 126). Ultimately, however, neither identified patient, family of patient, health care system, nor culture can rightfully be isolated as the locus of blame or exoneration. Rather, the portrait of chronic illness and disability offered here is one of a systems pathology that expresses core cultural values and conflicts.

As categories of thought and feeling, chronic illness and disability in American society play out a macabre social ballet in which the central drama is the embodiment and disembodiment of our worst fears and, at times, our deepest wishes. What the cultural mainstream casts out it then attempts to relocate in cadres of outcasts, those permanently marked by some affliction. The latter, in turn, adapt to a "condition" that is not entirely theirs. In a study of leprosy, Zachary Gussow and

George Tracy (1968) argue that stigma is the starting point for the formation of a "disabled" identity. Such an identity system reflects the lepers' efforts to minimize the severity of their condition and to prove that the disparaging label imposed upon them (and with which they may have unconsciously identified) is wrong. This dynamic is not unlike strategies adopted by numerous ethnic, racial, and other minority groups in the United States (see Stein and Hill 1977).

In a later study, Gussow and Tracy (1976) discuss the role of voluntary self-help groups in the management if not reversal of stigma: for example, Alcoholics Anonymous, Ephysema Anonymous, National Alliance for the Mentally Ill, Mended Hearts, ostomy clubs, stroke clubs, laryngectomy clubs, ex-cigarette smokers' clubs, and so forth. Self-help organizations, which are to an extent isolated by the wider society, often respond to rejection by repudiating those who have spurned them, thereby leading to even greater self-isolation and vindication by a turning inward. American age-grading, which takes such ubiquitous forms as ageism and the formation of academic and medical disciplines that specialize in the aged (gerontology, geriatrics), has created a dual image of youth as paradise and vitality and age as decline and handicap. This has inexorably led to the segregation and self-segregation of "the elderly" and the formation of such self-help groups as the Gray Panthers and the American Association of Retired Persons. (For a comprehensive overview of self-help groups, see Powell 1987.)

The Biomedical Value System

From the viewpoint of first-order biomedical values, caring, comforting, nondirective counseling, waiting, and "doing nothing" are anathema. Actively intervening, aggressively treating, controlling, curing, and fixing the patient are acceptable and are sources of increased self-esteem for the clinician. The latter core values preserve the illusion of distance between healer and patient. These other, virtually heretical approaches threaten to blur the role distinction, to make patient and practitioner more vulnerable participants in a common situation rather than one suffered only by the patient.

Intertwined with the values of activism and doing, and the core conceptualization of disease as a disturbance of inner organs and tissue, is the paramount significance given to visualization or seeing as a means of identifying what the pathology is and where it is located spatially. One could plausibly argue that culturally, technology follows and endlessly elaborates upon this visual mode of knowing. Technological imaging abounds utilizing X-rays, sound, radiation, magnetism, light, and inserted instruments as ways of attempting to see or visualize the inside of the body (for instance, optical and electronic microscopy, X-rays, computerized axial tomography [CAT scans], positron emission tomography [PET scans], magnetic resonance imaging [MRI], bronchoscopy, sigmoidoscopy, and the like). In such a clinical worldview, the potential virtues of listening tend to be minimized if not lost or narrowed to stethoscope-mediated listening. In short, various technologies of visualizing the body interior are means to the goal of locating and actively eliminating the pathology that is defined in terms of "internal" medicine (see Hahn 1985b).

Even the incorporation of various behavioral sciences (medical anthropology, medical sociology, clinical psychology, family therapy) into biomedical curricula during the halcyon years of the 1960s has done little to increase compassion and listening within medical professionalism. Rather, as I often observe, they have largely been assimilated into the doing and fixing model, providing biomedical practitioners with yet more of the same in their tool kit. In one department of family medicine, for instance, a psychologist/family therapist used what are termed brief, "strategic" therapy approaches, including paradoxical interventions such as "prescribing the symptom" (for example, telling an anorexic patient not to eat). For a time family medicine residents used a fad technique they called "zapping" patients with paradoxes. The residents concluded that because *they* felt more in control by having this technique, their patients must be benefiting from it as well.

Later, this family therapist introduced another technique, called "circular questioning," developed by the Milan school of family therapy, according to which approach clinicians pose a series of questions to various family members about how they think others would perceive the pertinent symptom, respond to it, and so forth. Many residents, at least for a time, were enthralled by the technique, seeing in it an endless bag of questions to ask virtually everyone in the family, to keep the residents in control of the relationship, and to prevent silences or too-freewheeling discussion. In anthropological terms, this illustrates ***cultural diffusion***, the process by which new cultural materials (such as from behavioral sciences) are selectively incorporated into older (and more established) cultural boundaries (such as from biomedicine) with the result that the new material conforms to the old premises (practitioner controlling, doing, maintaining social distance, and so on).

The specific localization of the site of pathology within the body and its subsequent treatment there are central to the biomedical value system. Heir to the body/mind dichotomy and to the split between the individual organism and the world, biomedicine explicitly conceptualizes disease, its cause, and its treatment in terms of the basic sciences. The central organizing paradigm of biomedicine is that of internal medicine. Robert Hahn writes that

> internal medicine is the mind, if not the heart, of "Western" medicine—Biomedicine. It is called simply "medicine." It is medicine's medicine, the generic and central specialty to which other specialties refer for the last word on our underlying ills, our "diseases." Internal medicine is perhaps the most rational of Biomedical specialties, advocating action by systematic calculation of the patient's internal pathophysiology, in preference to more direct, surgical penetration for unobstructed vision and intervention.
>
> While their techniques are often lethally and vitally powerful, internists are inclined to favor reason over force, and integral strategy over topical action. Medicine is thus known among fellow specialties as "conservative": To "go medically" is purportedly to intervene more cautiously, to act mainly from outside the body's boundaries, "non-invasively"; perhaps it is to respect more fully the body's constitutional and physiological processes. Yet even non-invasive medicine may be more or less "aggressive," actively intervening or forbearing entirely—"doing nothing," to allow a so-called "natural" course (1985b: 51–52).

Medical students, interns, residents, and practitioners feel that they are living up to their ideal of "real medicine" (biomedicine) when they have what they call "hands-on" contact with their patients. Given the physical, procedural emphasis on implementing the values of activity and mastery, the thought of just sitting and talking with patients and families is often disparaged and ridiculed. For centuries in the West, "listening" (to the chest, abdomen, with the invention of the stethoscope in 1816), palpating, percussing, and poking have been the stock in trade of physicians' hands-on assessment techniques from internal medicine. In recent decades, however, with the advent of high-technology forms of imaging (CAT scans, ultrasounds, and, of course, X-rays), direct touch, for diagnostic or therapeutic purposes, has been on the wane among biomedical practitioners. Roger Nosal writes that

> medicine, over the centuries, has involved the "laying on of hands" as both a means for diagnosis and especially as an adjunct to the healing process. Since World War II, advances in scientific technology and the enormous developments in pharmacotherapeutics have tended to force skills of manipulation, traction, and massage into the background of medical education. Recently trained students are provided with little formal introduction to this segment of practice unless they have extended exposure to physical therapy or perhaps the benefit of preceptorial experience with a clinician skilled in manipulative techniques (1987: 237).

Internal medicine represents the ideal of "physiological wholeness" (Hahn 1985b: 54). The cultural and medical extreme against which internal medicine compares itself is the specialty of surgery. Its emphasis is upon boundary-violating, invasive procedures, direct looking at and handling of the body's organs, and the virtues of aggressiveness, action, doing, mastery, conquest. Surgeons are both envied and ridiculed by their internist colleagues (including pediatricians and family physicians) for their prowess and often swashbuckling demeanor, dogged certainty, and commitment to decisive action. With envy and revulsion many family physician colleagues attribute to surgeons the aphorism "When in doubt, cut it out," the antithesis of watchful waiting. If internal medicine is the cultural and medical norm (both in the sense of official group ideal and statistical representativeness), surgery represents that norm of clinical ambition at its unrestrained extremes. Surgery is cast in the image of the dauntless Faustian frontiersman who takes nature into his own hands and fashions it to his will.

The distinction between internal medicine and surgery is one of degree rather than kind, for they share the underlying cultural theory of biomedicine, "according to which both pathogenesis and therapy are seen as essentially natural, biological, physiological and ultimately physical events" (Gaines and Hahn 1985: 9). Accordingly intervention in these events is guided by the central values of American medicine and its underlying culture. The biomedical cultural core is united in the view of pathology "as purely a disturbance in biophysiological structure of process" (Gaines and Hahn 1985: 6).

Allan Young (1976) distinguishes between "internal" and "external" medicine on the basis of *where* clients, practitioners, families, and communities *locate* the problem to be treated and thereby designate *what* or *who* is to be given treatment. Since the age of the great anatomists and dissectors—Andreas Vesalius, William Harvey, Leonardo da Vinci—internal medicine has been the touchstone for medical reality in biomedicine. Problems are to be looked for/sought out, located, defined, identified, isolated, and treated inside the human body—that is, physically on or under the skin. Improvement or cure is measured in terms of how the pathological tissue or organ compares with normal tissue or organ appearance and function. Further, in such internal medicine, the disturbance is conceptualized as always occurring within an individual human body. Within the division of labor of American biomedicine, two specialties personify the fundamental internal orientation: internal medicine, which is the more conservative with its focus on medication or "letting nature take its course," and surgery which is the more radical, taking to extreme the virtues of aggressive treatment, active intervention, and "masculine" prowess.

In external medicine, the cause, cure, and nature of the problem are situated outside the body. Far from being restricted to the symptomatic individual or presenting patient, the disturbance or pathology is identified by the practitioner as being embodied or caused by a broader context, which can range from disturbed relationships to environmental or occupational hazards to social pathologies (the nuclear threat). Biomedicine currently includes several specialties that at least in part embody external medicine in theory and practice: occupational medicine, sports medicine, community medicine, geriatric medicine, aerospace medicine, family medicine. The diagnosis and exorcism of "voodoo" possession and "root work" among some American black communities, nine-night Navajo coyoteway ceremonials used to cure illnesses, the contextual treatment of the "identified patient" in marital and family therapy, the seventeenth century witch trials in Salem, Massachusetts, and Hitler's effort to exterminate the Jews, who symbolized "cancer" and "vermin" in the "body politic" of Germany, are all examples of external medicine. (These two paragraphs benefited from discussion I had with Robert Like, M.D., November 1987.)

Despite their obvious manifest differences, both internal and external medicine share a tendency toward an artificially narrow focus. When this occurs in internal medicine (professional, folk, or popular), the whole of the problem may be taken out of the self and put altogether inside some part or parts of the physical body. Thus, for instance, in conceptualizing and treating cardiovascular disease, diabetes mellitus, or infectious disease, biomedical physicians tend to concentrate on adjusting or intervening in processes inside the body and give little consideration to matters of aggression, dependency, anxiety, and the like. In relation to these same diseases, practitioners of external medicine might examine the patient's disturbed relationships (family, work, church) or disequilibrium with the environment, practice divination to undo a possible "curse," or inquire into the patient's lifestyle for predisposing outer stressors. In external medicine, the whole of the problem is likewise extruded from the self and put into other people, relationships, behavioral habits, culturally expectable "life stress events" (for example, Holmes and Rahe 1967), and the like.

Medicalized meaning, both internal and external, may easily function for many professional and popular participants alike as an avoidance of personalized meaning. This assures that clinical discourse will be about some physicalized "it" rather than about the symbolic "I." Somatic reductionism thus serves as a personal, interpersonal, and cultural defense, thereby stabilizing the relationship while assuring that the psychosocial situation will not be addressed. Other professionals, such as clinic nurses or social workers, are often demoralized by the failure of their high-status medical colleagues (and administrative superiors) to acknowledge or to address the more personal, social aspects of the patients' distress, and by their tendency to delegate ("refer") this aspect or "part" entirely to "auxiliary" or "support" medical staff and exclude it from the physician-patient dialogue.

In American popular culture, for physician and patient to agree upon a medicalized diagnosis and treatment plan may help the patient to save face. Physician and patient tacitly agree to focus (and displace) attention from self to thing. For example, a 200 pound female had visited a number of physicians for medical assistance with her goal of weight loss, and had unsuccessfully tried dieting. Her mainstays included hamburgers, fried chicken, french fries, cheeses, beef and steak, eggs, and the like. She could not bring herself to cut down on these, no matter how hard she tried. She dismissed physicians' attempt to link her overeating with "stress."

Eventually, she found her way to an allergist, who conducted a $1,000 medical workup of food allergies. He presented her with an impressive display of computer printouts and graphs and gave a long, detailed list of the foods to which she was allergic; the list coincided with those foods she craved and consumed voraciously. He did not try to help her—or cajole her—to lose weight. He labeled hers a ***medical problem*** (food allergy), thereby relieving her of the fear, shame, and guilt of having a ***personal problem***. Other physicians had said she lacked will power.

Knowing now precisely what her pernicious "allergies" were, she diligently avoided them, eating instead the prescribed carrots, celery, fruit juices, boiled or broiled chicken, and the like. In a matter of months she lost eighty pounds and, instead of being miserable, was happy with her life. She did not need to think about her "self"; she directed her thought and action to her "allergies." In this case, which combines features of both the internal and external medicine models, the overlap between the professional and popular models permitted allergist and patient to collaborate on a face-saving, avowedly naturalistic approach and thus to avoid the debasing personalistic model that had been toxic to the prior clinical relationship.

What is most unfortunate about her original patient-physician relationships is that her doctors had relied upon a culturally standardized and stylized personalistic account according to which her weight problem was due to her lack of "will power" (a virtue that men are often held to possess and women held to lack). The original physician could not hear her story apart from a clinically personalistic approach that precluded information based on compassion and inquiry into the distress the woman's weight represented to her. In the least, her allergist evaluated her without judging her and treated her without (at least overtly) dismissing her. Ultimately, and paradoxically, the patient exercised her own will by going to the allergist, and the allergist achieved the coveted biomedical goal of a cure based on internal medicine principles. Yet, in falling back upon culturally conventionalized clinical accounts, both the initial physician and the allergist missed the opportunity to recognize their patient as a human being and elicit and work within the story they could not allow her to tell (I wish to thank manuscript editor Jan Kristiansson for her stimulating ideas about this case, many of which are incorporated into this paragraph.)

An interesting interplay between internal and external medicine can be found in the discipline of family medicine, founded in 1969 (see Stein 1987d; also Stein 1981b). In playing out the conflict between the image of generalists (those in general practice) and specialists (those who specialize in specific organ systems or smaller units are often called subspecialists), family physicians opt for a number of role resolutions. Some wish to demonstrate to themselves and to their competing medical specialist or subspecialist colleagues that they are equally competent at internal medicine. In so doing, they hope to elevate family medicine to a more bona fide, mainstream, legitimate status within the "family" of medical specialties.

Others, embracing the "biopsychosocial model" proposed by Engel (1977) and dissatisfied with the mechanistic, often reductionist thinking of "microbe hunting," seek to make family medicine into a broadly socially responsible, "contextual medicine." In this view, family medicine would encompass internal and external aspects of a complex system of meanings and processes. Still others are attracted to an emphasis on the external medicine aspect of family medicine and hope to legitimate the diagnosis and treatment of the family as if "it" were an "organ" of sorts. In this mode, family medicine practitioners would select the family as a focus for study akin to pulmonologists whose organ is the lung, cardiologists whose organ is the heart and circulatory system, gastroenterologists whose organ is the gastrointestinal tract, and so on. In a speech titled "Family Medicine: A Retrospective View," Jonathan E. Rodnick, M.D., laments, "I wish sometimes that we had an organ in the body called the family organ and then we could have had a discipline and specialty with no trouble at all. And we could have had an NIH [National Institute of Health] institute that way. But we don't, and we were instead born into the crisis of the biomedical mode" (1987: 3). At the fantasy level, Rodnick evokes the familiar issues of potency and gender insecurity (wishing for a "family organ," with "organ" commonly symbolizing the penis that is present or lacking) and anxiety about birth and about being wanted ("born into . . . crisis").

The genogram has become a widely adopted ideological as well as clinical tool of family assessment in family medicine. Briefly, the *genogram* (similar to an anthropologist's kinship diagram and popular genealogies) traces patterns of relationships in families during several generations (see Pendagast and Sherman 1977; Bowen 1978; McGoldrick and Gerson 1985). Several family medicine and family therapy colleagues have long expressed the wish that we be able to streamline, abbreviate, and package the genogram so that we would have a bona fide rapid assessment instrument analogous if not superior to those in other medical specialties. In one sarcastic moment, during a conversation with a physician colleague, I designated such an imaginary instrument a "fam-scan." The diseased or dysfunctional family system would thus become the organ that etiologically leads to internal bodily pathology in particular family members. Although family physicians would continue to practice internal medicine and make referrals to other internal medicine specialists, they would hope to demonstrate that the real and final cause of disease is the family unit.

Many family practitioners and family medicine academicians of this school reject the narrowness of internal medicine and zealously advocate the family systems thinking of external medicine. Ironically, however, the patient's, family's, and community's realms of meaning and feeling still tend to be excluded from clinical interest. As a result, in its underlying logic, much of family medicine's current family systems thinking and intervention resemble in cultural structure the very internal medicine model with which it has doctrinally quarreled. In short, within American medicine, the basis for inclusion, acceptance, and legitimacy of a *new* idea or modality is congruence with the overall *form* and its associated *values* of the American medical system.

Of course, momentous cultural distinctions do abound in medicine. In an article titled "Children, Families, and Mental Health Service Organizations," Helen Schwartzman et al. (1984) document how multicultural medical and mental health organizations really are. Different services, units, wards, and institutions have differing values, expectations, and perceptions from others, which result in organizational differences and conflicts that "perpetuate service delivery problems such as context replication and continue the practice of blaming the patient for differences that exist in the service system" (1984: 305).

Among the basic distinctions within American medicine that might already be obvious to the reader are those between technological, procedure-oriented organic medicine (often called "real medicine") and "talk" and other therapies; between surgery and medication regimen (or, in the conflict between physiatrists and surgeons, between traction and surgery); among psychiatry, clinical psychology, social work, family therapy, counseling biofeedback, and meditation; (within psychiatry) among biological psychiatry, cognitive psychotherapy, depth psychotherapy, family therapy, and group therapy; and among the labels "doctor," "physician," "therapist," and "counselor." In medical institutions chronic conflict occurs between those services whose functions are patient care and those whose functions are administration (a distinction that embodies the conflict between giving care and asking for payment for care received). Among medical (M.D.) and allied specialties (nurse, nurse practitioner, physician's associate, medical assistant), there is constant competition for legitimacy based on the authority traditionally ascribed to the physician. Moreover, although many family therapists and biofeedback technicians reject the medical model, they tend to appeal to the underlying cultural worldview they share with physicians. Further, they often seek to possess the authority and status associated with the physician whom they hope to displace. They vie for that authority by embracing and adopting the culturally high-status language of technology, hoping to persuade the prospective patient or client that theirs is a mightier technology.

Thus, biomedicine, while a unified cultural "whole" at one level of abstraction, is pluralistically multicultural and competitively so. Numerous biomedical specialties, together with their allied health, nursing, and physician's associate colleagues, not only cooperate with each other for the benefit of the patient but vie with one another for the patient as well. Even small differences mobilize vicious *clinical ethnocentrism* (the heightened positive valuing of one's own specialty and the devaluing of one's biomedical neighbors). Sciences, like ethnic groups, nations, and religions, all experience what De Vos (1966) calls "status anxiety" as they compare themselves with others, hoping to be superior while dreading inferiority.

Certainly, academic disciplines do not go so far as to kill for the sake of these group identities—that, at least, is done only in the name of religion, nation, ethnicity, and politics. But in relationships between medical cultures and institutions within biomedicine, no less than in international affairs, human beings everywhere create such gaps between "us" and "them" and create categories of "enemies" and "allies" to shore up their own cohesiveness and sense of self-worth (Stein 1985h, 1987b; GAP Committee on International Relations and Stein 1987; Volkan 1988). These universal group issues are every bit as real—and decisive in their consequences—as are the ostensible sources and foci of intergroup conflict and rivalry.

Therapeutic Activism

Throughout my experience as clinical teacher and supervisor, countless residents in psychiatry and family medicine have restlessly demanded, in word or in deed, "Just tell me what to *do* with the patient." As stated by Eisenberg:

> Doctors are trained to "do something." They believe that patients expect a consultation to have a tangible outcome: a pill or a shot. It requires the disruption of overlearned habits to change from doing to listening (and to come to recognize that listening is an important way of doing). It demands a shift in paradigms from disease to illness in order to change from prescribing to attending to meanings and to helping patients to examine options. Despite the fact that it is primary care physicians to whom patients with psychosocial disorders turn and from whom they get such help as they receive, most practitioners report themselves ill-trained for the task, uncomfortable with it, and reluctant to undertake it. Educated in tertiary care centers, they are poorly prepared for the problems patients present in primary care. . . . Physicians are rewarded disproportionately when they perform procedures in contrast to providing "cognitive services." One need not suppose that physicians are solely motivated by economics to recognize that it is difficult to resist the temptation to carry out a procedure, if only to confirm a clinical diagnosis, when it yields greater income and at the same time impresses the patient with its magical properties (1988: 208–209).

The dominant value orientation prevalent within medicine commits those in the healing professions to frequently unrealistic reliance upon one-way technique apart from the therapeutic relationship in which the technique is used. This orientation likewise leads clinicians to feel they have to do something (alleviate the pain, cure disease, remove the anxiety, change the family structure) in order to prove their competence. One of the principal motives behind and functions of the value of such therapeutic activism is to stave off the sense of depression, despair, and impotence in the physician.

Family physician James Mold, M.D., with whom I have co-authored two articles on clinical "cascades" that result from physician anxiety (Mold and Stein 1986; Stein and Mold 1988), points out to me that physicians often become overly involved in the care of patients poststroke—for example, in ordering and adjusting medications and in ordering Foley catheters (which commonly lead to urinary tract infections). For him, stroke rehabilitation is not, for the most part, a medical problem but a rehabilitation problem. Occupational therapy and physical therapy should be quickly involved in the poststroke rehabilitative care of the patient. For him, stroke is not a physician problem, but because physicians want to do something, they often stay involved and thereby complicate matters and delay the process of rehabilitation. He recommends instead that physicians "resist the urge to do!" (Mold 1988).

In his article "The Ailment," Thomas Main (1957) describes the emotional responses of hospital personnel to difficult patients. Main's description of what physicians and nurses view as the ideal patient corresponds to Parsons's portrait of the "sick role" (1951). Unfortunately, this ideal rite of passage through sickness to restored health—with its phases of separation, transition, and reincorporation into society (Van Gennep 1908)—is more often exception than rule. Whether in biomedical or mental health institutions, patients often do not respond according to practitioners' timetables or recover to the degree clinicians hope and expect. Failure to achieve a "cure" or a "fix" often precipitates an attempt by the clinician to restore his or her sense of self-esteem: "If human needs are not satisfied, they tend to become more passionate, to be reinforced by aggression and then to deteriorate in maturity, with sadism invading the situation, together with its concomitants of anxiety, guilt, depression and compulsive reparative wishes, until ultimate despair can ensue" (Main 1957: 129).

The physician's self-blame often vacillates with recrimination against the patient (see Klein 1946). The flight from despair can lead to relentless activism, ostensibly on behalf of the patient, to protect the physician from depression. Main argues that this "refusal to accept therapeutic defeat can . . . lead to therapeutic mania, to subjecting the patient to what is significantly called heroic surgical attack. . . . The sufferer who frustrates a keen therapist [or physician] by failing to improve is always in danger of meeting primitive human behavior disguised as treatment" (1957: 129).

The concept of acting out is crucial for understanding the underlying dynamics of much medical decisionmaking and the value given to action. In introducing this concept, however, I must first explain how I do *not* intend it to be understood. In popular, folk, and common medical usage, "acting out" is used synonymously with such disparaging descriptions as "impulsive," "lacking self-control," "immature," "too openly sexual or aggressive," "bad," "noncompliant," "seeking immediate gratification." This is the widespread image of the allegedly instinct-ridden psychopath who cannot stop himself or herself and delay gratification like the rest of us normals! This is not how I use the term.

Ralph Greenson defines acting out as "a repetition in action instead of words, memories, and affects" (1967: 68). Often persons must symbolically enact feelings, fantasies, and traumas that they are unable to express verbally. Acting out represents what Roy Calogeras calls "motor symbolization," a kind of "motor memory" (1982: 487), a reliving of the past without conscious awareness of what one is reexperiencing. Ira Stamm identifies three common, specific forms of counter-transference acting out in psychiatric hospital treatment settings: "(a) premature discharge of the patient from the hospital; (b) inappropriate expression of anger and sadistic impulses toward the patient; and (c) sexual involvement with the patient" (1987: 7).

From my observation, the first two expressions of countertransference acting out are especially common among biomedical hospital physicians, their staff, biomedical outpatient clinics, and their staffs. When the hoped-for acute-care conquest of disease becomes instead the dreaded chronic care, the physician often feels emotionally overwhelmed and betrayed—by the disease or the patient or both. Rather than accept the new situation and adjust (lower) his or her expectations, the physician may well act out aggressive feelings and fantasies (Main 1957). The patient becomes a target of the physician's anger, which may take the form of abruptness, discourtesy, passive-aggressive lateness, and referrals or consultations that have as their purpose riddance of the troublesome patient.

Therapeutic activism is often a valid, reality-based necessity in medicine. Decisiveness is a virtue in many life-threatening situations. In medical practice, the strength of the need to act, to take charge, together with the inaccessible meaning of that need, is rationalized by medical training and group consensus (and pressure) as being for the patient's good. Only rarely (see Chapter 7 for examples) does the physician reflect on the obligatory, compulsory nature of the act. The compulsion to act is rarely recognized as a repetition and an attempt to master developmentally early traumas and unconscious conflicts that are not yet integrated in the physician's ego. The "repetition compulsion" (Freud 1920) dimension of clinical action is masked by the medical training that legitimates it and the professional practice that institutionalizes it. Such behavior is virtually required to sustain the relentless aggressive treatment that physicians are taught patient care requires.

The compulsive aspect of activism often manifests itself in intensive care unit (ICU) situations in which the patient is dying. Many physicians and ICU medical staff are reluctant to discuss "do not resuscitate" orders with the patient or with family members because they firmly believe that the function of health practitioners is to preserve life and reverse the path to death to the fullest extent possible. One family physician remarked about how many of his medical colleagues approached respiratory alkalosis (a chemical imbalance that may cause lightheadedness or fainting) among elderly patients in the ICU: "That's where the fun begins. They're thinking about manipulating the sodium and potassium levels, doing some short-term adjustments, but they don't look down the road that they're really going nowhere."

Through what Balint (1957) calls a "collusion of anonymity," they "avoid looking at their own death issues . . . and give it to someone else, or try to put it aside in a bunch of tests and manipulations of fluid levels," as this physician colleague put it. To a large degree, the global picture of life and death is discarded, and discrete, circumscribed procedures become the focus of attention. The challenge, excitement, and fun of manipulating various individual bodily functions and processes quickly supersede addressing the patient as a person and his or her experience of the disease—or of the final moments of life.

Often the challenge and fun of often endless small adjustments become virtual ends in themselves. Then the patient-as-person serves as the medium through which therapeutic activism can be conducted and through which mastery can be demonstrated. At a deeper level, such activism can serve as a means for the physician to bind anxiety and diminish guilt, to discharge sadistic wishes, to avoid feelings of loss and depression, and to postpone feelings of intolerable passivity, helplessness, and hopelessness associated with the imminence of death. A sense of personal relatedness and responsibility to the patient is overridden by a sense of responsibility toward one's supervisory medical colleagues or members of the medical team and by the prospect of being able to demonstrate one's biomedical prowess in some narrowly circumscribed area. As one physician consoled himself after his patient had died: "I lost my patient two hours later, but at least I got her potassium level up."

Control as a Value in Medicine

No domain of biomedical practice, training, and culture is exempt from the wish for and value of control. The highest virtue is to be able to bring patients' pathologies under control. Its obverse side is self-control, the hallmark of professionalism. As increasingly large portions of all social life are medicalized, there is a reciprocal, symmetrically escalating relationship between the public's magical expectation for medicine to bring everything under scrutiny and control and medicine's eager compliance—and its quest to exact greater compliance from patients. Medicine serves up higher and better technological procedures to achieve such control.

Biomedicine's preoccupation with patient compliance assumes that the patient's hierarchy of values and sense of locus of control should correspond with those of the physician. But physicians' values of individualism, future orientation, mastery over nature (see Parry 1984), and *internal locus of control* (the perception that one is in charge of one's own life and destiny) are often at variance with patients' values. For most health professionals, health itself is the preeminent, if unspoken, value (a value held, I hasten to add, in behalf of patients because physicians often fail to keep their own health as avidly as they pursue that of their patients). For many patients, however, values such as family, occupation, or religion may supersede health (see Stein and Pontious 1985).

An occupational medicine physician and family practitioner born in west Texas described a widespread attitude of "white," Euro-American patients in the cowboy culture of the Great Plains:

> "Who made 'health' the central issue of our life?" they ask, when the physician is too heavy-handed about compliance or patient education. "The point of my life," they'll say, "is to be a rancher. I only want a doctor when I can't break my bronco and my bronco breaks me." Physicians are always thinking of longevity: "How can I help someone to live longer?" But for these ranchers and farmers in west Texas, medical care is not their first priority. Men often don't make themselves available for elective surgery or for an angina test. Doctors usually have to make their appeals [for the patient to come in for treatment] through the family.
>
> The man is the figurehead, even though it's a supposedly patriarchal culture. The woman is the one who organizes the rural farm family. In west Texas and

> Oklahoma, farmers' logic is, "The horse needs broken; break it." "I'm sick; cut it out." It's just like "I'm a broken fence; fix me." Medical care's got to be tangible.
>
> A patient of mine had cancer of the colon. During harvest he was passing blood and ignored it. For him, the whole world stopped until the wheat was in the bin. He'd take the chance of tearing himself up more. It's the same in the oil patch. A guy who's fallen and broken bones you've set—no sooner is he on his feet than he goes back to work and falls again. In the oil field, there's this initiation experience. A new guy is a worm; he's got to prove how tough he is, how much pain he can take, how banged up he can be so he's a real man like the others. In our area, doctors and PAs often have different expectations and goals from those of patients.

In proposing a contractual approach to patient care, Timothy Quill (1983) argues that the clinical relationship is negotiated and consensual rather than obligatory from the practitioner's or the patient's side. Although this view of clinical reality has gained some recent acceptance as an ideal that functions to decrease a physician's often enormous sense of responsibility and potential guilt feelings, in practice the hierarchical compliance model has scarcely been eroded. Doctor, patient, family, medical staff, and society often feel that the clinical bond is obligatory and implicitly define it as such. Why else is there such a pandemic of malpractice lawsuits if patients or families did not feel that physicians failed to live up to their assumed obligations? Physicians often feel that patient compliance with their advice, judgment, and will is an obligatory aspect of the often unstated therapeutic contract. They feel responsible, if only in a technical sense, for the outcome of an illness and therefore feel obligated to control the patient somehow. They ask with exasperation, "If the patient is not going to try to get better, why did he or she come to the doctor in the first place?" Frustrated by the fact that many of his pregnant (obstetrical) patients gained considerable weight, one physician sarcastically snapped that his solution would be to "sew their mouths shut." "Control" often means "behave"; little wonder that clinical relationships have been relabled "patient management" and many doctors now view themselves as "case managers."

In considering the clinical issue of compliance, it is important that we not omit the larger cultural and historical ambience in which it occurs, for the issue of compliance does not take place in a social vacuum. In American biomedicine, compliance is an official value and clinical goal that occurs within a mélange, if not articulated system, of other values and goals. These include, inter alia, patient satisfaction, the decline of the "professional sovereignty" (Starr 1982: 389) of the physician in the clinical relationship, heightened expectations of medicine occurring at the time of the decline of religious convictions, the sanctity and privacy of the physician-patient dyad (institutionalized in the code of confidentiality), the conflict between the physician's role as patient advocate (autonomy) and as social policeman in behalf of social control (conformity), and so forth. Medical and wider social contradictoriness in values, and ambivalence as well, makes the topic of compliance a highly complex one. Doctors, patients, families, and society at large are not always consistent or of "one heart," which is in part why compliance is both a perennial and a seemingly unresolvable issue.

This constellation of core biomedical and wider cultural values sets the stage for what James Mold, M.D., and I call *clinical cascades* (see Mold and Stein

1986; Stein and Mold 1988). In a typical medical cascade, physicians feel powerless to stop what is experienced as a cumulative succession of worsening problems and inadequate solutions. The physician cannot accept even temporary inaction and reflection as a solution. In clinical cascades, only immediate and decisive action feels "right" and "enough." The individual physician's anxiety and need to do something often precipitate identification of other medical team members with him or her. Reciprocal identifications intensify the anxiety and press for action.

The sequence of the anxiety cascade can be visualized as a "loop" in which (1) the fear of loss of control leads to (2) the attempt to gain control, which (3) fails—because control of complex systems is often impossible—and leads to a stronger sense of loss of control, which leads back to (1). George Devereux (1980a) in a different context discusses this sequence in terms of the "vicious cycle of psychopathology" in which anxiety, defense, secondary anxiety, secondary defense . . . spiral. The cycle cannot be interrupted and can only be intensified so long as participants continue to struggle for control without taking the time to inquire into the meaning of control and loss of control in the first place.

Florence Kluckhohn and Fred Strodtbeck (1961) and John Spiegel (1971) identify "mastery over nature," "future time orientation," "doing," and "individualism" as stable, first-order core American values. Additional, more specific, values that enact or implement these core values in medical decisionmaking and treatment include control, certainty, completeness, lack of ambiguity, power (omnipotence), knowledge (omniscience in the form of "facts"), goodness (omnibenevolence). So long as a physician is able to exercise and fulfill these values, he or she feels competent, successful, good, validated, and vindicated as a physician. Should these values fail to be fulfilled, the angry rebuke of conscience—and often of colleagues, administrators, patients, and families alike—usually ensues.

In medical practice, the physician is vulnerable to disappointments in his or her own self-expectations in patient care (Balint 1957; Davidson 1986; Katz 1984a, 1984b; Stein 1985g; Stein and Apprey 1985). In the face of patients' demands, these self-expectations often recapitulate and rekindle the physician's own childhood anxiety (which is heightened in medical training), and such feelings are now displaced and projected onto the current doctor-patient relationship. Failed control evokes the self-castigating feeling of being incompetent, helpless, a failure as physician. The fear of medical (= personal) failure through lack of success (= technological cure) provides a frequent pall, if not a free-floating atmosphere, of anxiety in which the prospect of loss of control launches the increased quest for greater exercise of control by physicians and by other supporting medical personnel. The cascade serves both as symptom of and putative solution to the widespread obsessive-compulsive character style of medicine.

The premium placed on control may help to account for physicians' often stereotyped affinity for the sport of golf. One physician explained as follows, when asked what attracted him to golf:

> When you're in [medical] practice, it's hard to get away from patients for any long period of time. When I'm playing golf, to be any good at all it takes total concentration. So even if I'm away only for an afternoon, I forget about the fact that I've got so many responsibilities. It's like being away on a short vacation, yet you've never really

left town. On the golf course, there's a lot that's in your control, if you've got the skill to do it. There's nothing between you and the hole, if you play the course right. It's you against yourself. It's a way you can relax, because nobody's standing over you.

Through the years, I have heard accounts similar to this from other physicians. I infer that through the leisure "sport" of golf, many physicians feel able to realize more fully than in medical practice those values that biomedical culture espouses: success through visual-manual coordination and finely honed motor skill, personal control over situations, lineal planning and decisionmaking, individual autonomy, self-reliance, disciplined and decisive action.

Sociologist Renee Fox (1959) and psychoanalyst Jay Katz (1984b) separately show that peremptory clinical activism, which implements these core values and their deeper meanings, serves as a defense against uncertainty. It sustains and ritually creates "dogmatic certainty" (Katz 1984b) through the exercise of power and skill. Not only do individual physicians' anxieties foster clinical cascades, but the medical training process (professional socialization) itself induces such anxiety and institutionalizes cascades as "solutions" to it. For instance, a common teaching technique called pimping, analogous to the learning by degradation in military boot camp, creates an interpersonal or group atmosphere of terror as a means of teaching clinical content and attitude.

Pimping, which occurs throughout medical school, internship, and residency, subjects the young doctor to verbal attack from his or her superiors, who often try to humiliate the young physician in the presence of other medical colleagues by relentlessly searching for his or her "weak spots" in knowledge or technique. The fear of being "one down," at the mercy of another—a patient, a supervisor, another physician, an administrator—leads to perpetual vigilance, to the revenge-tinged attempt always to be "one up," and to aggressive action when the clinician winds up in the "passive" position. The dread of helplessness and uncertainty helps seal the identification with the aggressor and with it the professional attitude. This dread may later trigger clinical cascades in patient care.

Gender Issues as Values in Medicine

Much of biomedical thought and action is implicitly if not explicitly couched in the idiom of gender. Despite medicine's avowedly nurturing role (health *care*), its language is unabashedly male. "Hard science," "real medicine," "aggressive intervention," the "cure" and "conquest" of "real disease" are all idealized idioms of masculinity. "Soft science," "psychological medicine," "passive treatment," "talking," and "listening" are the more dissociated idioms of femininity. Without "hard facts," "hard data," many biomedical practitioners feel naked and impotent to act. The wish to be as virile as possible is realized through the language of accurate diagnosis ("being right") and successful action in patient care. This contrasts with the fear of being less than virile, feminized, as associated with passivity or inadequate action (being diagnostically wrong or unsuccessful in treatment).

In the twelve years I have worked with PAs, jokes among them have abounded about the sexualized notion of their role as "physician extenders." Allusion is made to various penis enlargers advertised in the popular culture to give men a bigger organ, presumably to enable them to perform better sexually and to look more virile to women. PAs bristle at the notion of being extenders of others' organs or selves and want to have their own identity and its associated potency. A popular PA bumper sticker in the early 1980s read "PAs Do It Better Under Supervision"—the medical denotation of "doing it" being secondary to the sexual connotation. PAs express the struggle between an independent and a dependent identity and function in sexual terms: a boast that their manly prowess is even greater under a physician's watchful eye. Although out and out Oedipal (son against father) revolt is averted, the mocking tone hints that the enforced dependency is felt deep down to be unnecessary, especially because PAs claim as much as 80 percent "substitutability" (a loaded term) for primary care physicians' roles. The bumper sticker is a humorous protest not only about a medical division of labor but about its gendered connotations as well.

As mentioned earlier in this chapter, in family medicine many practitioners and academics wish they possessed a family organ that was accorded equal potency and status with the organ systems that are the hallmark of established specialists' identities. A family medicine specialist often feels inferior and denigrated as a generalist who lacks a true organ. This castration fear to some extent underlies the chronic concern many in family medicine have about their potency as practitioners, teachers, and shapers of public policy.

Let me offer a somewhat more extended example of how biomedicine is metaphorically gendered. Some years ago, a university department of family medicine moved from an assortment of office, clinic, and converted house-type buildings into a single multistory facility. The department occupied two floors and included family physicians, administrators, various behavioral scientist teachers and researchers (with Ed.D. and Ph.D. degrees), PAs, secretaries, and clinic/departmental business staff. Although physicians had offices on both the third and fourth floors, the view quickly congealed that the third floor was the physicians' floor and the fourth floor was the behavioral scientist researchers' and PAs' floor. The third floor ("three") was perceived as the location of clinical practice and departmental administration, whereas the fourth floor ("four") housed those designated to "service" the physicians. Three became identified with "hard science," while four became identified with "soft science."

A number of faculty with offices located on four bitterly joked about the word "service." In its official meaning, it referred to patient care, to orientation toward the community, and so on. In its unofficial meaning, it evoked the world of the female prostitute who is summoned to cater to the sexual whims of the men who hire her. This "family myth" of the psychogeography of the department governed mobility between floors. Many physicians on three studiously avoided going to four, and some adamantly refused to participate in meetings if they were scheduled for the conference room on four. Many medical students and residents only dimly knew that four was a part of departmental office space. Four was not officially presented among the available repertoire of roles to be incorporated into the family physician's professional self-image.

One physician, however, violated these implicit rules. Housed on three, he collaborated on several research projects with a social scientist on four and constantly went up to four for meetings. A jovial man, he often stopped and talked or joked with the personnel on four. Soon, faculty on both floors began to label him, albeit facetiously, as "bifloral" and "an interfloor floater." Three was the "male" floor, and four was the "female" floor. The two were supposed to be segregated. This physician's violation of the implicit rule (and gendered role) elicited gender anxiety, and as a result the offending physician was branded as symbolically bisexual, rather than as an unambiguously "real" man.

I have observed that many women physicians have eagerly taken on the mantle of biomedicine as a symbol of masculine identification and hoped-for prowess and status. For these, the need to prove oneself (through patient compliance, cure, and so on) is at least as great as among male physicians—who cannot take their masculinity for granted but must reaffirm it through clinical work. During the last decade or so, *male* physicians (and males generally) have been struggling to relinquish some control over patients and have been ambivalently attempting to incorporate what might be called softer, "feminine," aspects of the biopsychosocial model into their thinking and practice. Many *female* physicians, reared early in their families to be generous hostesses and to fulfill others' wants, find themselves seeking in and through medical training to acquire the authority and skill to exercise more influence and control over their own and patients' lives. The institution of medicine and the practice of medicine become the testing ground and proving ground for these (not only medical but culturewide) gender conflicts. (See Table 1.2 for a condensation of genderized images in medicine.)

In medical education and practice alike, clinical roles, knowledge, skills, and theories are compartmentalized according to culturally widespread categories of gender. As affective, cognitive, and behavior-directing sets, they are internalized and become embodied as inner splits that take the form of "me" and "not me." In the context of biomedical practitioner roles in which the masculine is both dominant and the cultural ideal, this means that male *and* female practitioners, who identify with this ideal and join the medical power structure, can with little anxiety and guilt disavow whole areas of more vexatious, because personal, clinical reality.

Professional Role Identity: A Matter of Focus

The quest for role clarity and conceptual closure often sacrifices what is potentially clinically significant for what is primarily anxiety alleviating (see Devereux 1967; La Barre 1972). This compartmentalization is one of the primary cultural functions of biomedicine. Disembodiment of features essential to human life occupies the core of medical education and of clinical diagnosis and treatment. The fearsome unknown is, through rationalization, rejected as irrelevant. The culturally known, knowable, and worth knowing are safe and constitute acceptable, reliable, replicable truth. What one avoids and excludes from consideration within one's clinical professional role reveals what is most threatening to one's sense of identity and

TABLE 1.2

MASCULINE/FEMININE DUALISM IN BIOMEDICAL CULTURE

Masculine Images and Values	Feminine Images and Values
Active	Passive
Doing	Being, becoming
Technological intervening, having a procedural orientation, prescribing medicine	Listening, talking
Control	Out of control
Cure, fix	Care, "hand-holding"
Doing to, manipulating, palpating, performing lab tests	Doing with another, touching
Physician, doctor	Therapist, counselor, nurse, social worker[a]
Biomedical science and technology	Social/behavioral science, social work
Science	Nature
"Hard science"	"Soft science"
Doctor	Patient
Individualism and "line of authority" or "chain of command"	Decision by consensus
Taking charge of situations	Waiting, "going with the flow," making decisions in a situational basis
Internal locus of control	External locus of control
Future time orientation	Past or present time orientation
Military, sports, business, and technology metaphors	Interactive metaphors, such as support, nurturance
Death as unnatural, but to be conquered	Death as natural, an inevitable part of life
Surgeon as epitomizing image	Psychiatrist, psychologist, family therapist, pastoral counselor[a]

[a]Although these professionals are viewed by higher status biomedical professionals as "feminine," members of these mental health or biopsychosocial specialties have in recent years been striving to divest themselves of the association with "feminine" values. Psychiatry has to a large degree attempted to disassociate itself from behavioral science and become more biologically oriented. Much psychotherapy has become focused on symptom removal and short-term effectiveness. The structural, strategic, and family-of-origin schools of family therapy (Salvador Minuchin, Jay Haley, and Murray Bowen, respectively) tend to be directive. As Nora Krantzler (1986) points out, American nurses are attempting to become associated with physicians' image of manipulators of technology.

to the boundaries that maintain it. In medical education and practice one attempts to manipulate manifestations of core cultural conflicts rather than to resolve them by identifying their deeper sources. One is thus able to evade indefinitely those out-of-control, out-of-awareness sources of conflict by acting as if they do not exist because the real (internal medicine) problem lies elsewhere.

Consider, for instance, the increasing value accorded in the past decade to such behavioral treatment therapies as biofeedback. Biofeedback has been defined as a "clinical technology" that is instrument oriented and that functions as an instrument-mediated intervention. The locus of the problem is the "biological" system. The solution to organic-specific dysfunction consists of gaining "voluntary," "conscious control" over "internal physiological responses" through biofeedback technology (Green 1976). The frequency of the use of the term *control* in discussions of biofeedback suggests that term's overriding significance as a philosophical issue and value orientation. Behind the specific goal, such as decreasing blood pressure, the philosophical intent is to increase a person's self-control, control over his or her own life and body functions, and sense of autonomy.

After a prescribed number of training sessions, the client is expected to associate internal physiological cues with their visual representations, to autogenically lower his or her blood pressure in stressful situations while maintaining conscious control, and to further generalize the experience to interpersonal relations. Practitioners take enthusiastic pride in the sophistication of biofeedback technology, which allows not only accurate "objective" representation of physiological change but (presumably) avoids contaminating factors of clinician subjectivity. In the behaviorist approach to hypertension, only the fact of elevated blood pressure is a relevant datum. Moreover, the clinician remains far removed from what is occurring in the doctor-patient relationship and therefore must impose this removal on the client. Thus, biofeedback training involves learning to observe and monitor external representations of internal bodily states. But what occurs inside must be mediated, indeed replaced, by what is visible or audible on the outside. By concentration on the physiological, one can avoid the emotional and the interpersonal.

In the biofeedback laboratory the client is prevented in numerous ways from recognizing the potential role of emotional, familial, or occupational issues in hypertension. In fact, all attention is diverted from this realization: first, by the spatial-technological design of the clinical setting; second, by the exclusive, explicit focusing of attention on specific physiological states (as visualized on technological apparatuses) at the repeated instruction of the presiding clinician; third, by the fact that the client is directed to recognize such states outside herself or himself (on a television monitor, voltmeter, and other means of feeding back visual or auditory cues that represent physiological change); and, finally, by the paradoxical fact that the client learns to deal with a problem (that is often induced by emotional overcontrol and self-constriction) through a therapeutic regimen whose goal is relaxation through a substitute form of self-control.

The clinician's anxiety about his or her selfhood finds expression in the way he or she deals with the otherness (not-selfness) of the patient or client. What could be a safer coping strategy, supported by scientific and cultural doctrine, than to protect and insulate oneself behind a rigid clinical method (biofeedback) and to be armed with a simplified conceptualization of the problem (hypertension = elevated blood pressure)? Therapies are inseparable from clinical ideologies; the latter are often externalized expressions of personal conflicts and their resolutions (see Erikson 1958, 1959, 1963a, 1968, 1974).

Exclusive attention to technique safeguards against the possibility (and vulnerability) that emotional involvement will occur. In biofeedback training, methodological orthodoxy serves as a culturally sanctioned rationalization for interpersonal distancing. In deed if not in word, the presiding clinician declares to the patient that neither their relationship nor the patient's emotions or story need be involved. The problem is defined so as to render them extraneous or irrelevant; they would only contaminate the purity, rigor, and structure of the procedure.

Contemporary American society embraces technological symbolism (from medical to military) in order to borrow from it omnipotence and security, to merge with it in quest of perfection, and to embody disavowed aspects of ourselves. From the *Star Wars* movie series of the late 1970s to the proposed Star Wars (Strategic Defense Initiative) antimissile defense shield of the 1980s, American culture seems to need in art and in technology real "influencing machines" (Tausk 1948) for our fantasies to be realized in and through external objects. In discussing cultural facets of the nonhuman environment, Harold Searles writes:

> It seems to me that the members of our culture (and, likewise, the members of cultures in the other highly technological nations, including Russia) tend to *project* the "nonhuman" part of the self and perceive it as a nonhuman thing which threatens the conscious self with destruction; it is too threatening to let oneself recognize the extent to which the nonhuman environment has, as it were, already invaded and become *part of* one's own personality (1960: 397).

He later adds:

> I believe that our culture fosters, actually, an unconscious *identification with* the ingredients of our nonhuman environment, to such a degree that we are barred from experiencing either the fullness of the realization of our own uniqueness or the rich sense of relatedness with that environment (1960: 398–399).

In a subsequent reformulation of "nonhuman phenomena," he writes that

> the importance of the nonhuman environment in its own right (i.e., over and beyond, or apart from, the influence of any other person in the normal child's or schizophrenic adult's environment), now appears as a displacement—of some increment of the child's essentially mother-directed feelings (of love, dependency, and so on) over to the nonhuman realm—a displacement which cannot be sustained as one pushes on into a deeper personal understanding of this subject (1965: 29).

An current example of this technomorphic identification is the cultural elaboration of Peter Drucker's (1954) management by objective (MBO) approach to administration. (It was preceded a half-century earlier by the "scientific management principles" of Frederick Winslow Taylor [1911].) Variations on this management style have been widely adopted in industry, corporations, medicine, and academia.

On the face of it, this approach would seem to foster clarity and consensus through the sharing of explicit goals and avert hierarchical capriciousness by having all participants working toward a common goal. Nevertheless, the cultural elaboration of MBO has led in other, unanticipated directions. When taken to its extreme, this approach to human relations ***does not contain persons at all, only functions that people perform*** in the service of realizing the objective through routines and protocols.

Personal judgment and responsibility, as well as reality testing, diminish as superego functions (conscience, judgment, responsibility) are ceded to the organizational structure and are in turn reinternalized and experienced as one's own standards. Among the paramount cultural values embodied in MBO's corporate ego approach are harmony, smoothness of operation, conflict avoidance, pragmatism, utilitarianism, efficiency, performance, objectivity. Having identified with and internalized the machine as image and value, MBO's practitioners and advocates recreate the machine in their values, organizational relations, and structure. The organization apparatus "works" only so long as potentially disruptive relationships remain sufficiently depersonalized. Everything must be in its place, apportioned, balanced, subordinated to the objective. As the fictional culture hero of the 1970s, Archie Bunker, begrudgingly declares, "Them that works, eats." I suggest that this connotation of functionality is one of our most positively valued cultural symptoms and that any hint of dysfunction, and the dreaded dependency associated with it, is one of our most negatively valued cultural symptoms.

The new "organization man or woman" (medical or not) is a quintessential team player, harnessed to the corporate machine with which he or she is identified. Further, as Erik Erikson puts it, to esteem only what "works" makes "'functioning' itself a value above all other values" (1963a: 322). Pared down to functions alone, people become unwitting functionaries of other people's machinery and corporate enterprises. As life becomes increasingly devoid of depth, it fragments into mere "lifestyle." Concern for meaning dissolves into urgency about the mechanical correctness of role-playing.

In a recent book on the tragic history of diethylstilbestrol (DES), which is associated with breast and gynecological cancers, vaginal adenosis in DES daughters, and infertility in both male and female offspring, Roberta Apfel and Susan Fisher argue that DES can be seen

> as a paradigm of the peculiarly modern phenomenon in which large-scale destructive consequences of a medical or technological innovation emerge unexpectedly as much as a generation after a benign or inconsequential beginning. A second, even more far-reaching aspect of the DES story is that it encapsulates in a quite remarkable fashion the whole complex history and structure of modern medicine in relation to modern life (1984: 3).

This is the sinister side of the fact that biochemistry- and microbiology-based medicine has improved human life enormously. When scientific progress is conducted in the service of cultural impatience, the quest for total control, and the compulsion for therapeutic activism and immediate results, the act ultimately subverts the very science it invokes and claims to represent. The mistrust and horror of technology run amok resonate in the success of the media genre exemplified by Stephen King novels and films of the 1970s and 1980s.

In a haunting passage, Apfel and Fisher discuss a recurrent response by virtually all audiences to their findings regarding DES:

> The people to whom we described our findings always failed to grasp what we were saying at first. They wanted to know who was responsible for the disaster—who profited by it, either in money or reputation or public honors. They wanted to know who had deceived the public and why. They wanted, in short, the secret, inside story of how the scandal occurred. We had to tell them that there was no inside story, no significant heroes and villains; that the scandal is intrinsic to the very structure of modern medicine (1984: 8).

The widespread fantasy of sinister malevolence and its obverse side, utopian benevolence, constitute the dual cultural faces of technology within and beyond medicine. In their somber concluding chapter, Apfel and Fisher remind us that "the enormous growth of the medical research establishment, supported and promoted by the government, the public, the drug industry, and the academic medical profession, has accelerated and systematized the development of new drugs and medical technology" (1984: 127). So long as unexamined interests and popular passions govern public policy discussions about the development and use of technology, we will continue to define every problem as a technological one and prescribe solutions in terms of narrow technique devoid and denuded of context. Sometimes a culture's most cherished values are not in its best interest. Sometimes they become a dead end. Apfel and Fisher write that

> new technical developments and improved institutional arrangements will not get at the problem of the continual recurrence of iatrogenic disaster. What is needed, rather, is a shift in the character of the participants. We already have an abundance of technical virtuosity and theoretical sophistication. Now we require a special kind of human excellence or, to use an old-fashioned word, virtue. . . . Whatever name it goes by, it refers to a developed human capacity to make independent, autonomous judgments about urgent practical matters for which there are no general rules (1984: 128–129).

In the language of psychoanalysis this could be read: Where peremptory id (drive, wish) and raging superego (driven conscience) were, there shall ego be. Apfel and Fisher counsel a capacity for reflection, delay in action, moderation, and wisdom that is profoundly at odds with one of the principal culturally shared mental functions of technology:

> Prudence focuses not only on what we know and can do but also on what we do not know and cannot do. We need to remember our ignorance and our clumsiness as well as our knowledge and our skill. We need to be aware of our zeal for truth

> and for healing, not only as sources of power, but as passions that can lead to self-deception and errors of judgment (1984: 129).

But such zeal, self-deception, and error of judgment rest upon core cultural values that assure future imprudence. A similar tale is told in the next chapter, which considers the symbols or metaphors that underlie and direct the course of medical culture.

TWO

Medical Metaphors and Their Role in Clinical Decisionmaking and Practice

HAVING IDENTIFIED KEY VALUES and widely shared images of biomedical healers, I now turn to those key organizing metaphors that embody and express these American values and images. I forewarn the reader that we will be journeying in unfamiliar territory. Conventional wisdom holds that the stuff of medicine is real and practical, hardly grist for symbolic interpretation. Not long ago, a senior biomedical researcher and administrator, struggling to understand my approach, quipped, "What's a meta for?" In that spirit, I ask the reader's forbearance.

Cultures and ages leave their footprints through the metaphors their members live by. *Cultural metaphors* consist of one or many images in widespread use within a society that condense, organize, and consciously represent what it feels like to be a member of a group at a particular time (see deMause 1982). Cultural metaphors are anchoring points, grand symbolic condensations by which people organize their meanings, their lives, their view of the world, and their actions in the world.

A cultural metaphor is the conscious aspect of a group fantasy the society shares about itself and about the universe in which it exists. In highland New Guinea, the tambaran serves as such a dominant metaphor. Among the Ilahita Arapesh of New Guinea and widespread throughout Melanesia, the *tambaran* is a male secret society, yet it is more than an individual institution. As an organizing metaphysical principle of maleness (see Tuzin 1980), it pervades many Melanesian societies like a symbolic and everywhere ritualized group conscience. To grasp it is to grasp the central meanings of the culture for which it is essence and cynosure. For centuries in the West, the church served as a vast metaphysical condensation of countless individual symbols into a single image of the world. From the mid-1960s through the mid-1970s, the pluralist image of ethnicity reigned as a chief national metaphor in the United States. In the early 1980s, many Americans, following President Ronald Reagan, imagined the Soviet Union to be an "evil empire" and voracious "bear" ready to devour vulnerable America (Stein 1987b).

Cultural metaphors influence how we feel about our bodies and about ourselves, what we believe our bodies and lives to be and mean, and the kinds of relationships and actions that take place in our world. A metaphor not only conjures a compelling image of humankind but also serves as an ideal of what a good, healthy person, family, group or society *ought* to be like. In short, the metaphor draws upon a shared value toward which many collectively aspire. Theologian Abraham Heschel writes that

> statements about man magnetize the inner space of man. We not only describe the "nature" of man, we fashion it. We become what we think of ourselves. . . . A theory about man enters his consciousness, determines his self-understanding, and modifies his very existence. The image of man affects the nature of man. Any attempt to derive an image from human nature can only result in extracting an image originally injected in it (1965: 7–8).

Speculation about human nature is not inevitably and hopelessly projective or utterly distorted. Not all theories and images "magnetize" equally. When they become felt and experienced as obligatory, theory becomes dogma and image becomes idolatry. Heschel's warning about the confusion of theory with reality, what I call the often largely unconscious motivation to impose one's favorite ideology upon reality and subsequently confirm it, is the central epistemological and clinical issue of this book.

Within anthropology, there has been a tendency to divide those facets of culture that are adaptive to the natural world from those facets that are symbolic. Alfred Kroeber distinguishes between "reality culture" and "value culture" (1952: 152–166). Weston La Barre (1972) distinguishes between ego-oriented "secular" culture and superego-oriented "sacred" culture. Countless others in the social sciences have employed a distinction between the "instrumental" and "expressive" realms of culture (for example, Bennett 1982: 17–18). Yet American farmers use their combines both to harvest their wheat crop and to flex their virility, assert their independence, and feel a sense of power and control over recalcitrant nature (Stein 1983c). There is no a priori reason scientifically designed machines may not be used toward irrational ends, not only by individuals but as shared representations of entire groups. Anyone who has ever driven an automobile on the highway knows this full well. The Nazi use of gas chambers, fueled by the insecticide Zyklon B to exterminate whole populations as vermin, is an especially sinister example of the symbolic uses of modern technology within a powerful and prevalent cultural metaphor.

Cultural metaphors objectify shared inner worlds and at the same time make claims about the nature of the world held in common. Metaphors help us to organize our thinking through the use of symbols. They may also obstruct our thinking when we mistake the symbol for the reality we are trying to grasp (that is, when we take metaphors literally rather than figuratively and playfully).

When whole groups live out their metaphors as though their lives depended on them, there is little that is playful or figurative in the burden such concrete metaphors assume. Few metaphors feel to their devotees to be "merely" a metaphor. Rather, metaphors tend to carry the persuasive ring of conviction; they feel palpably real. This, in fact, is much the role of cultural consensus anywhere: to persuade believers that shared fiction is fact, that the world could not be otherwise, and that the world must not be perceived otherwise.

Metaphors are reference points that serve as mental "lighthouses" in our navigation through life. They condense manifold ideas and fantasies around a very few symbols. They highlight dominant cultural values. Metaphors greatly simplify explanatory and decisionmaking processes, reducing complexity and ambiguity to consistent images. Projecting our metaphors upon the world, we experience the world as though the metaphors were really "out there." We then use them to confirm our assumptions about the world. With our metaphors, we increase in confidence and decrease in accuracy.

Because we often ascribe to our metaphors the quality of reality, we cannot receive corrective feedback that would increase our accuracy. Certainty is achieved at the price of flexibility. It is difficult to learn from mistakes when the indispensable metaphor is likewise a source of error. We become overconfident in our metaphors because these metaphors are inseparable from our very selves.

In *Metaphors We Live By*, George Lakoff and Mark Johnson (1980) argue that metaphors are indispensable scaffolding in communication. We must, after all, speak in some language, imagine in some image. Yet, as Alfred Korzybski long hammered on his semantic anvil, "The map is not the territory" (1941). Our maps mislead us and endanger us when we confuse and conflate our metaphors with the very stuff of life, when we employ our maps as unyielding guides to life's elusive territory, when we act not as though they *might* be true (or false) but as though they *must* be true. In using them, we conform the unexpected or the surprising to the expected, the predictable, the known, the reassuring.

We assess the future, the unknown, on the premises of the past. Through metaphors we unwittingly transform play into necessity. To the extent that metaphors feel like facts rather than symbols, to that degree we conflate fantasy with reality and diminish adaptation. When the validity of group metaphors becomes more compelling than the accurate assessment of reality, we cannot have access to the deeper meanings, feelings, or fantasies that underlie and sustain those metaphors.

We can fathom the depths of metaphors when we can acknowledge that they are only metaphors. Metaphors in medicine and elsewhere are symbols, like the ghostly tracks of radioactivity in a Wilson Cloud Chamber, of often frightening, forbidden aspects of the self (see Stein 1985a; Stein and Apprey 1985, 1987; Stein and Hill 1986). In this chapter I explore both the surface picture and the underlying dynamics of medical metaphors, and I discuss their clinical sequelae or consequences in medical practice.

Cultural Metaphors in Medicine

Lakoff and Johnson (1980) persuasively argue that people inhabit symbolic worlds organized by key themes and images. American medical culture's dominant metaphors are those of business or economics, technology or man as machine, sports, and war. Other, more subsidiary metaphors include the family, the life cycle, religion, health/disease, freedom, and time. (See Table 2.1 for examples.) In *The Physician's Covenant: Images of the Healer in Medical Ethics*, William F. May (1983) identifies five core metaphors for the physician in the contemporary West: parent, fighter, technician, teacher, and covenanter.

TABLE 2.1

METAPHORS WITHIN WESTERN MEDICINE THAT SYMBOLICALLY ORGANIZE AMERICAN CULTURE

Military/war: attack, aggressive, invasive, magic bullets, defenses, resistance, bureaucratic overkill, killer cells

Sports: team, huddle, score, punt, turf, a different ball game, win, lose, game, coach, in their court

Technology/engineering: input, feedback, mental apparatus, machinery murmur, that doesn't compute, efficiency, getting revved up, grease the wheels, leverage, cash flow, organization as a well-oiled machine, driving force

Family: parent organization, sister company, organization as family, paternalism

Life cycle: birth pains, infancy, adolescence, maturity, decline, death, rebirth

Religion: save a patient, lose a patient, the symbolism of white

Health/disease: AIDS, obesity, anorexia nervosa, cancer, cardiovascular disease, wellness, and so on

Economic/business: the bottom line, potassium saving and wasting, patient as consumer, the health care industry, patient management, marketing your practice, therapeutic contract

Freedom: medical advertisement with visual images of the Statue of Liberty, eagle, bird of prey in flight, man in the saddle or in the car

Time: clock, watch, race, not enough time, time is running out (3 minutes to midnight), time is money

> The physician's freedom with first names and body contact signals a parental understanding of the healer's role. The white coat points to the scientific origin of medical authority and hints at the technician, the body mechanic, at work. The title "doctor" from its root implies teaching, while the term "professional," in root, suggests the notion of a covenant, a declaration or vow to be faithful for something to someone. Finally, the language of war dominates the modern understanding of disease and shapes the professional's [fighter's] response (1983: 17).

One could adduce further meanings, even changed ones, to these images and terms and thereby hint at how multiply textured and overdetermined they are. For instance, the color white also denotes purity and the sacred: The technical-scientific role is enveloped with the mantle of the sacred in our largely secular society. The term *doctor* has accrued overtones of omniscience, omnipotence, and omnibenevolence, one who is less a teacher than a doer and one who, even in the language of "patient education," attempts to find ways to cajole or threaten the patient into doing (complying) as well. In the language of bureaucracy, a professional is less one who professes an inner vision of the world and more an "organization man"—or in the sports metaphor, a "team player" for the "corporate mission." Nonetheless, May draws our attention to the emotional, cognitive, and behavioral significance of clinical metaphors that, albeit imperfectly, organize the public and professional image of the physician into recurrent patterns of attitude and expectation.

One can gain access to the symbolic organization of culture from ordinary sources. One can, for instance, elicit cultural themes by scrutinizing medical advertisements in the literature that biomedical practitioners read. Cultural dynamics can be "gathered" in virtually any cultural context. It only requires the wit and courage to peer beyond the official cultural agenda (Stein and Hill 1984).

Pharmaceutical firms spend prodigious sums of money on colorful advertisements in American medical journals. The ads rarely describe only the pharmacokinetic properties and precautions of the medicine. The symbolism or iconography associated with each ad is meant to be a hidden cultural persuader. In a sense the metaphor is the message; it is the "metamessage" that frames or qualifies the explicit scientific message.

For instance, in one current ad a massive bank vault illustrates the principle that "it pays to save potassium" (economic metaphor). Two variants of an advertisement for a cough/cold medicine offer pictures of a World War II P-47 Thunderbolt and a B-17 (military metaphor), both headlined "famous fighters in the upper airways." In an ad for a medicine for urinary tract infection, a slim, youthful, slightly clad woman is depicted jumping outdoor hurdles, all of which is headlined "a proven winner in recurrent UTI [urinary tract infection]" (metaphors of sports and outdoors). Two recent advertisements employ variations on the Statue of Liberty, thereby illustrating the implicit message that the medication is a path to freedom. In one ad for an anti-itch medicine, Liberty is scratching her itchy back with her left hand; in an ad for a decongestant, Liberty is depicted with congested eyes, icicles dangling from her torch, and a box of Kleenex held in her left hand.

In an ad for an asthma medicine, a man's fist is depicted as decisively grabbing the defective portion of the lung (the metaphor of aggressive, macho medical control of disease), offering a powerful mental representation of how the medication is supposed to work. Another ad pictures a space capsule in the foreground and a space station in the background and runs a headline that reads, "Cough/cold relief that's as modern as tomorrow" (capitalizing on the cultural themes of modernism and technology). An ad for an antihypertensive drug pictures an outdoor winter scene with a man vigorously skiing and is accompanied with the headline "Because the hypertensive shouldn't have to compromise" (an ad that addresses the cultural themes of vigorous activity, outdoorsmanship, and the manliness of no-compromise solutions to problems). Countless medicines are advertised in terms of outdoors and/or sports scenes, captioned by the promise of helping the patient to regain unrestricted activity. Medical advertisements are a treasure trove of cultural themes that supplement if not subliminally overwhelm the strictly scientific biomedical appeal.

In the past decade or so in American culture, the organ most associated with the definition of the presence or absence of life has shifted from the heart to the brain. Cessation of heartbeat has given way to brain dead electroencephalogram readings. This shift has been accompanied by a dramatic change in the metaphoric center of the self, and with it the sense of what constitutes this self. To say that this change in organ choice signifies a certain schizoid "heartlessness" not only within biomedicine but within wider cultural currents is more than an exercise in poetic license.

Indeed the culture has in fact moved considerably toward a more detached, depersonalized, aloof, left-brain metaphorized conception of clinical relationships and responsibilities. The widespread image of the mind, certainly the brain, as a computer capable of registering only the facts suggests a cultural dynamics of heightened autism, psychopathic qualities, and superego drivenness. Further, our language implies that we are impelled by a conscience that has been split off from the sense of self and relatedness. Through the metaphorical permissiveness of the brain-computer image of the human self, relationships—clinical ones included—can legitimately become matters of calculation, accountability, technological procedure or intervention, cognitive or behavioral operation. We are comparatively free of the unnecessary messiness of those subjective qualities (in addition to patently mechanical ones) once associated with "having heart."

Although technological symbolism has existed for several centuries in the West (for example, the medieval clock), its current popular appeal as metaphor is as a counterpoise to the "softness" and vulnerability associated with the preceding epoch in American culture history. Pleasure has given way to penance, indulgence to abstinence, pluralism to new absolutism. We have instituted a dour internal cultural counter-reformation to erstwhile libertine excesses. The style of long billowing hair and electric "Afros" has given way to close-cropped haircuts. Erstwhile men of flab aspire through austere "fitness" or "wellness" regimens to become men of steel (Stein 1982f). Our answer to the 1960s' outpouring of polymorphous sexuality is neopuritanism and homophobia. Shakespeare counseled that "ripeness is all." We now seem to contend that toughness is all. The gauge of outer steel, however, bespeaks inner vulnerability.

Another use of metaphors in medicine is associated with the ubiquitous imagery of competition and conquest. In academic and community-based medical environments, I note the extent to which (the official, naturalistic, biomedical model notwithstanding) medicine is taught and practiced as if it were a football contest and an act of war (see Burnside 1983; Caster and Gatens-Robinson 1983). Clinical training and conference room folklore are steeped in the language of "team," "huddle," "game plan," "quarterback," and "carrying of the ball."

Sports metaphors in medicine center around themes of winning and losing, on the need to have team players and sound quarterbacking to prevent loss. Famed football coach Vince Lombardi's epigram is applied to virtually all things medical, from patient care to competition in the medical marketplace: "Winning isn't everything; it's the only thing." There are winners and losers, and nothing worthwhile in between. Relationships with colleagues and patients alike are phrased in the sports idiom.

Many colleagues in family medicine strive ambitiously to be "number one," both in their own eyes and in those of other specialists with whom they are relentlessly compared. This competition often is phrased in the language of baseball: the wish to "play in the major leagues" but the fear of being relegated to "play in the minor leagues all our lives." Family medicine residents and interns training at the academic medical center frequently lament, "With us, every game is an away game," which is to say that not only are they spending much time on other specialists' medical services (outpatient and hospital alike) but that they are handicapped with a disadvantage throughout medicine because of it. Part of family medicine's wish to serve as "gatekeeper" for the health care system (that is, be the "point of entry" for patients on the "ground floor" of the health care pyramid) is to be able to position itself so as to assure a "win" over other specialties.

Physicians repeatedly describe themselves as being "on the front line" and in need of "getting aggressive with this patient." Moreover, just as in the military, new, young recruits sent to the front lines are called "grunts," third and fourth year medical students, and especially interns, fresh out on the wards, are called grunts as well. Medical situations supposedly call for "shotgun therapy," "a blast of antibiotics," "our biggest guns," and wished-for "magic bullets." Hospital emergency room and ICU work is medicine "in the trenches" (allusion to trench warfare). Those just completing medical school want to start hospital internship "hitting the ground running" (allusion to marines arriving at a beachhead or paratroopers invading from the sky). Medical training is rife with continued images of combat: "They're killing us on this rotation"; "You never know when an attending [faculty physician] is going to drop a bomb on you"; "As an intern we mostly learn to dodge bullets."

Cholesterol is among the latest on the cultural enemies list. A letter dated October 28, 1988, from James H. Sammons, M.D., executive vice president of the American Medical Association (AMA), sent to members, begins with a call to arms:

> In an unprecedented initiative aimed at reducing the incidence of cholesterol-linked CHD, the AMA has declared war on cholesterol. With immediate effect, we are launching a major multifaceted, multimedia cholesterol-lowering offensive.
>
> In the first phase, we will provide physicians with the latest information needed to combat hypercholesterolemia. In the second phase, we will deploy an intensive educational campaign to alert the general public to the risks and treatment of high blood cholesterol, encouraging them to consult their family physician.
>
> To accomplish these ends, we will mobilize every resource at our disposal (1988: 1).

Throughout medical training and practice, war is waged against the *clock* (monochronic, lineal time, which can easily and quickly run out), against *disease*, against practitioner *loss of control*, against *death*, and (should these be insufficient to quell the practitioner's anxiety) against the *patient* himself or herself. If medicine is a military campaign in which there are winners and losers, and if to be a loser is often a fate (of humiliation, guilt, inadequacy) worse than death, someone or something must bear the burden of blame for the defeat. The practitioner may have the depressive's and compulsive's tendency to internalize the cause of defeat ("I missed something," or "We killed the patient"); or such internalization can quickly reverse into the search for "external" causes of defeat, blame, and vindication.

One physician described the aggressive treatment of disease in the language of demonology. In a lecture on soft tissue infection, a vascular surgeon admonished his medical audience that "With a patient in septic shock, you (physicians) go on a witch hunt for the bacteria or the patient dies. . . . It's a witch hunt. You gotta find the infection." Earlier in the presentation, he declared dramatically: "We (physicians) often have one shot left, and if we lose, we belong to the bacteria." Using humor to illustrate his point, he projected onto the screen a Gary Larson "Far Side" cartoon, depicting three elk or antelope in a hollow and a hunter in the distance. The caption, in which the elk are the speakers, reads, "He's got one shot left, then he's ours." Part of the medical urgency of the situation is a consequence of the blurring of the boundaries between patient and practitioner. If treatment fails, the physician implicitly fears that he, not only the patient, will "belong to the bacteria." Fear of the patient's death merges with the half hinted at fear of one's own. The menace of surgical infection, necrotizing fascitis (the death of inflamed fibrous membranes that cover, support, and separate muscles), and multiple infections is no longer an exclusively natural disease, but a personalized, anthropomorphized enemy who must be eradicated with scientific counter-witchcraft, lest—at least in fantasy—both physician and patient be consumed by its vile power.

At its deepest, the war medical practitioners wage is for the self-esteem that accompanies the demonstration of mastery and victory, proof that they (as men *or* women) are indeed "real men." What Alan Dundes refers to as the "homosexual battle paradigm" (1985: 125) of competitive games and war can be discerned in the latent content of the language of medical practice. Dundes concludes that "if (1) the language of warfare is sexual, and (2) the participants in warfare are essentially exclusively male, then warfare, like football, presumably represents in part a ritualized form of homosexual combat" (1985: 126). Sexualized aggressive competition within medicine takes culturally idiomatic forms of expression. I have heard countless doctors say, often when referring to the practice of "defensive medicine," "In medicine you spend a great deal of time covering your ass." Medical health care teams, clinical departments, and professions commonly represent themselves as a football team competing with other similar units. Clinical supervisors repeatedly remind their charges that the wise doctor knows "when to try to score and when to punt" (that is, when to do a diagnosis or procedure oneself and when to obtain a consultation or make a referral to a presumably more knowledgeable or skilled practitioner).

La Barre's remarks on masculine body-experience and sports also translate well into the meaning and experience of medicine for males. The sports metaphor goes with the territory to be conquered.

> Every male game—and athletics are quintessentially masculine—shows this projection of body image and emulation. The runner and swimmer must go faster than competing males; the javelin and the shot-put must go farther; the boxer knocks down his opponent; the wrestler pins the other under him in submission. In baseball, the man with the bat stands up against the whole opposing team; in golf, the champion hits the ball harder and farther and more accurately toward the hole, and with fewer strokes. In all team games one group of males tries to press another

> group shamefully backward, to force the symbolic ball into enemy territory or into his goal. And the winning team can dismantle the goalposts in football; in basketball it can clip off the net from the basket. The very form of games is male in body-image: to be the active invader, to avoid the passive fate of being invaded. Thus, the mistake made by the male who overvalues maleness is to demean a female for being different. It is not necessarily demeaning to be the receiver of love (1971: 48).

In medicine, the homoeroticism among team players is directed into a variety of ritualized roles. In pimping, junior physicians are put "under the gun" (as many describe it) of a barrage of questions about their knowledge of medical facts, differential diagnosis, treatment plans, medication levels, outcomes, and contingency plans. The style and language that many associate with the drill are in keeping with a homosexual combat substrate. Many medical students, interns, and residents say that the worst thing one can do is to admit "I don't know" in the sight of one's medical peers and superiors, for when one feels "caught with your pants down, you're made to feel like you're nothing but a pussy" (that is, a female's vagina). The latent purpose of the pimping ritual is for the teacher to try provoking the junior partner into defending and hardening his or her "manhood" while trying at the same time to expose the younger clinicians' vulnerability and "really stick it to them." The ritual is a way of making a man out of the apprentice by menacing him or her with the prospect that he or she is but a woman in a medical world of men.

At medical case conferences and departmental faculty meetings, conflicts between one clinical department and another and between medical faculty and residents are commonly expressed in a sexualized idiom: "What we're seeing is the wimp syndrome. And the way we'll solve it is by putting the screws to [the resident, the competing clinical department, and so on]." Many medical situations are experienced as emasculating, feminizing, against which feelings and fantasies physicians recoil by resuming the active sexualized position to recover their sense of virility and potency (compare Shapiro 1987).

Further, latent homoeroticism is directed toward shoring up the physician's active, masculine image through palpating, percussing, poking, and penetrating the patient, who becomes the passive, feminized object. Patient care can thus become the medium and focus of the battle for medical male supremacy. Although treatment has multiple levels of meaning for the male physician, it is in part a ritual in which he attempts to demonstrate and reassure himself of that masculine supremacy. For the male physician the struggle to control the patient's insides may become in some measure the struggle to reassure himself that he is still a man. Moreover, the physician's abhorrence of clinical failure, loss of control, or loss of mastery-activism represents the feared identification with the passive, feminized patient upon whom invasive procedures are performed.

In one aspect, the role "doctor" implements a defense against the role "patient" (passive homosexual position). As a defense mechanism, *reaction formation* consists of the transformation of an unacceptable wish or drive into its opposite (for example, the wish to hurt as converted into altruistic or unctuously solicitous behavior). If medical practice implements reaction formations against passive homosexual stirrings and fears, it is understandable why physicians should have such great difficulty in discussing their patients' feelings. Moreover, given the emphasis throughout medical education and practice on "being tough"—an emphasis resonating with a strong current throughout American culture history (see Wilkinson 1984)—physicians' preference for and trust of "hard" science and mistrust if not contempt for "soft" behavioral and social sciences become comprehensible.

Medical Metaphor as a Discourse of Control

In her classic analysis of metaphor, Ella Freeman Sharpe writes:

> My theory is that metaphor can only evolve in language or arts when the bodily orifices become controlled. Then only can the angers, pleasures, desires of the infantile life find metaphorical expression and the immaterial express itself in terms of the material. . . . First of all the discharge of feeling tension, when this is no longer relieved by physical discharge, can take place through speech. . . . Speech secondly becomes a way of expressing, discharging ideas (1948: 275–276).

In metaphor, therefore, "the displacement is from physical to psychical and not *vice versa*" (1948: 275). On the one hand, the conscious meaning of the word differs in part from the original source of the physical experience signified by the word. On the other hand, in feeling tone, no matter how disguised and abstract the thought, the acquisition and lifelong cultivation of the power of speech does not and cannot leave behind the experience of being a human body: because the human body is not only what we have, but what we are. As modes of control, sphincter and speech are forever affectively linked, no matter how far the mind soars from its body, and irrespective of the degree to which the function of a current idea has changed or progressed from its original aim.

> The activity of speaking is substituted for the physical activity now restricted at other openings of the body, while words themselves become the very substitutes for the bodily substances. Speech . . . becomes a way of expressing, discharging ideas. So that we may say speech in itself is a metaphor, that metaphor is as ultimate as speech. . . . Many a skilled exposition on science, art, politics, philosophy occurring during an analytic session serves the same unconscious purpose as . . . more obvious defenses. Only when the analyst can find that these discourses serve the same purpose as a stream of urine, a smoke screen, flatus, bleating, is he able to get behind words to the unrecognized, unfelt anxiety. . . . The verbal imagery corresponding to the repressed ideas and emotions sometimes found even in a single word will yield to the investigator a wealth of knowledge (1948: 276–278).

Metaphor thus bridges present-day emotional states with past psychophysical experience (1948: 281). The language of metaphor can inform us of the shared "body image" (Schilder 1950) and the "body ego feeling" states (Federn 1952) that make its cultural symbolism compelling.

Health and mental health practitioners in American society feel not only that they are skilled at their healer role but that they should be able to effect a cure.

The language of discourse in medical group decisionmaking often suggests the presence of medical "explanatory models" (Kleinman 1980) that deviate from the naturalistic biomedical one (see Stein 1986c). For example, at medical teaching conferences, the presenting physician and other participants (faculty, residents, interns, students) may stigmatize a particular patient as a "troll," "wimp," "sissy," "gomer" (get outta my emergency room), "a real loser," "problem patient," "albatross," "worm," "crock," "whiner," "crybaby," "jerk," "dirtball," "sleezebag," "scuzzbag," "spos" (subhuman piece of shit), and the like. These images might alternately designate a patient who has failed to be compliant on medical regimens, a patient who has not been found to have an organic lesion (equated in the medical lexicon with "real disease"), a patient who has been especially difficult or demanding personally, or a patient who seems to be virtually identical with patients previously seen who occupy a disdained category (such as, Veterans Administration [VA] patients who are dependent, manipulative, demanding).

Often the use of the moralistic label enables the clinical group or physician to presume he or she knows more about the patient than is warranted by actual experience with the patient. In turn, the physician might overlook or dismiss complaints and symptoms, perform a more cursory physical exam, omit the ordering of laboratory tests, and the like. As a result of discounting the possibility that a more serious disease process might be present, the physician may miss a medical diagnosis because it has been superseded by a metaphorical one.

The converse of this is also common, as in medical argot that describes a person as "the gall bladder in hospital room 276," "a tricky berry aneurysm who came into the ER," "an interesting squamous," "a pretty mangled femur" (who just arrived at the hospital), "small cell carcinoma," "schizophrenic," "manic-depressive," and the like. "Person" here collapses as a category into disease or organ system. At a typical case conference or hospital tumor board (at which the cancer is "staged," that is, its stage of severity is the main issue under discussion), the presenting physician might begin with, "The patient is a fifty-two-year-old, white, married female who presented with such and such physical complaints." In stereotypic fashion, the patient's age, "race" (a cultural category that divides all Americans into white, black, Hispanic, Oriental or Asian, and Native American), and marital status are entered into the evidence but are rarely used as clinically relevant. From this point onward, interest centers on the disease entity and/or the pathological organ system.

Here, the biomedical diagnosis is sought and perhaps confirmed, but it expands and in turn reduces the ill person to a metaphoric image of a presenting symptom or disease. In all these examples, the ill person is reduced to a metaphoric image. In the earlier example, a moralistic metaphor ("troll") dehumanizes; in the latter examples, disease itself becomes a metaphor that dehumanizes. In both instances, the purpose of the metaphor is to increase social distance between doctor and patient, a process that is rationalized and enhanced by medical group consensus.

Given that language used in medicine is often not limited to the biomedical model, it is useful to explore other standards of evidence in day-to-day episodes of medical decisionmaking. Metaphors serve as powerful organizing principles in group process. A content analysis of medical meetings reveals that much of emotional consequence for patient care bubbles beneath the surface of the biomedical model. For instance, consider the following sentences and phrases taken from a variety of recent medical conferences:

1. "You ought to fire him [the patient] if he doesn't follow orders" (business metaphor).
2. "Sometimes you'd like to drop-kick a patient into the end zone, but you can only make a lateral referral to somebody else's service" (sports metaphor).
3. "He tackled the real difficult patient. He handled it aggressively. But he got shot down [by a faculty physician] a couple of days later" (sports and war metaphors).
4. "In the clinic, I hit her with everything (antibiotics), but she still came in the hospital door" (sports/military metaphor).
5. "We've got to get in there and blast away with the biggest guns of steroids" (war metaphor).
6. "It's cheaper to keep a person healthy than to fix him after he's broken" (mechanical metaphor).
7. "This resident has the skills of plugging into people" (electrical metaphor).

Although one might be tempted to dismiss all these metaphoric statements as gratuitous, as mere figures of speech, they indeed articulate underlying, if disavowed, agendas and implicit ways of viewing the subject matter of medicine (see Burnside 1983; Caster and Gatens-Robinson 1983; Hayden 1984). According to Ella Freeman Sharpe, "Words both reveal and conceal thought and emotion. In psychoanalytical treatment our task is often that of getting through barrages of words to the sense experience and the associated thoughts. But words too can reveal the union of these and we are greatly helped if we believe this and can recognize the revealing phrase. Metaphor fuses sense experience and thought in language" (1948: 274).

As indirect speech, metaphor can be a valuable access to feelings, or it can unnecessarily cloud meaning. The observer, teacher, or clinician who works within individuals' and groups' metaphors can enhance rapport so long as indirect communication is not used defensively. Mark Nichter, Gordon Trockman, and Jean Grippen note the need to identify "a patient's prominent idioms of distress (Nichter 1981) considered in respect to culture and interpersonal context" (1985: 74). (For a discussion of metaphors by other writers in the psychoanalytic literature, see Aleksandrowicz 1962; Arlow 1979; Carth and Ekstein 1966.) In discussing metaphorical communication with psychiatric patients, Nichter, Trockman and Grippen write that "the dynamics of metaphorical communication and team care plan goals must be well understood if metaphorical reference is to be used as a technique for enhancing rapport. This includes an appreciation of when metaphorical reference is being used as a means of increasing cognitive distance from problems, and when it is being used to enhance interpersonal or cross-cultural communication" (1985: 77).

At times the emotionally charged language of metaphors may overtake the explicit agenda of a meeting. For example, at one recent conference I attended on future health care systems, a presenter spoke as follows while discussing his proposed plans and strategies in family medicine: "We'll either come out on top or be a part of a food chain. . . . It'll be a battle in the streets. . . . [We need to avoid being in the role of] feeding hospitals. . . . You can sit around and rearrange the deck chairs on the Titanic all day." The word "competition" was frequently used during the presentation. Themes of oral aggression and cataclysmic fantasy clearly emerge in the metaphoric language of these excerpts. (For an extensive description and illustration of the technique of "fantasy analysis" of group materials, see deMause 1982, 1984; Stein 1985f).

I wish to make two points here. First, in *all* groups, unconscious fantasies and wishes parallel if not affect, sustain, and direct group thought, practical action, and evolution (Anzieu 1984; Bion 1959). By paying close attention to the language and metaphors of a group, one can discover that behind the ideal or official values lie implicit, operant ones (Spiegel 1971). Behind the consciously expressed aims may lie those unconscious ones that the observer has deduced (Richards 1956).

Second, there is often a resonance or interplay between the fantasy agendas of small groups and those of the larger cultural or national group (see Stein 1980d). The aggression-violence-catastrophe imagery in the preceding small group corresponded significantly with the dominant cultural group fantasies in the contemporary national group. The language of war has been pervasive throughout American culture in the 1980s (see, for example, deMause 1984). (See Chapter 4 for an examination of the influence of military metaphor within medical group dynamics.)

Attention to the use of metaphors in medical meetings reveals what a conversation or conference is ultimately about. During a 1987 presentation I attended on the future of family medicine, a family physician-academician spoke repeatedly in terms of "industry indicators," "what increases productivity," "product line management," "fixed price, limited choice" in health care, and the need for "decisions in rationing medical care." Earlier in 1987, in a private discussion with him about family medicine goals and strategies, I had used the phrase "medical education." He objected to the term, replacing it with "manpower training" as the locally and nationally acceptable phrase. For him, the business metaphor had clearly supplanted earlier family medicine images of "quality of care," "person-centered medicine," "holistic health care," and the like. The subject of his discourse was profit.

Since the late 1970s, when the current era of corporate medicine was inaugurated, one has repeatedly heard such phrases as "cost-effective care," "resource management," "competitive positioning," "managed care systems," "market strategies," "capturing of market segments," and the like. These exemplify the language of what Harry Kormos (1984) terms the "industrialization of medicine." According to this recent metaphor, economic and technological metaphors are now fused or merged into economic reductionism, which is epitomized by the phrase "the bottom line." This corporate medicine era formally came into being in 1983 with the first set of DRGs.

DRGs, government-mandated hospital reimbursement mechanisms for Medicare patients, exemplify a whole style of cultural thinking in corporate medicine. There are currently nearly five hundred DRGs. Each diagnosis has an associated fixed dollar amount for which Medicare will reimburse the hospital. Whether the patient stays in the hospital one day, only a few days, or many days, the hospital will receive the same reimbursement for that patient's care.

The official purpose of the DRG system is to lower the cost, not the quality, of hospital care. But change in care is a frequent by-product of the conflict between physician loyalty to the patient and to the hospitals (and more widely, to other corporate/medical organizations). Ideally, DRG rules set up incentives that lead to the modification of behavior in accordance with those incentives. Although earning a living has always been a part of the practice of medicine, income production, for oneself and for the organization, has never been so explicit and highly ranked as a goal of medicine. Nevertheless, corporate medical and administrative colleagues commonly explain the DRG system in a language that attempts to remove the direct, cause-effect relationship between increased income generation and decreased quality of patient care. One physician-administrator emphasized that

> hospital length of stay is not directly governed by DRGs. The ceiling is a *by-product* of profit considerations. . . . Hospitals want it both ways. Hospitals want to fill beds. But as soon as the patient is in the hospital, there is the incentive to get the patient out as soon as possible because the hospital is going to get the same amount of money no matter how long the patient is in or what they do to the patient. . . . Since the hospital pays for all the patient's care, the hospital has an incentive to get the patient out earlier.

Physician peer review organizations (PROs), private organizations that are mandated and sanctioned by Medicare, enforce physician compliance with the DRG system by policing other physicians and are used by hospitals to achieve administrative goals. A language of euphemism displaces the profit motive and makes decisions ultimately appear to be the responsibility of individual physicians. Physicians are corporately set up to enforce organizational policy, to be the "henchmen" of their peers, thereby disculpating administrators and clinician-administrators from the onerous decisions they are asking to be made.

Since the mid- to late 1970s, a broad consensus in American society has been reached about the need for dramatic cost containment policies in biomedicine. Medical economics has rapidly become one of the most influential features of medical practice and public policy. Yet, as Kormos points out, the medical crisis is at least partly a definitional one:

> The level of current expenditures for health may in fact be intolerably high. Such a state of affairs does not however immediately establish the existence of a *medical* crisis. Until and unless it can be shown that there is something wrong with health care, the cost of that care can indeed make for a politico-economical problem ("who should pay") but there is not *ipso facto* a crisis in medicine. Conversely, if there is something wrong with medicine, then that should be looked into, regardless of whether a great deal or very little money is involved. As it stands, those who write about the crisis in medicine rather indiscriminately invoke the fiscal problems surrounding medical care as obvious proof that medicine, rather than society, has a problem (1984: 324–325).

A widely shared group fantasy (deMause 1982) about an avowedly medical crisis displaces attention from other disturbing, and far more expensive, social enterprises that spiral out of control. I refer specifically to the resurgent nationalism, militarism, and nuclear armaments escalation that began in the late 1970s (B-1 bomber, Trident submarine, Strategic Defense Initiative, and so on). A generation ago, Jules Henry (1963) noted how Americans seemed to specialize more in death than in life. Current priorities in national expenditure seem to account for this deeper function of the economic metaphor.

Economic reductionism thereby joins ranks with traditional biomedical reductionism in which attention is focused upon disease entity or pathological process rather than upon whole persons. Since the late 1970s, American culture has seen the revitalization of the biomedical model, which has supplanted the more holistic model introduced during the 1960s. In the view of the prevailing economic and industrial model, people are treated and conceptualized as part objects instead of as whole persons. This is hardly vitiated by the euphemistic, if not deceptive inclusion of the word "care" in the names of several health maintenance organizations (PruCare, Health Care Plus, Takecare Prepaid Health Services, Pacificare).

Coincident with, and a direct expression of, the corporate medical ethos is the burgeoning of interest by medical and nonmedical personnel in (more efficient and profitable) clinical decisionmaking (Ritzer and Walczak 1986). Mathematical "critical appraisal skills" and "formal decision analysis" are now offered in many medical school curriculums. A scientific society devoted to formal medical decisionmaking now exists. In practice, if not in theory, these tools are often used to justify the bureaucratization and technologization of medical education and practice.

What is true of the flight in language from richness to minimalism via the technological metaphor is likewise true in scientific research methodology. Contemporary American culture commonly mistakes research rigidity for rigor. Moreover, culturebound "experiments" can only "prove" (and reprove) what they already assume. One may seek what one wishes to find and find only what one is capable of observing. The defensive and consensus-maintaining function of prevailing theoretical and research paradigms is a little-discussed factor in scientific method.

Decontextualization is a preponderant model in government and foundation-sponsored research. As ethnographically and depth psychology–oriented investigators can attest, the so-called soft sciences can attract comparatively few research dollars in comparison with the hard and basic sciences. The return to narrower research paradigms in biomedicine and its sustaining basic sciences suggests the presence of a bona fide "crisis cult" that is as fundamentalistic and nativistic in its psychology as are the more obvious political and religious movements of the time. In considering our cultural rules in scientific and medical investigation, La Barre writes:

> Compulsive quantification does not make the communication of an anthropological complex more exact; on the contrary, it crowds out of observation numerous subtle qualitative contexts and ingredients that alone give the real event its coherence and meaning. Numbers denude contexts of their significant meanings. . . . Discovery itself is always high-contextual serendipity. Hence in the hungry pursuit of intellectual veridity and Truth, we sacrifice the validity of fact, by a kind of Heisenberg Principle, and we can only prove what we already believe (1977: 784).

Images in American Medicine: The Altar of High Tech

Today, the symbol of technology serves as a unifying self-image for much of American culture. The language of technology has not only become a formal system of communication about technical matters and a professional argot; it has also become an increasingly widespread language for describing and expressing the self. Through that language we reveal who and what we feel we are, how we should relate to others, and the status of that language in relation to other idioms of discourse that express our identity and our relationships. Through that language, too, we reveal what kinds of information about ourselves and the world are worthwhile and what other kinds of information are worth less—or worthless. The cultural language of technology can be used as a kind of self-designed group Rorschach or Thematic Apperception Test that offers a key to our collective autobiographical themes.

Technological symbolism and the theme of human mastery extend to the remote past of Western culture, if not to biblical history itself. René Descartes is widely recognized as one of the earliest exponents of the mechanical symbol of the body. In 1748, Julien Offray La Mettrie published *L'Homme Machine*, and in 1817 Mary Wollstonecraft Shelley published her novel *Frankenstein: Or the Modern Prometheus*, a work that subsequently became a mythic template for countless folktale variants that recount our lingering ambivalence and fears about technology.

Peter Morley gives a succinct historical overview that identifies Descartes's role in the emergence and consolidation of the body-machine equation and reductionism:

> Although it is true that Socrates, Plato, and Aristotle established the dualistic tradition, it was Descartes who, in the context of his rationalist philosophy, set the stage for the present debate. It was his revised dualism that shattered the notion that the human species could be viewed holistically. The Cartesian division of body and mind may be seen as a shibboleth, but it is important to recognize that as a view of the world it was seized upon by medicine as a way of organizing and applying the profession's *materia medica*. . . .
>
> The body conceptualized as a machine is no doubt an overworked metaphor, but it is essential nevertheless to grasp the intrinsic meaning of this precept in order to fully understand the tradition of medical knowledge as rooted in empirical science. For the anthropologist, this task is no different than that involved in the description and interpretation of any group's belief system and world view. The perception of the body as a complex machine certainly facilitates the physician's comprehension of structure and function and of inner homeostatic balance. The key word is inner, however, for the physician is essentially concerned with a closed system rather than with a much wider equilibrium encompassing culture, nature, and the human species.
>
> The Cartesian disjunction enabled biology to develop a preoccupation with physiological and pathological mechanisms. Although the new biology unquestionably generated a wealth of knowledge that furthered the medical quest, it paradoxically assumed an exclusionary role in the history of medical ideas, becoming narrow in focus and scope (1988: 16–17).

Descartes's radical declaration of independence, "Cogito, ergo sum" ("I think, therefore I am"), at once decreed the legitimacy of an exclusively cognitive psychology (and philosophy) and surgically severed the human animal from nature. At once human and nature were demystified and human separated from nature. The heroic mental exercise of "Cogito" expelled angels and demons alike from the new science. In turn the disembodied human being became reembodied as a machine. As the object of veneration, the once-important soul was supplanted by the now all-important body. The naturalism and systems holism of the new philosophy, however, were a sacred illusion; the new objectivism quickly excluded all those potential "facts" that the "Cogito" could not assimilate into the body-machine image. The irony of the new naturalism, devoid of animism, was how unnatural and lifeless it really was. Devitalized nature, in essence, was now dead, and life became a mere matter of mechanistic functions and entities. Descartes's and his followers' banishment or trivialization of "the soul" made problematic a definition of what human life contained. The culture history for which Descartes served as founding rebel, father, and hero at best drew a boundary around what his followers found interesting and significant. In biomedicine, a Cartesian offspring, one of the clinical consequences was that the practitioner performed diagnosis and treatment as if the patient as sentient creature were dead. Little wonder that the corpse, the cadaver for anatomical dissection, is usually the first patient whom a student meets in medical school.

The Western intellectual history of the thoughtful criticism of science and technology is a rich one. It began with what Alfred Whitehead describes as the "romantic reaction" (1925: 70–90), one whose focus was nature and "a conscious reaction against the whole tone of the eighteenth century. That century approached nature with the abstract analysis of science, whereas Wordsworth opposes to the scientific abstractions his full concrete experience" (1925: 78). In a similar vein René Dubos describes the eighteenth century Age of Reason's unbridled optimism, "According to the Encyclopedist, science not only was an instrument of progress but would soon bring about the millennium" (1959: 27).

The eighteenth century rationalists' utopian dream of progress through science was quickly dissolved into a dystopian nightmare by the romanticists who followed. "We murder to dissect," Wordsworth's famous protest, reflects the romantic quest to recapture a lost wholeness and stands as an accusation against science for disrupting that wholeness. The romantic protest against the technomorphizing of human life, relationships, and medicine has recently been variously expressed by such writers as Jacques Ellul (1964), René Dubos (1959), Lewis Mumford (1971), Ivan Illich (1976), Stanley J. Reiser (1978), Robert F. Morgan (1983), and Sherry Turkle (1984). I do not question the obvious merits of science and technology—their progressive, ego-oriented aspects, their playfulness and creativity, their adaptive function for humankind. They may be used to expand human consciousness, to increase a sense of awe and wonder, and to confer on us a new and widened perspective on the place of *Homo sapiens* in the universe. Science and technology will surely play a vital role in the emergence of an enlarged, planetary sense of humanity.

Nevertheless, identification with the machine images offered by science and technology restructures our experience of ourselves and our relationships with others and with the world. Following Viktor Tausk (1948), and Margaret Mahler

(1958), Harold Searles argues that where regression and *dedifferentiation* (the failure to distinguish perceptually between self and other, inside and outside) have occurred and ego boundaries therefore have been lost, "identification with machines serve[s] defensive functions, i.e., attempts to cope with the concretized and projected inner impulses" (1960: 77). Rudolf Ekstein argues that "the 'influencing machine,' then, represents both the wish to return to an undifferentiated, symbiotic phase and the lonesome struggle against the loss of precarious identity" (1966: 209) (for further discussion of the "influencing machine," see Tausk 1948; Searles 1960; Elkisch and Mahler 1959). In describing psychotherapy with an adolescent, Beulah Parker (1962) notes the restitutional (reorganizing) function of the patient's identification with machines: to overcome loneliness and thereby to maintain contact with the world, yet to remain independent of people whom he feels are unreliable.

In writing of her observational and clinical work with psychotic children, Mahler (1968) inquires how the experience of the self, the body, and the world as a machine becomes an emotionally plausible if not compelling solution. She describes "the compensatory or restitutive *animation*, *'machine-ization'* of the inanimate object world" (1968: 59), observing that

> one could reconstruct this acute, step-by-step failure of the perceptual-integrative capacity of the ego, which is eventually relegated to becoming the passive victim of the defused, rapidly deneutralized instinctual forces. The ego tries to ward off the onslaught of the two sets of stimuli, from without and from within, by a number of psychotic mechanisms, the outstanding of which are massive denial, displacement, condensation, and dedifferentiation. Complex stimuli, particularly those that demand a social-emotional response, are massively denied, autistically hallucinated away, so that ego regression may not halt before a level of perceptual dedifferentiation is reached at which that primal discrimination between living and inanimate . . . is lost (1968: 57).

In search of adaptation, the disintegrating ego regresses to such mechanisms as dehumanization and *reanimation* (that is, remachine-ization of the inanimate object world). Through negative hallucinations—that is, the hallucinating away of the mother, the world—the child or adult psychotic creates a stimulus barrier against the mother, who in turn is the first representative of the outside world (1968: 64–65).

> In the wake of this kind of negative hallucinatory psychotic denial, inner percepts, saturated with aggression, gain ascendency. Such inner excitations cannot be denied; they force themselves into the sensorium. . . . The psychotic ego tries to dedifferentiate, to deanimate them. Emotions are equated with motion, via the perception of motor innervations, and are also equated, it appears, with mechanical movements. These inner sensations of one's own body and of other life phenomena are then projected onto and confused with machine phenomena. The split of the ego into an intentional part and an experiencing part is frequently clearly discernable. The body image thus appears to be mechanically put together in a mosaiclike way, by fragments of a machinelike self-image (1968: 63).

The psychotic child, in turn, projects this mechanical experience of the body onto the world, perceptually fusing it with the world. Dynamics, not analogy, is the bridge between the bizarre, frightening inner world of child psychosis and the sometimes reassuring, sometimes menacing, social metaphor of high technology.

In mutually fashioned culture, as in individual psychosis, once the machine image is used primarily as an identity image, the integrity and perfection associated with it—in inner and outer worlds—must be maintained at all cost. Thus, in biomedicine potentially disruptive subjectivity is repudiated as "unprofessional." In this distorted application of technology, life must be devoid of sentiment in order "to get the job done." By becoming merged with machine as a collective ego ideal, one in turn becomes no threat to that "machine"—and to those who control it—and need not feel the threat of abandonment or separation because oneself and the machine are united. As illustrated by the following vignette, technology becomes a metaphor of our disconnectedness—to our selves, our feelings, others, and the world.

A medical team was treating a hospitalized seventy-five-year-old man dying of cancer. The oncologist, however, was jubilant because an X-ray and a CAT scan showed evidence that an irradiated tumor in the patient's chest cavity had shrunk considerably from the oncologist's skillful application of therapy. When the family physician mentioned to the oncologist that the patient was nonetheless dying, the oncologist replied, "That's not my department. It's somebody else's problem. You can see clearly, however, that this tumor we've been treating has shrunk." In another instance, a family physician voiced frustration about the care received by his elderly patient. He complained that medical specialists in one organ system had paid no attention to disease process in another system: "They said they're lung doctors, not heart doctors. They spiffed up her lungs, but ignored her pericardial effusion."

Compartmentalized focusing of clinical attention protects practitioners and staff from disturbing thoughts and feelings that would emerge if they considered the whole. The defense mechanisms of isolation (the splitting off of feelings from thought and perception) pervade the clinical division of labor. Significantly, it is to the so-called softer, supposedly less objective, medical and behavioral sciences that highly specialized biomedical physicians turn to take up where their own emotional range leaves off.

When anxiety becomes too great to say "self," we say "thing" instead. We withdraw empathy (identification) from another person or even from some facet of ourselves. Identification with machines is a symbolic way of reaffirming our need to depersonalize ourselves and others. It helps us to keep a safe distance from inner pain (Stein and Kayzakian-Rowe 1978). G. Gayle Stephens, M.D., a leader in the family medicine movement since the late 1960s, notes that many biomedical physicians seek to establish all clinical work on "an objective therapeutics, quite apart from the person of the doctor and the patient" (1984d). Ironically, of course, this ostensibly objective therapeutics is subjectively grounded in the technological metaphor of "man."

As metaphors pervade all institutional settings, their "reality" comes to be experienced as indisputable. Since the early 1980s, informatics and cognitivist, computer ideologies (in the form of theories and methods), like the mechanical ones that preceded them during the past three centuries, have rationalized a collective self-image that feels not only right but necessary. Psychodynamically speaking, such metaphors are akin to the secondary, conscious elaboration of a dream.

In a tongue-in-cheek article titled "What's in a Name? 'Mechanical' Diagnosis in Clinical Medicine" (1984), Gregory F. Hayden, M.D., abundantly illustrates how replete contemporary medical diagnosis is with mechanical allusion. He discusses "diagnoses named after various machines or tools on the basis of structural or functional similarities between the physical findings and the mechanical instrument" (1984: 227). Even in limiting himself to the cardiovascular, nervous, and musculoskeletal body systems, he offers a lengthy list: water-hammer pulse, machinery murmur, sawing-wood murmur, water-wheel murmur, canon-shot noise, cogwheel rigidity, scissors position, jackknife epilepsy, pendular nystagmus, clasp-knife phenomenon, hammered skull, hammer toe, mallet finger, typewriter finger, funnel chest, screwdriver teeth, and silver-fork deformity.

Physicians are not alone in their use of mechanical diagnosis and treatment terminology. Patients, too, often describe themselves and their expectations in mechanical terms to doctors: "I just came in to have my wiring checked out"; "I'm run down"; or "I need my annual tune-up" (see Scheper-Hughes and Lock 1987). The American cult of immediacy, with its search for rapid, instant, and disposable solutions, has had its influence on the therapeutic relationship, both in causing greater directedness on the part of the clinician and in legitimating expectations of quick cure on the part of the patient. Writing of "the symbolic equation of humans and machines" in modern biomedicine and society, Scheper-Hughes and Lock describe our "body alienation" (1987: 22):

> We rely on the body-as-machine metaphor each time we describe our somatic or psychological states in mechanistic terms, saying that we are "worn out" or "wound up," or when we say that we are "run down" and that our "batteries need recharging." In recent years the metaphors have moved from a mechanical to an electrical mode (we are "turned off," "tuned in," we "get a charge" out of something), while the computer age has lent us a host of new expressions, including the all-too-familiar complaint: "my energy is down" (1987: 23).

The medical use of mechanical metaphor when thinking about and describing the human body has had widespread "circulation" for generations. The very origin and development of science would have been impossible had human and nature not been partly disenchanted of their animistic, mystical, and anthropomorphic attributes. Analogy, however, has often decayed into more concrete thinking and literalism. With the internalization of such imagery, people come to perceive and experience the body to be a machine rather than merely to be machine-like. Marshall McLuhan argues that "man's answer to a machine world is to become a machine" (1967: 102). Erikson writes:

> If we detect in [the ego] a tendency to mechanize itself and to be free from the very emotions without which experience becomes impoverished, we may actually

> be concerned with a historical dilemma. [Child-rearing customs] have begun to standardize modern man, so that he may become a reliable mechanism prepared to "adjust" to the competitive exploitation of the machine world. In fact, certain modern trends in child training seem to represent a magic identification with the machine, analogous to identifications of primitive tribes with their principal prey. . . . If, then, the ego itself seems to crave mechanical adaptation we may not be dealing with the nature of the ego, but with one of its period-bound adjustments as well as with our own mechanistic approach to its study (1959: 46).

Ernest Becker similarly observes that

> our belief in the efficacy of the machine control of nature has in itself elements of magic and ritual trust. Machines are supposed to work, and to work infallibly, since we have to put all our trust in them. And so when they fail to work our whole world view begins to crumble—just as the primitives' world view did when they found their rituals were not working in the face of western culture and weaponry (1975: 9).

American culture conceives of the human organism in machinelike terms, complete with replaceable parts. Recent "miracles" of heart and kidney transplants would have been impossible without this orientation. The same is true of the lifesaving "tubes" and "valves" that are grist for Ivan Illich's (1976) critique of "medical nemesis." But such an appetite for fragmented parts can be voracious and can consume (and thereby invalidate) other understandings of ourselves and our sicknesses. American culture views treatment in the image of the automobile body shop (Zborowski 1969). You take your body, like your car, into the shop for periodic checkups and for repair when it is not operating optimally.

Consider, for example, the now common use of biofeedback as a treatment of hypertension, a condition medically defined as a dysfunction (elevated blood pressure) in need of repair (a decrease in blood pressure) (Stein and Kayzakian-Rowe 1978). An earlier holistic psychoanalytic paradigm of hypertension (F. Alexander 1950) has been discarded in favor of a culturally reductionist definition, etiology, and treatment based on a mechanical view of the human body and human life. Biofeedback exemplifies a treatment mode that is an extension of what Lewis Mumford calls "the myth of the machine" (1971). The language of behavior modification and biofeedback is one of exclusive attention to outer states or observable behaviors, not to self-reported feelings. To behaviorists as to many physicians, the self is an unreliable instrument.

This unreliability is corrected through the language of the computer and the machine (see Stein and Kayzakian-Rowe 1978).

> biofeedback is the use of monitoring instruments (usually electronic) to detect and amplify internal physiological responses, in order to make this ordinarily unavailable information available to the individual and feed it back by way of electronic or electromechanical devices. *Biofeedback training* is the clinical or therapeutic use of the information for the purpose of teaching a person to gain voluntary control over such physiological processes or responses. . . . Biofeedback is a special case of the general feedback method of control, where the system is a biological one and where

> the feedback is artificial, mediated by man-made detections, amplifications and display instruments (Green 1976).

Fragmentation, compartmentalization, and isolation are inherent and essential to biofeedback therapy. The therapist goes to considerable lengths to separate himself or herself from the client. The use of space subtly communicates the kind of human relationships that are permitted (see Bateson 1972; Watzlawick, Weakland, and Fisch 1974). The very spatial, technological, and impersonal arrangement of the therapy expresses and embodies the cultural problem of ambivalence about human relatedness, even as it ostensibly enhances the client's healthy relationships with others.

With affect unacknowledged, attention is displaced to a preoccupation with physiological functions or dysfunctions, and the somatic (body) and the intrapsychic (meaning and feeling) are severed. Biofeedback thereby partakes of the Cartesian radical separation of mind and body and is congruent with the need to defend against relationships involving human intimacy, commitment, trust, responsibility, vulnerability, limitation, and loss.

Because of its rootedness in American folk-scientific medicine, biofeedback training is a culturally "appropriate" therapy in which physical complaint is more acceptable than is the expression of inner and situation-induced emotional distress. In a sense, the experimenter-clinician "aids" the client in the continued repression of emotional conflict. In a culturally relativistic sense, I acknowledge that biofeedback probably "works" or will prove to work for hypertension (as it has for headache, migraine, and so on) so long as the problem is defined as a matter of faulty learning. But one cannot separate what it means for a treatment modality to "work" in American culture from the underlying view of personhood in this culture. For it to work requires that unconscious aggression and anxiety, often underlying the elevated blood pressure, be ignored as superfluous.

But Franz Alexander (1950) proposes that elevated blood pressure functions precisely as a somatic "defense" against the anxiety associated with aggressive impulses.[1] Simultaneously it expresses a constant vigilance that perpetuates the very core conflict from which relief is sought. While teaching a "relaxation response" to replace the *visible* "anxiety response," biofeedback training of hypertensive patients fails to come to terms with the underlying problem of anxiety. Even as new findings about the contributions of diet, exercise, body fat, and so forth complicate the etiological and treatment picture of hypertension, a truly holistic approach would not automatically "rule out" aggression and anxiety as potential issues.

High technology comes the closest of anything in our secularized society to being consistently vested in the mantle of the sacred and imbued with its mystique. We credulously overlook the fact that the truths we ask our machines to pronounce are only those that we told them in the first place or that we read into them with the sweat of our own inferences. Our modern solution to the problems of sexuality, aggression, loss, body integrity, and mortality is to technomorphize the human body and human relations. Uncertain of anything in the next world beyond death, we attempt to make this world flawless. Because our flaws now lie in our mechanical operation, we call upon a still greater machine to eliminate them. By becoming extensions of machinery if not machines ourselves, we hope to achieve secular salvation.

Many professional medical groups in American society have embraced the new high technology. The "higher" the technology, the more elevated the status. Even among medical scientists, the influence of the technological metaphor may spell the difference between real and false progress. As Lewis Thomas, M.D., writes, "the researcher may be led down the garden path by his equipment. If he is in possession of sophisticated instruments of great power, and if he is being assured that whatever other new instruments he can think of will be delivered to the door of his laboratory tomorrow, he may find it difficult to stop himself on a dead road of inquiry, even if he knows it to be dead" (1983: 91).

At a regional meeting for nursing educators held in Kansas City in the early 1980s, speakers addressed the issue of technology for the 1990s in teaching, patient services, and research. Several nurse educators spoke glowingly of the coming technological revolution as it would affect students and patients: individualizing instructions, eliminating classrooms in favor of a computer terminal, freeing faculty for individual scholarly pursuits, assisting nurses in assessing and monitoring hospital patients, providing self-instructional video packages for patient education, and substituting computer programmed psychotherapy for traditional psychotherapy to meet the growing demands for these services more economically (and to assist the hospital in creatively responding to the declining demand for inpatient services). Not voiced at this meeting was any expectation that the new high technology would somehow elevate the status of nurses and their work (see Krantzler 1986). In fact, a number of nurses privately lamented the decline of "total care" and its substitution by a more aloof attitude toward patients, more focused attention to physical symptoms alone, and increased preference for performing technological procedures rather than for interacting with patients. (This example was provided by Hill 1983.)

The medical education of osteopathic physicians, which originally emphasized hands-on diagnostic and therapeutic skills (and which allied osteopaths in spirit more with chiropractors than with allopathic practitioners), has in recent decades acculturated considerably to the mainstream American biomedical model. As in nursing training and practice, the erstwhile distinction between therapeutic touch and therapeutic technology has diminished with the use of high technology in patient care. In both cases, the cultural diffusion of the ideology of high technology has permeated and reordered the doctrines and practices of disciplines once far apart in their clinical ideologies.

The status issue is far more explicit in the recent writings of medical specialties, especially family medicine. Although in its original reformist ethos, it was largely person centered and as concerned with a patient's life situation as with his or her disease, family medicine has already considerably acculturated to the technological metaphor and the corporate-industrial model as a means of relieving if not eliminating what many in family medicine call their "inferiority complex." Thomas L. Schwenk, M.D., concludes his article, "Family Practice and the Behavioral Sciences: The Need for Technology," with a call "to elevate the understanding of the psychosocial diseases toward the elegant simplicity of high technology and thereby provide family practitioners with highly sophisticated behavioral science technologies. One of the many important tasks facing family practice is to create a high technology of behavioral science" (1982: 19). Through his appeal to the technological metaphor Schwenk hopes to enhance the status of family medicine—to rescue it from insecurity and to raise it to parity with if not superiority over other medical specialties. Similarly Donald A. Bloch, M.D., describes family therapy as "an important technology [that] has taken the systemic paradigm farther than most other disciplines have. It is the technology on which medicine can rely for much of its needed ability to intervene in clinical systems" (1984: 123). As in Schwenk's passage, the idiom and image of technology are the persuasive rhetorical devices.

In an article titled "Media Images of Physicians and Nurses in the United States," Nora Krantzler (1986) uses advertisements from the *American Journal of Nursing* and the *Journal of the American Medical Association* to explore key beliefs and values held by and about American biomedicine. She notes that although "the white lab coat and stethoscope have predominated as identifying symbols" (1986: 934–935) of the activity of medical science,

> yet as one examines the most current issues of the *Journal of the American Medical Association*, the most startling thing is that depictions of actual physicians-at-work are no longer necessary to [address areas of uncertainty in medical practice and provide ongoing socialization to medical professionals]. In current advertisements, physicians are manipulators of technology behind the scenes. They are rarely shown talking to patients, more rarely yet talking to nurses or to each other. . . . The tendency is to show brightly-colored, high-tech imagery, such as computer simulations, and to focus on scientific evidence of efficacy. . . . This is a significant trend, reflecting the growing dominance of technology in biomedicine (1986: 937, 939).

In the conclusion of their study of the history of DES, Apfel and Fisher write that

> most of the enormous power of contemporary medicine derives from the extraordinary interplay between its technical capacities and its theoretical understanding. There is a synergy between these two in that new technical developments make greater scientific understanding possible, and scientific understanding frequently leads to the creation of new techniques. In its fascination with these twin sources of its power, medicine is in danger of forgetting that our understanding is and always will remain profoundly limited and that our technical abilities are always subject to profound misuse and error (1984: 129).

This crucial point has likewise been made by Jay Katz (1984a) in his study of the reluctance of physicians to discuss with their patients their own—and science's—limitations, complexities, and ambiguities. Moreover, the *unconscious purpose* of the widespread cultural overinvestment in technical capacities and in narrowly defined (context-free) scientific understandings is *to help us to forget* that our understanding is and always will remain partial and that our techniques will always be imperfect.

Technological symbolism serves the dual role of "screen memory" and "screen fantasy" (that is, memories and fantasies that hint at, while displacing attention from, more affect-laden and disturbing recollections and ideas) (Ekstein 1966: 337). In warning of the extremes this symbolism can take, John Mack writes of "our blind faith in the capacity of technology to solve all human problems" (1986b: 278).

> The Star Wars program (SDI, BMD) represents a coming together of ideological extremism and blind faith in technology. Through this extraordinary technology, we are told, we may become safe behind a kind of heavenly astrodome. . . . Star Wars is a bizarre, apocalyptic cosmic fantasy in which American space-based satellites, radar sensors, and laser beams (good) carry on a war by proxy against Soviet ground launchers, missiles, and decoys (evil) (1986b: 279).

The danger, however, is that "faith" in our defenses could imperil us the more. We might convince ourselves that we can survive nuclear war and nuclear winter—so that the war is worth the gamble. In biomedicine, we might come to believe that CAT scans and X-rays are enough, that the doctor-patient relationship itself is superfluous.

Medicine did not single-handedly invent the technological metaphor. Nor has it oppressively imposed the metaphor on society. Although a participant in the ethos, medicine is not its source. David Hilfiker, M.D., remarks that "most people—doctors and patients alike—harbor deep within themselves the expectation that the physician will be perfect" (1984: 119). Little wonder that all Western medicine is so embattled by the cultural paradoxes it lives out. The public demands from its doctors and their machines what they once asked only of their priests and gods. The medical community, with its broad retinue of ancillary services and vendors, tries to comply with public insatiability by providing technological omnipotence of its own. One may scarcely decry medicine as a "nemesis" when medicine's constituency has enthroned and enshrined its technological wizards with a mystique that befits the sacred. Technology, too, is heir to the disillusionment and rage that surface with volcanic fury and seek an object when its putative magic fails to live up to practitioner, patient, and public expectation. We are ambivalent about all our gods, sacred, secular, and profane.

Disease as Metaphor

In their book *The Psychological Autopsy* Avery Weisman and Robert Kastenbaum (1968) draw the valuable distinction between the disease a person dies *with* and the disease that person dies *from*. The disease a person dies with may well be an extension or culmination of those deeper personal, family, and life struggles that have prepared the way for disease symptoms. Besides their physiological reality, diseases are also symbols if not fulfillments of often unspeakable life courses (see Dale 1987; Feder 1978). Diseases may likewise become powerful social symbols, metaphors of whole cultures and ages. These metaphors, if not their associated diseases, are themselves the outcomes and articulators of whole historical epochs. When diseases become organizing metaphors, their bearers become social *cynosures* (La Barre 1956)—categories of people who are given considerable social attention and visibility.

In *Illness as Metaphor*, Susan Sontag (1978) discusses the nineteenth century through an analysis of tuberculosis (TB) as an organizing metaphor and the twentieth century through an analysis of cancer as an organizing metaphor. She contends that disease can serve as a "social text" that society and historians interpret (see also Stein 1979a). For Sontag, "TB was a disease in the service of a romantic view of the world. Cancer is now in the service of a simplistic view of the world that can turn paranoid" (1978: 68).

TB was the apotheosis of beautification in a romantic age of hysteria. The victim of TB was a heroic ideal imbued with pure spirituality. Possessing an angelic, fragile countenance, such a person was above sensuality. At the same time, to have TB was license for libertinism, an indulgence of the passions that could be attributed to the illness. Death from TB was thus a fulfillment of spirit and a restitution for surrender to desire.

Cancer now conjures an unending Orwellian nightmare of foreign intrusion, unsuspected terror that overruns, controls, consumes, and destroys—all with the compliance of the host whose very machinery is used for its own self-destruction (Sontag 1978: 35). The prevailing image of cancer is of a mechanized body that has lost complete control of its own machinery of life and is overtaken by an alien force that consumes the body. Cancer is the most durable metaphorical vessel for our paranoia.

In the February 1984 issue of *Reader's Digest*—a monthly known to be a superb barometer of social preoccupations—Lewis Thomas, M.D., writes, "Cancer is feared by everyone. And this fear is reaching epidemic proportions. Not the disease itself—there is no such thing as a cancer epidemic. . . . But the fear of cancer is catching, and the country stands at risk of an epidemic of apprehension. The earth itself is coming to seem like a hugh carcinogen" (1984: 142). The terror of cancer extends far beyond the disease. In an article titled "Cancer and Death in the Promethean Age," Ellen Golub writes that "cancer becomes a screen upon which we project our anxieties about our own power. . . . Cancer is, for us, a metaphor of our powers gone wild. . . . Autonomy, power, and will: these are the core of meaning with which this metaphor is 'awash'" (1981: 728–729).

Until the early 1980s, American medical culture was dominated by two diseases as metaphors. Cardiovascular, or "heart," disease was the "positive" disease; it was the outcome of heroic achievement (itself metaphorized into the "Type A personality") and could in turn be "beat" by heroic determination (multiple bypass surgeries, heart transplants, compulsive jogging). Cancer (the spectrum of malignant neoplasms) was the "negative" disease; it was the outcome of a life somehow wrongly lived that was destined to end by wasting away.

> The modern age has complicated our desire to control and made us ambivalent about our powers. We invest cancer with the negative aspects of that control and, of all things, heart disease with the positive aspects. . . . Although heart disease is the number one cause of death in this country today—although it kills twice as many people each year as cancer—we fear it less because it offers us a sense of autonomy and independent choice. The lone runner, with but a pair of shoes, controls his body's development of muscle tone, stamina and fitness; he appeals to us as a lithe and organically tuned human instrument. While the cancer victim, host to a

> parasite gone wild in its development, is yoked to machine for detection and treatment and provokes in us our deepest dread and our darkest dreams (Golub 1981: 730).

In an article on cardiovascular disease and the construction of time in Western culture, Cecil Helman (1987) argues that the model of Type A behavior (time urgency, drivenness to capitalist success, ambition, anxiety, maleness; see also Friedman and Rosenman 1974) reflects key moral values. On the one hand, the model represents a symbolic fulfillment of Western values realized through the image of linear, monochronic time marching from past to future, the drummer beating time for the mythic Horatio Alger success story. On the other hand, the Type A model is antisocial. For Helman, the heart attack (myocardial infarction, or MI) that is the putative outcome of Type A behavior symbolizes the turning point in a morality play, when good triumphs over evil and the deviant Type A person is redeemed and integrated back into society (if he lives, that is) by becoming more Type B (friendly, people oriented, less competitive, dependent, female). I would add that this conflict between good and evil cannot be too far resolved in favor of good, whether for the person with cardiovascular disease, the family, the medical practitioner, or the society. For the process of treatment and rehabilitation is designed *not* to challenge the cultural status quo but to reaffirm the pulse of the cultural clock. The lessons of Type A must not be learned too well.

In a brilliant analysis of the clock as ikon of monochronic time in the West, Ebel seeks to explain the ubiquity of the clock metaphor.

> The invention, perfection and progressively more pervasive distribution of clocks and watches in Europe—and eventually to Europe's colonial dependencies—was the natural outcome of Europe's Christian "clock-mentality," whose roots can be traced to the pages of the Old and New Testaments. The arrival of Christianity in northern and western Europe, over a period of many centuries, helped to bring its formerly barbarian believers to the very advanced state of mind enjoyed by Jews and their sympathizers in the Mediterranean society of 500 B.C.–500 A.D.: a frame of mind in which guilt and anxiety about one's shortcomings in the eyes of an all-seeing ever-present God could be successfully handled only by "making every moment count" and rigidly organizing one's outer and inner life accordingly. By the time watches and clocks became normative accoutrements for even average people—in the nineteenth and early twentieth centuries—Everyman and Everywoman can be said to have reached the point explored by Saint Paul and other revolutionaries two millennia before.
>
> To be technologically progressive in the relentless European mode requires a "clock-personality" widely and even universally diffused. . . . The father of Prince Andrew in Tolstoy's *War and Peace*, like many characters in the novels of Dickens, suggests that the problem posed in the proto-Freudian years of the nineteenth century by the rigid, completely time-ridden personality, was also the secret of Europe's capacity to dominate the planet (1984: 418–419).

I have quoted Ebel here extensively because, through a brief discourse on clocks, he has inadvertently shown how profoundly entwined the image of cardiovascular disease is with theology, values, imperial expansion, and relentless guilt and anxiety.

Not only is the human body increasingly being used as a metaphor, but ***illness and disease, too, are becoming widespread metaphors of our time,*** which is in keeping with the increasing medicalization of personal, social, and political issues. In a discussion of anorexia nervosa as cultural metaphor Vincenzo DiNicola writes that

> it is possible that the prevailing fascination with anorexia nervosa is another aspect of our Western infatuation with our own individual self-definitions, a turn inward, "down the spiral staircase of the self" as Montaigne put it. For example, rather than applying to ourselves metaphors from the natural or physical world (as in "cancer"—from "crab," "articulation"—from vine joints), today the world is being increasingly described in terms of our own bodies and behavior. Illness metaphors have even reached architecture (the *New York Times* "Architecture View" mentions "anorexic skyscrapers" and "bulimic buildings") (1988: 51) [See however, Stein 1982c, for an interpretation of how autistic features of our culture have become embodied in widespread architectural styles].

The consequences of medicalization, whether of metaphors appropriated from nature or projected from the body, can be devastating to those who bear their brunt, just as they appear to be healing to those who purchase their integrity at the expense of others. I think, for instance, of the political use of the "cancer" metaphor in describing threats (Jews in Nazi Germany, kulaks in Stalin's USSR) to the "health" of various "bodies politic." Whole categories of people are depersonalized, stripped of their humanity; they become "part objects."

Sontag passionately argues against the construction of any other than biomedical meaning around disease. In her view, metaphorical construction damages the patient's perception of herself or himself, the clinicians' perception of the patient, and society's perception and behavior toward people diagnosed with symbolically burdened afflictions. She argues for the deconstruction of meaning to make treatment more humane and concludes that "illness is *not* a metaphor. . . . The most truthful way of regarding illness—and the healthiest way of being ill—is one most purified of, most resistant to, metaphoric thinking" (1978: 3). Having recovered from cancer, Sontag bristles at the oppressiveness that results from the imputation of psychological or family factors in the etiology of the dread disease. Better, she contends, that all disease be regarded as personally meaningless, biomedical events (a position adapted toward schizophrenia by the National Alliance for the Mentally Ill).

The trouble, of course, is that *any* etiological account and treatment plan are full of meaning. The search for one exclusive kind of meaning is more often than not the search away from and defense against another type of meaning. The distancing and self-disculpating dynamics of "blaming the victim" are distinct from the search for the causes of disease and other forms of suffering. The "fact" of the metaphor is one thing; the meaning and mental function of that metaphor are separate matters (F. Alexander 1950; Stein 1979a).

We can hardly resolve problems when we are unwittingly committed to their misdefinition, when cultural treatment is "designed" to assure that the whole story will not be told. When the social "duty" of a symptom is great, it is the duty of the treatment to fail, even if it appears in the short run to succeed. The wider the boundary of the symptom, the more closely metaphor and disease are fused, the more compromised the treatment. Until we can address the symbolism that enshrouds seemingly intractable social problems, we will continue to put forth our best effort to misdiagnose the problem and thereby work at solving the wrong problem.

Consider, for instance, the relationship between cultural meaning and AIDS. Together with testing for human immunodeficiency virus (HIV-) positive blood, AIDS has become a pernicious, if not lethal, metaphor. Since the early 1980s, the spectral image of AIDS has overshadowed even cancer. The public as well as medical response suggests that many feel AIDS is invading and threatening to consume the United States—as if the counry were a single organism under attack.

In their article "Medical Students' Attitudes Toward AIDS and Homosexual Patients," Jeffrey Kelly et al. summarize their 1986 study of 119 second and third year medical students (University of Mississippi School of Medicine) by remarking that the authors

> did not anticipate that medical students to such a great extent would believe AIDS patients were more deserving than leukemia patients of their illness and more deserving to die, to lose their jobs, and to be quarantined. The students reported strikingly less willingness for even an everyday, casual interaction (such as having a conversation) with an AIDS patient than with a leukemia patient. . . . Prejudice against and stigmatization of AIDS patients and homosexuals are a social issue among the general public. In the case of medical students, however, such stigmatizing carries implications for health care quality, the comfort of patients with physicians, and the comfort of physicians with their patients (1987: 555).

They argue that most medical students' fear of contracting AIDS can be quelled by accurate information about HIV transmission. Yet, "the fact that homosexual patients and AIDS patients were stigmatized in a nearly identical way suggests that bias related to sexual preference is also present" (1987: 555).

That AIDS, people with AIDS, and people with HIV-positive blood tests are powerful metaphors for our time can be gleaned from a review article on anorexia nervosa by DiNicola (1988), who further comments that "there is no necessary relation between the root cause of the illness and the metaphoric reading given it as a critique. For example, a moralistic reading of AIDS would see it as a symbol of the wrongfulness of promiscuity and homosexuality; as to causality, this argument would point to a moral problem in the vectors of transmission, but would not comment on the virus itself" (1988: 52). Here, the disease is a "sign" used metaphorically to judge sexuality. At the same time, this symbolism allows room for a dispassionate, technical understanding of the disease process and for some degree of empathy toward the sufferer of AIDS. Using illness as a metaphor differs, however, from merging the metaphor with the disease so that it is absorbed into the disease's very reality. "A moralistic approach would argue that AIDS is the result of distorted sexual relationships, and not because of some incidental details of anatomy leading to higher risk; there would be a conceptual blurring of the two groups, people with wrongful sexual practices and AIDS patients" (DiNicola 1988: 52).

DiNicola's interpretation points to a more general question: How much (if it could be quantified), or which aspects, of AIDS (or any disease) are metaphorized? Among many biomedical practitioner colleagues (physicians, nurses, PAs), AIDS has become a virtually *living metaphor* in which those suffering the disease have nothing and no one to blame but themselves for their morally opprobrious drug-related and/or sexual behavior. Many colleagues describe AIDS as "a disease 'of' and 'for' homosexuals" that is somehow earned or deserved because of immoral behavior. In the view of these practitioners, such patients should be isolated and quarantined on something like Alcatraz or Devil's Island. They should be treated humanely but not given extraordinary efforts to prolong their lives. Although these colleagues are willing to discuss the AIDS virus (still questioned by some, see Schmidt 1984) in a neutral, scientific way in the abstract, as soon as they consider it in the context of a specific HIV-positive patient or one diagnosed as having AIDS, homophobic panic, revulsion, condemnation, stigmatization, and withdrawal of empathy often immediately ensue.

It is difficult to be comforting and compassionate and to function as a healer toward people who embody and bear the brunt of society's revulsion and fascination. Pariahs are kept at a safe distance. The entire society's evil is symbolically placed "inside" whole categories of despised, discountable, superfluous persons (see Lifton 1986; Bock 1988). World history is replete with whole populations who have been stigmatized and sacrificed for purity's sake: Christians, Jews, blacks, Native Americans, gypsies, kulaks, witches, Aztec prisoners of war. Current medical and popular literature about AIDS abounds with metaphors of war (see, for instance, Burda and Powills 1986). The Canadian airline steward who was traced as a source of much spread of AIDS among homosexuals in North America was labeled "patient zero," a term that evokes the image of nuclear war ("ground zero"—the place where the bomb is dropped and contamination with radioactive material is heaviest). War against the disease may easily merge with war against those who have the disease.

In a grim sense, as a symbolic plague, AIDS serves for many as a solution. Those with the HIV complex become the focus of attention and a convenient target upon which to lay all blame for their predicament. Societal ambivalence and guilt about sexuality are displaced and played out on the stage of AIDS. Such defenses as projection, externalization, and rationalization enable those without AIDS to feel good, righteous, and justified in withdrawing a sense of shared humanity toward those with it. AIDS is but the most recent, and most foreboding, image of modern, medically phrased apocalypse.

Since the late 1970s, American society has become increasingly obsessed with various "poisons in our national bloodstream"—tobacco, ethanol, cocaine, heroin, sodium salt, cholesterol, triglycerides, sucrose, asbestos, industrial products such as benzene, to name but several. Episodes of individual and group acting out have "confirmed" this paranoid ethos. The mass suicide through cyanide-laced Kool Aid that ended the People's Temple in Guyana in 1978 was succeeded by a rash of over-the-counter drug poisoning scares. The genital herpes epidemic of the late 1970s signaled the end of the previous era of sexual liberation and was welcomed by many as a harbinger of deserved punishment. As an external object, AIDS culturally arrived at the "right" time to validate the hysteria and vindicate the paranoia (see Schmidt 1984; Hocking 1987).

In domains of life ranging from medical education to public policy formulation, offering accurate information about the transmission of AIDS is not enough. Any thoroughgoing program of public education dealing with AIDS must address the hysteria, the paranoia, and the often unbridled contempt intrinsic to the AIDS epidemic. We must have the courage to understand why scapegoating is so widespread a response to AIDS and what aspects of ourselves we deny by isolating those with AIDS and pointing a clinically self-righteous finger at them. Ultimately, what we accuse "them" of is a secret we keep from ourselves. Perhaps it is time for us to examine honestly our own complex, ambivalent, frightened sexuality. If we can, we will have less need for AIDS to be so lethal a metaphor, and those with AIDS will bear less of society's self-recrimination and self-destruction.

The Medicalization of Life

Medicalization and *somatization* (the channeling, experiencing, and labeling of feelings and conflicts as physical ones) have become powerful American metaphors among the professional, folk, and popular cultures. Scheper-Hughes and Lock write that

> illness somatization has become a dominant metaphor for expressing individual and social complaint. Negative and hostile feelings can be shaped and transformed by doctors and psychiatrists into symptoms of new diseases as PMS (premenstrual syndrome) or Attention Deficit Disorder (Martin 1987; Lock 1986a; Lock and Dunk 1987; Rubinstein and Brown 1984). In this way such negative social sentiments as female rage and schoolchildren's boredom or school phobias (Lock 1986b) can be recast as individual pathologies and "symptoms" rather than as socially significant "signs." This funnelling of diffuse but real complaints into the idiom of sickness has led to the problem of "medicalization" and the overproduction of illness in contemporary advanced industrial societies. In this process the role of doctors, social workers, psychiatrists, and criminologists as agents of social consensus is pivotal. As Hopper (1982) has suggested, the physician (and other social agents) is predisposed to "fail to see the secret indignation of the sick." The medical gaze is, then, a controlling gaze, through which active (although furtive) forms of protest are transformed into passive acts of "breakdown" (1987: 27).

In *Medical Nemesis* (1976) and in a series of articles (1974, 1975, 1982), Ivan Illich criticizes the "medicalization of life," which has collapsed all human suffering into a technical problem to be surmounted. Drawing his argument and critique from a Greek drama and mythology that he rejuvenates, Illich argues that human envy of the gods and their prerogatives (the most unreachable being immortality) calls forth nemesis (retributive justice). The hero's transgression—such as Prometheus's greed, which leads him to steal fire from the gods—evokes "inescapable cosmic retaliation" (Illich 1974: 918). Western man's "'tantalizing' hubris" (1974: 919) has led him to crave technological ambrosia, to expropriate death from nature and from the gods, which leads to industrial nemesis.

As a result, "the sickening technical and non-technical consequences of the institutionalization of medicine coalesce to generate a new kind of suffering—anaesthetised and solitary survival in a world-wide hospital ward" (Illich 1974: 920). For Illich, the solution is not greater access to the health care system but greater reliance upon self-care and reduction of "professional intervention to the minimum" (1974: 921). Moreover, "the medicalization of health inevitably tends to degrade the art of living, of suffering and of dying, an art that has permitted thousands of unmedicalized cultures to cope with their reality" (1982: 466). Contrary to the popular sacred myth of biomedicine, he concludes that "The true miracle of modern medicine is diabolical" (1974: 921).

Central to Illich's critique of biomedicine and of industrial society is a false dichotomy between the natural human and the technology-dominated human. Illich's dissenting voice is valuable, but his invidious distinction between Western society and an idealized, simpler, more authentic primitive society does not hold. All cultures have their admixture of "naturalistic" and "personalistic" (Foster 1976) etiological and treatment models, their secular and sacred domains of problem conceptualization and problem-solving. Other societies' health behavior is as ritual ridden as ours. The Navahos, for example, are surely as health and death obsessed (C. Kluckhohn 1944) as is mainstream American popular (lay) and professional (biomedical) culture. They have lengthy, expensive communal healing rituals ("sings").

Research within or outside medicine is in many respects a search influenced, if not driven by, a wish. Science would not be so encumbered with methodology if scientists did not recognize, if only subliminally, how readily data could be manipulated to conform to hypothesis. What Devereux refers to as "the blurring of the frontier between reality and the imaginary" (1980a: 227) is certainly not limited to medical science.

> Culture-historically, the existence of this dividing line is a relatively recent discovery. In most primitive societies the dream is essentially consubstantial with reality. . . . The *fact* is that the primitive acts realistically most of the time; the *trouble* is that he does not know that he is acting realistically when he bandages a wound but unrealistically when he tries to cure an illness by offering a sacrifice. . . . The Greeks were among the first to differentiate between reality and the imaginary *as categories*, yet in practice they—and Plato in particular—often treated certain of their cherished fantasies as real and treated as fantasies certain things they chose not to believe—just as we do (Devereux 1980a: 227)!

Driven by anxiety, we inadvertently sabotage our finest achievements and seek refuge in frightened ignorance of ourselves and of the world (see Henry 1971). Jules Henry writes that "in order to be accepted in a culture one must accept or adopt an uncritical attitude toward its customs and its fears" (1963: 122). In our case, such acceptance may irrationally undermine the scientific enterprise from within medicine itself. The issue is not technics versus a romanticized art of living and dying. Rather, our cognitive and emotional investment in the "wonders" of medical technology and in scientific research is often of a magico-religious kind. Witness the durability of such popular terms as "magic bullet," "wonder drugs," and "miracle cures."

In interpreting and criticizing the dominion of the technological metaphor in American medicine and culture, I do not oppose technique per se; I oppose technique disembodied from the physician and patient (and wider culture) as persons. Let me explain by borrowing from another idiom. Some of the most profound interpreters of the symphonic literature—among them conductors Arturo Toscanini, Otto Klemperer, Fritz Reiner, Erich Leinsdorf, Erich Kleiber, George Szell, and William Steinberg—were prodigious technicians. By comparison, many of the currently popular orchestra conductors often turn out technically flawless virtuoso performances that fail to inspire. It is not accidental that the age of high technology, in music as in medicine, has selected against depth of feeling and for superficiality of encounter.

Technology is not necessarily or intrinsically evil, destructive of human dignity and wholeness. Technology can as much express curiosity and creativity (Volkan 1986: 18) as it can express schizoid withdrawal and grandiosity. Franz Alexander writes of Prometheus: "The punishment of Prometheus for teaching mankind the secret of fire was a miscarriage of justice. Not Prometheus, not the scientist, is the culprit, but mankind, which abuses the knowledge it receives from its intellectual pioneers" (1960: 148).

When metaphors become more compelling than reality, when life imitates metaphor, we are apt to become hopelessly lost in our own forest of symbols. If technology is to become more a tool of our adaptation and less a parasite on that adaptability, American society will have to differentiate more clearly between its symbolic uses and its reality dimensions. As we increasingly animate the world with our mechanical, computational, sports, military, and business metaphors, we sink more deeply into a cultural dreaming from which, if we are to survive, we must now awaken.

Having identified and explored the most pervasive values and metaphors in biomedicine and American society, I turn now to one of the main functions or social tasks to which biomedicine is appointed: that of social control. Despite the professional value of objectivity and nonjudgmentalism toward patients, biomedicine's task of social control rests upon a moralistic foundation.

Notes

1. From an evolutionary point of view, Rycroft writes that "anxiety [is] a specific form of vigilance, neurotic anxiety [is] a special form of anxiety which arises as a by-product of the tendency of man to internalize his environment, and defenses [are] responses which can be evoked by internal as well as external stress . . ." (1968: 138).

THREE

Medicine, Moralism, and Social Control

Beneath the official medical ideology of scientific neutrality, rationality, professionalism, objectivity, empathy, moral commitment to patient care, and (in the past two decades) treatment of the whole person if not the whole family system run deep and swift moralistic currents. In this light, the chapter describes and interprets the meaning of informal clinical taxonomies such as "good" and "bad" patients; the physician who cures as a "success" and the physician who cannot cure as a "failure"; patients who are truly sick and therefore deserve compassion and patients who are not "really" sick and therefore deserve contempt and ridicule; and patients who are compliant and patients who are noncompliant with physicians' advice. The split between libidinal attachment to certain categories of patients (liking good patients) and aggressive *object relations* with other categories of patients (disdaining and rejecting bad patients) is documented with numerous examples drawn from the author's clinical work and discussion with colleagues in rehabilitation medicine, Veterans Administration hospitals, and preventive/wellness programs.

Object relations, a concept widely used in psychoanalytic thinking, refers to the fact that all human relationships—including clinical ones—are mediated and constituted by the inner significance the relationships have for the participants. "Object relations" denotes people's mode of relating to the world, mediated by their mental representations of themselves and of others, representations that are fueled by libidinal and aggressive drives, as these in turn came to be structured early in life through relationships with emotionally significant people (objects). The moralism that often enflames adult relationships is heir to residues from the primitive splitting of early childhood that readily peopled the world with absolutely "good guys" and utterly "bad guys" (Laplanche and Pontalis 1973: 277–281). Moralism is not only a consequence of values and metaphors intrinsic to the culture of medicine. It is likewise induced from the wider society in terms of the

Portions of Chapter 3 were published in Howard F. Stein, "'Sick People' and 'Trolls': A Contribution to the Understanding of the Dynamics of Physician Explanatory Models." *Culture, Medicine and Psychiatry* 10(3)(Sept. 1986): 221–229.

social control role medicine is expected to play; that is, it is part of the object relation based division of labor between physicians and their public. Physicians are to a large degree expected to restore order to a society that many experience as out of control. The aspect of medicine as morality play is illustrated by the contemporary symbolism of ethanol, sodium salt, sucrose, red meat, and so forth as medicalized social evils. Finally, the psychosocial dynamics of the wellness movement, now a decade old, is a medicalized expression of the wider ethos of social Darwinism, survivalism, minimalism, narcissism, and militarism, according to which the "fit" survive and merit admiration, whereas the "unfit" do not.

Good Versus Bad Patients: The Moralistic Model

In a series of works, Kleinman (1978, 1980, 1983b) discusses the influence of the doctor's and patient's explanatory models upon the clinical relationship. Kleinman's concept is an effort to formalize the fact that all participants to a sickness episode (physician[s], patient, family, nurse) bring certain understandings of what is taking place and what is to be expected. All have criteria for a good or bad outcome. Explanatory models entail all participants' notions of the etiology of the problem; explanations that account for what the problem is, why, and when it occurred; and expectations about the proper course of treatment and outcome. (In a number of works I explore the influence of unconscious emotional factors within the physician on medical decisionmaking and treatment [Stein 1982h, 1983b, 1985c, 1985g; Stein and Apprey 1985].)

Kleinman writes that "doctor-patient relationships can be examined as transactions between different systems of medical knowledge that frequently produce tacit conflicts in views of clinical reality" (1978: 429). I wish to add to this formulation only that physicians' own EMs are often far from monolithically scientific in practice. In fact, physicians often bring multiple, competing systems of knowledge and feeling to the clinical encounter. These systems frequently produce tacit conflicts within physicians' own views of clinical reality and in turn generate conflicts in the doctor-patient relationship.

During a discussion about a patient who had died (the patient's history included diabetes, hypertension, schizophrenia, and long-standing asymptomatic resting tachycardia [a rapid heartbeat]), a family physician said:

> It's not just this patient. It happens to all of us. It's not just a medical issue. [I asked, "What bothers you the most?"] Something you do or do not do that contributed to her death. She was my favorite patient. . . . There's a feeling that I killed her. It will happen in the future. The terrible retrospectoscope, it's our worst torturer. . . .
>
> Specialists can give you bad advice. You massage your conscience. Should you know everything? . . . How do you forgive yourself when your patient dies? The courts don't always forgive you. When should you "go" with your own feelings versus when to take the consultant's advice?
>
> [I asked, "Did you let the patient down?"] Family doctors want to please a lot of people. Good patients like you; bad patients don't, or they die. I wish I could

> do something more to fix her. I was not confident in the assessment. I could have gotten a CAT scan. . . . I am grieving over the loss of a *real* person. I didn't expect her to die. Some physicians avoid this involvement. It's protection. How do you not be overconcerned about omissions and commissions? How do you forgive yourself for not being a master computer? I don't want to get complacent. As long as I get close to people, their dying is going to hurt.

As this physician's agonized account attests, the ingredients of physicians' explanatory models are often profoundly complex. For instance, the use of empathy, the struggle against becoming overwhelmed by it, and the resistance against experiencing it altogether, are powerful—if frequently unacknowledged—motivators of medical knowledge and action. Israeli psychoanalyst Rafael Moses writes that

> empathy is that faculty which enables us to feel with another human being, to cognitively and effectively put ourselves into his or her place, and therefore to become aware of the other's feelings, needs, and wants. . . . There are some "helpers" who become aware that their empathy serves as an obstacle to their helping function. They overidentify. A doctor of excellence once confided in me that he could not let his patients talk to him about their worries and problems, because they moved him so. He felt he just could not afford this degree of exposedness, of vulnerability. Sometimes, then, what may be "too much" empathy must be prevented from exerting a harmful effect. Thus the function of dis-empathy is, in certain circumstances, a protective one for its holder. This is so either when the individual is particularly sensitive; or when the task to be carried out requires it; or last, when there is much suffering around us. . . . When empathy becomes dysfunctional, when it is necessary to hurt someone to achieve a goal considered "right," empathy is shunted aside. For most "helpers," an excess of empathy becomes an encumbrance because it causes too many painful feelings in them. And even when empathy is exercised—and when its exercise is vital—a price is often paid in pain, in uncomfortable introspection, and in some inhibition of action (1985: 135–138).

In biomedicine, contending models exist within and between specialty worldviews (Blumhagen 1980; Hahn and Gaines 1982), and within practitioners (Stein 1981a, 1985g; Stein and Apprey 1985). This is so because, to use Kleinman's distinction, physicians bring "illness" as well as "disease" models to the clinical encounter. Moreover, their "ideal" model may diverge from their "operant" model as well (see Spiegel 1971). For instance, components of the ideal biomedical model include (1) biomedical rigor in diagnosis and treatment (a rigor that different specialties define differently) and (2) compassion and empathy toward all who suffer. In practice, however, compassion and empathy are often extended more toward (1) patients who evince "real disease" (true organic change) and (2) patients whom the physician regards as unable (rather than "unwilling") to control themselves and make themselves better.

At a family medicine grand rounds, a resident presented the sad case of a fifty-year-old white married male. He had a history of well-controlled hypertension and well-controlled diabetes. The physician(s) liked him and admired him, his work ethic, and his family. They regarded him as compliant with diet, medications, and so forth. Then he had several days of slurred speech, a sensation of extra saliva, and dragging of his left foot. The resident diagnosed him as having had a "stroke." One of the faculty physicians insisted that "stroke" was a lay term: What was the likely cause of his symptoms? An aneurysm (a localized abnormal dilatation of a blood vessel)? Cerebral ischemia (local and temporary reduction of blood to the brain due to obstruction)? What explained the intermittent nature of his symptoms in the hospital?

At first, all discussion centered around the ***differential diagnosis***, that is, all possible diseases that could produce the patient's symptoms were suggested, and then most were carefully ruled out in extended discussion. I asked what his and his family's mood was through all this. One resident replied, "He's been the type to go with the flow. Tries to keep upbeat. But he's now down." Another resident interjected, "It's not fair. He's a likeable patient. He's the type who's taking good care of himself, follows the doctor's orders." Another protested, "Why do these things happen to good people? He's been living right and he still gets sick." A faculty physician said, "It could make you cry."

Physicians and other biomedical practitioners, in addition to functioning according to an official, scientific diagnostic schema (disease-entities), operate according to an unofficial, moralistic taxonomy of types of patients. There are good patients and bad patients, successful physicians and failed physicians. Emotional investments in either conceptual framework can interfere with biomedical rigor and empathy. The physician's view of the illness can in fact prevent him or her from identifying the disease.

Good patients are those diagnosed with bona fide organic disease and who are not held responsible for the control if not cure of that disease. Exceptions to this classification are patients whose lifestyles doctors hold responsible for "bringing the disease on themselves": for example, lung cancer, chronic obstructive pulmonary disease, and heart disease among smokers. Good patients are those who respond quickly to physicians' efforts to alleviate their suffering, who accept and understand the physician's model, who submit to and enthusiastically comply with the physician's treatment recommendation. Good patients obey the physician's "rule of silence" in not disagreeing with or contradicting the physician and take up little of the physician's time (Wright 1987). The good patient is one who affirms the self-image of the "good doctor" and makes the physician feel successful, competent, in control, powerful, a "winner" in the battle against disease.

The bad patient may or may not have a bona fide biomedical diagnosis and is held responsible for the control of his or her disease. The bad patient, often called the "difficult" patient (Anstett and Collins 1982), is one who makes the physician feel unsuccessful, defeated, a failure, out of control, powerless, incompetent, or a "loser." The bad patient is refractory rather than compliant, seeks to control the physician, and refuses to relinquish his or her symptoms (which could be done through self-control or greater exertion). According to this view, the bad patient is the legitimate object of clinician aggression and as a result is often "turfed" to other medical services.

As discussed earlier, physicians and other biomedical practitioners have developed a rich lexicon of ridicule and disdain to describe those patients who undermine their self-esteem. A splitting of affect also characterizes the attitude of other health care personnel, who divide patients into "sick people" and "trolls." Sick people evoke and merit compassion; trolls evoke and deserve contempt. Hate for trolls is not only permitted but encouraged in the clinical portion of medical education, whereas hate for truly sick people is proscribed and condemned.

Physicians' sense of incompetence, impotence, and inadequacy in diagnosis and treatment is to a degree alleviated by the translocation of fault to the patient. Physicians elevate and restore self-esteem by diminishing the image of patients. Some images go even further: Patients become small, sinister nonhuman forces, even feces, so as to eliminate from the physician's self-image the possibility that the physician might be "shit." The affect-based bifurcation of patients into good and bad is a protective maneuver by which physicians place outside themselves the source of positive and negative feelings about themselves and the physician role. These two categories of patients literally embody idealized and devalued attributes of clinicians themselves.

During a recent family medicine grand rounds, Dr. A presented the case of a white, male army veteran in his sixties, who was hospitalized in a community hospital some 100 miles from a VA facility and complained of low back pain and the inability to walk. At the time Dr. A was on emergency room duty and admitted this patient of a local community physician. Dr. A spoke frustratedly about the patient and the management problem:

> This guy looked like everybody I saw in the VA and I hoped never to run into another one [what physicians call the VA syndrome—of dependent, hostile, manipulative, demanding patients, whom doctors may see as paid and treated not to improve functioning]. I tried to order him to walk, but he said he couldn't walk. I thought he was refusing to walk, that he wouldn't walk.
>
> While I was taking his history, he told me that some time ago a doctor told him to keep himself cleaned out. He said he took a teaspoon of Clorox [a chlorine bleach] and a teaspoon of Lysol [a disinfectant] to keep himself cleaned out. He acted like a real troll. I wanted to prove he could walk so that we could get him out of the hospital. I had written him off as a real troll. But later I talked with Dr. X [the community physician] who told me that he [the patient] was schizophrenic and probably could be diagnosed as having polymyositis [widespread muscle inflammation, producing weakness, that may become chronic and produce severe disability]. I realized I had a sick guy that I'd thought was a jerk [said in a disgusted-with-himself voice]. He has long lived alone and is a hard-working, respected carpenter.

Self-indulgence turns to horror when a physician discovers that a patient previously branded as a troll, a worm or real jerk turns out to be a sick guy with a "real disease" for which he is not responsible. Contempt for the patient boomerangs into self-contempt. The confusion of categories and resulting perceived mistake on the part of this physician unleashed profound shame, guilt, remorse, and disgust. To mistake a sick guy for a jerk was medically unforgivable. Where the physician had difficulty forgiving the patient for being so recalcitrant, he subsequently had difficulty forgiving himself for having vented about, if not upon, the wrong kind of patient.

Later that day I talked further with Dr. A about this case. I said that I felt he might have some unfinished business about this patient. He acknowledged this.

He talked about his ambivalent and guilty feelings toward the patient: "How can you resent a guy who's got a real disease? I hadn't realized he was schizophrenic, too."

We discussed the cultural stereotype of schizophrenics ("schizophrenics are always acting crazy"), the fact that many schizophrenic patients do not act symptomatic all the time, how the patient was evidently a well-compensated schizophrenic much of the time, and that his paranoid tendencies were most likely to come out in situations such as hospitalization (in which the doctor and nurses suspected his motives, did not trust him to really tell them what he was capable of doing, "confirmed" and heightened his own mistrust, and so on). Dr. A recognized that this patient had not deserved his initial wrath and somewhat heavy-handed approach. I said that this was the kind of patient whom one may easily "make up your mind to hate and suddenly discover that you can't, or you mustn't." I also pointed out that all of us, to different degrees, are "compensated" for some inner hurt or flaw, and that numerous schizophrenics, depressives, and borderlines are not visibly troubled much of the time. I said that from his case presentation the only tentative "red flag" toward a diagnosis of schizophrenia I had seen was the patient's rather concrete way of dealing with the earlier doctor's advice that the patient "keep himself cleaned out."

We further discussed patients who are assigned to categories of disliked people. I said that even VA patients have meanings and reasons for what they do. Moreover, the VA syndrome of dependency and manipulation is not altogether the patient's doing; the institution also fosters it. Nevertheless, I acknowledged his disdain for patients who "refuse" to try being independent, responsible, or cooperative—all values that he and his family of origin deeply held. In addition to encouraging him to elicit and accept the patient's EM, I accepted his EM and the feelings associated with it.

Finally, I encouraged him to ask himself, "Have I ever been made to feel like a troll?" in order to have a better sense for the sources of his feelings toward patients whom he regarded as trolls. I suggested that he might try to "compensate" when a patient seems to be like all his previous ones in a despised category by asking himself, "In this patient's behavior or physical findings, can I find one or two exceptions to the kinds of expectations I have for patients like this?" This kind of "test" may hold in abeyance the tendency to stereotype the patient according to a category in which he or she does not belong. (See Figure 3.1 for a schematic of the multiple contexts that contributed to the construction of this physician's EM in the foregoing case.)

Among the contributors, in addition to the official biomedical disease model, to physician EMs are the resident's own family/cultural models for sickness behavior; emotional factors that are expressed in countertransference (Stein 1985g: Stein and Apprey 1985); specialty models (family medicine, internal medicine, surgery); experiences and models from prior medical institutional settings; role with patient vis-à-vis the medical institution (admitting physician only, rounding on patient in hospital, outpatient clinic only); extent of a physician's urgency to arrive at a diagnosis and treatment plan; degree of familiarity with patient and patient's family; and perceived "character" or "type" the patient represents. In sum, physician EMs

FIGURE 3.1
SCHEMATIC REPRESENTATION OF SOCIAL SYSTEM IN CASE EXAMPLE

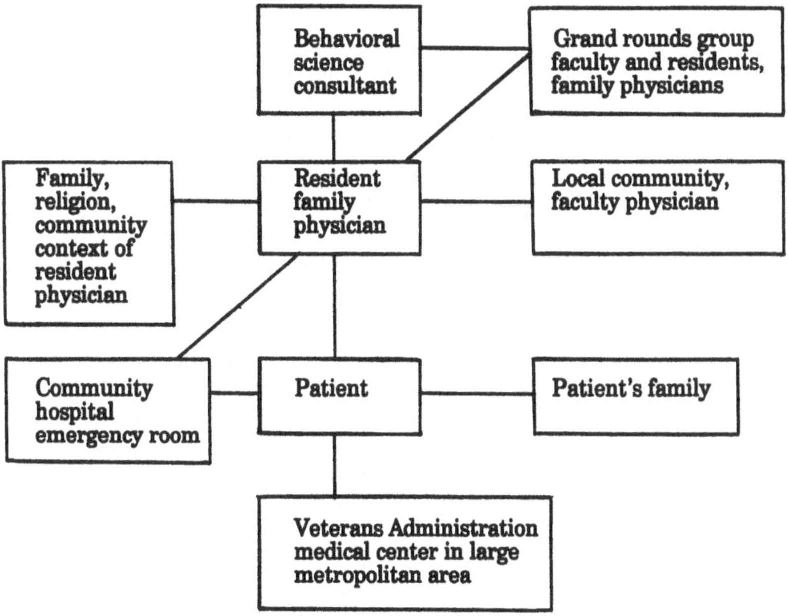

are not only biomedical and situational; they derive from the culturewide system of mainstream values, attitudes, and stereotypes.

Recently, I discussed the notion of good and bad patients with several community-based, male family practitioners in the rural Great Plains. For them a good patient is one who comes to the doctor "when he's (or she's) really sick." Such patients "downplay their pain and take it like a man." "Wimps" and "whiners" are the obverse of the good patient. These are people who "bother the doctor when there's nothing really wrong with them," "people who take up your time, who call you when they don't need to, and who don't do what you've told them, even though you've explained many times to them they're not sick," "people who make a lot of noise and complain about their pain." Wimps are men, and women, who are not stoic, who do not have the pioneer spirit and work ethic, who become emotional rather than adroitly practical about their diseases and injuries. The group of rural physicians then contrasted, with ridicule, their practices with the health maintenance philosophy of an urban training clinic. One physician said sarcastically:

> They bring in these rich folks when they're perfectly well for regular health maintenance checkups. I've seen them [patients] in the clinic down there and never figured out what we're supposed to say or talk about. They've got no symptoms. They're not sick. So why are they at the doctor's when they should be working or

in school? We're supposed to sit there and talk about lifestyle. I guess that rich people who don't have anything better to do need to come in to the doctor to go over the fact that they have no symptoms. Out here in rural farming country, people are too busy working to bother about lifestyle. Out here, if you made regular appointments with your doctor like that, you'd have to be a real wimp. A doctor out here who tried to build a practice around health maintenance would be laughed out of town. They wouldn't come to you as a patient if they weren't real sick.

As I am familiar with both rural and urban clinical settings, I added that I would find it hard to single out these patients for blame—the teaching and practice style of the urban training clinic in a sense cultivates this kind of patient health awareness and care.

According to a powerful nonofficial but nonetheless normative biomedical model, one category of patients is justified in taking the sick role, whereas another category of patients is not justified in so doing. The assignment of patients to one category or another is as much (if not more) based on an assessment of the patient's "moral character" as it is based on the severity or threat of the diagnosed disease. Assessment of moral character in turn affects how rigorously or aggressively a clinician pursues further biomedical diagnosis and treatment.

At a year-end (December) "wrap up" discussion with a group of residents, I asked them to suggest themes or topics that they would like to have addressed in the near future at one of our conferences. They avidly replied that they would like to hear a talk on smoking/obesity/overeating. There ensued some gallows humor about female patients who called them in the middle of the night during the holiday season tearfully complaining that they had just realized they were fat. What could the physician do about it in the middle of the night? they asked mockingly. In their anger and frustration, these physicians demanded greater patient accountability and wished for some weight-reducing treatment that worked and was income producing.

I briefly commented on the timeliness—in fact the annual recurrence—of this issue and frustration among physicians and patients alike. Between Thanksgiving and New Year's (or Superbowl Sunday?), people tend to engage in eating and drinking binges, only to feel guilty, ashamed, and uncomfortable afterward. Then they often turn to their doctors for magical solutions or a regimen (penance) to undo the indulgence. Many who "let themselves go" during the holiday season desperately elicit the physician's help in regaining self-control.

In January, however, few residents attended the eating disorders lecture that they had requested. I postponed the formal lecture until mid-February and continued case discussions until then. When I finally did present the formal lecture, they collectively *thanked* me for not having talked about the topic of overeating during the Thanksgiving–Christmas–Superbowl Sunday period (even though they had asked me to do so). They had wanted to feel free themselves to eat and drink during the cultural saturnalia. Their agitation with patients had been partly due to their attempts to control in patients what they had little success controlling in themselves. I used this timing to talk about culturewide ambivalence about self-control and self-indulgence, their ambivalent role as societal policeman, their wish to be out of control yet to control others, and the timing of these issues in the annual cycle. The ostensible issues of conference scheduling and difficult patients were revealed to be physician issues as well.

Mistaken Identity: Moralism in Patient Care

Participants at a family medicine case conference had been discussing the case of a hospitalized asthmatic eleven-year-old boy whose father had virtually refused to believe that his son was really in distress. The presumed delay in bringing the boy to the hospital led some of the physicians to suspect child abuse. From the father's ruddy face and long hair some of the physicians concluded that the father was an alcoholic and a hippie. Other physicians cautioned against jumping to conclusions, to avoid being judgmental, especially when a family seems "hysterical" and inappropriate during a crisis. "It's easy to get wrong impressions at first. I've been burned before when I acted on those first impressions. Keep your cool when everyone else is in crisis."

A number of younger physicians in the group spontaneously began to discuss the case of another young patient who had a febrile seizure on the floor of the emergency room. The group erupted with raucous laughter. One physician said, "I think I'll seize myself!" Another added, "We'll have a seizure party." A third commented, "Soon we'll all be down on the floor." The first physician interjected, "We're always the ones taking charge and keeping our cool. Let me off this train. I'd like to get down on the floor myself!"

The case conference burst out of its earlier serious discussion about maintaining decorum and self-discipline while others are seemingly regressing and enjoying themselves. The sudden humor expressed the presence of a powerful *wish* to be out of control, to regress, in fact to abandon if only temporarily the physician role and assume the role of patient. This illuminating example of projective identification with a patient shows what practitioners often hold at bay through professional demeanor. It also illustrates the temptation for practitioners to view patient behavior projectively, through the "eyes" of their own wishes, thereby diminishing the likelihood that they will understand the meaning of the symptom or disease for the patient. For example, if to the group of physicians, the patient's seizure represents the eruption of license to act regressively and irresponsibly (which they cannot themselves do), it is likely they will not inquire deeply into the meaning of the seizure for the patient and family.

Medical humor, especially when sadistic in tone can be, at least in part, a manic defense that serves as a "safety valve" against the sense of depression and despair that identification with patients evokes. Aggressive humor is an attempt to keep one's own depressiveness at bay (compare Segal 1955). It is not surprising that the physician's own illness experience may be a valuable tool that transforms revulsion and ridicule into empathy (see Hahn 1985a). Consider these vignettes.

Vignette 1

A physician friend was hospitalized for life-threatening abdominal surgery in a tertiary care center. Specialists from immunology, surgery, and gastroenterology, each with a different EM, strenuously "fought" over her treatment—often in her presence. During recovery, a gastroenterology resident came by her room late in the afternoon ("rounding") and said humorously to her, "Now I don't want you to go dying on me. I need to get some sleep tonight. You promise you'll make it through the night?" The patient replied, with a bewildered look, "I guess." After he left the room, she said to me, "What am I supposed to do? I thought I'm the patient. But he's asking me to take care of him. If I die, I've let him down." She also realized how emotionally demanding she could be on patients, as if reversing patient and caretaker roles.

Vignette 2

A resident detested any patient who demanded Vistaril (hydroxyzine pamoate, an antianxiety drug) and regarded anyone who made such a request as weak, irresponsible, dependent, giving unnecessarily in to pain. Having grown up in a highly religious, rural, self-sufficient west Texas town, he respected patients who looked after themselves and who rarely complained. Toward the end of his residency, he and I were sitting alone in the conference room prior to the beginning of the behavioral science lecture. He said to me:

> You know, Dr. Stein, I've come to have a different view of folks who ask me for Vistaril. I always figured people could put up with pain, that they do their work without needing medication. Well, I just had some surgery to have nasal polyps removed, and I never realized how painful something could be. I tried to tough it out, but it was excruciating. I couldn't stand it. So I wrote myself a prescription for Vistaril and felt a lot better soon. Maybe I won't be so quick to write off every patient who comes through complaining of pain.

Physicians' frequent use of the pronoun "we" in doctor-patient interaction is a key to physicians' perceptions of self-other boundaries and to their assumptions about authority, power, and control. In clinic examination rooms and in hospital rooms and wards, physicians often say for an opening line or early in the interview, "How are we doing today?" or "How are we feeling today?" Inquiries into whether the patient is taking the prescribed medication often take the form, "Are we taking our medicine on schedule?" In a teaching conference, a faculty physician similarly quizzed a resident, "Have we taken a chest X-ray on this man [the resident's patient]?" A common inquiry made by faculty physicians to interns and residents at clinical teaching conferences dealing with obstetrical care and pediatric care of the newborns is, "How's our [the possessive of "we"] mom doing?" or "How's our baby in the NICU [neonatal intensive care unit] doing?"

When, more than a decade ago, I first heard such commonplace questions, I thought that such a way of thinking and acting was patronizing (or matronizing!) and condescending. I soon discovered, however, that the use of the first person plural pronoun, and of its possessive, conveyed a great deal about how physicians perceived themselves in relation to their patients and in turn what they expected their role, and their patients' role, to be. The use of we-our often expresses personal concern for, if not unconscious identification with, patients. At the same time, the physician consciously maintains professional distance from the patient.

Nevertheless, the phrase may have the odd effect of obliterating the distinctiveness of the patient.

Many physicians use the pronoun "we" to convey a profound concern for their patients' condition and welfare—as if to say that their own well-being is deeply bound up with that of their patients. Other physicians use it more as an expression of the wish to control the patient, whom these physicians experience as extensions of themselves (we = myself in you as well as the speaker addressing you). Here, the observer misses the crucial blurring and confusion of boundaries if he or she notes only the attempted exercise of power, authority, and presumed status over the patient. We-our conveys the message "I do not experience you or your reality or needs as distinct from my own" and attests to the inseparability of the self-representation of the physician from his or her inner object representation or image of the patient. "We" also consciously affirms the tacit dictum that "a doctor is not a patient" through the physician's effort to control the patient.

In the past decade, a considerable literature in biomedicine has developed challenging the attitude of exacting compliance from patients. Some physicians have developed terms such as "adherence" and "concordance" in an attempt to describe the doctor-patient relationship as more mutual, as less one-sided or authoritarian than before. A kind of laissez-faire minimalism has developed among many physicians ("The patient will do whatever the patient will do; I am not responsible for changing the patient, only for serving as an adviser") in place of the earlier, overbearing maximalism. Nonetheless, euphemism and word replacement do not obscure the goal of compliance to which most physicians still adhere.

Perhaps no single concept save compliance can take us so quickly to the heart of contemporary American medicine. Recent euphemisms and revisionisms—adherence, congruence, patient advocacy, explicit therapeutic contracts, patient satisfaction, consumerism, patients' rights, and self-regulation—only attest to the tenacity of the notion of compliance within the medical world and in the wider culture. Political scientist Amitai Etzioni, for instance, defines compliance as "a relationship consisting of the power employed by superiors to control subordinates and the orientation of the subordinates to this power" (1961: xv). In an article on "the logic of non-compliance" among epileptics, James Trostle, W. Allen Hauser, and Ida Susser argue that compliance connotes "submission and powerlessness" (1983: 52), so that "the study of the relationship between a 'doctor's orders' and a patient's compliance is akin to the study of domination" (1983: 53). Patients who consult familial and extrafamilial personal networks in fact exercise far greater control of the treatment process than the dominance/submission image would suggest. Yet, within medicine it remains a compelling wish, image, and expectation.

In the words of Lorne Becker, M.D., a family physician and family medicine teacher, "When a lack of concordance occurs, the traditional approach has been to attempt to find ways to force patients to alter their behavior" (the medical advice, it is usually assumed, needs no alteration) (1984). Physicians search for "some therapy which makes non-compliance impossible, such as the use of long-acting injectable medications rather than pills to treat strep throat, gonorrhea, or chronic schizophrenia" (1984). When such "closely supervised" therapy is not feasible or fails, physicians search for other means to achieve the same end. Often patient education, for instance, "seeks to arouse the fear of the dire consequences of failure to comply" (1984). The goal of control remains paramount. Psychiatry and family medicine residents frequently ask me to provide a definitive answer to the question, "How can I make my patients take their medicine?"

In a recent critical review of Kleinman's "negotiation model" (1978) in clinical practice, Michael Phillips reminds the reader of

> clinicians' discomfort with being more sensitive to the concerns of patients and more democratic in making treatment decisions. Another problem of the negotiation model is that many patients, particularly those from non-Western cultures [and I would add many ethnically traditional members of Western culture], do *not* consider education and negotiation part of the normative interactions of patient and healer. Thus the clinician has the difficult task of altering patients' entire conception of the therapeutic interchange before it is even possible to engage them in the process of negotiation and education—many patients (who may be emotionally distraught because of the illness episode) are unwilling to make such a major change in their expectations of the clinician (1985: 32).

Thus, although many of the more recently trained physicians may embrace—at least avowedly if not half-heartedly—the negotiation or self-regulation model, they will often encounter patients who refuse to abide by what Thomas Szasz and Marc Hollender earlier termed the "mutual participation" (1975) approach. This latter style is more adult-adult than the compliance model and emphasizes the autonomy and mutual responsibility of all participants to the clinical relationship. However, many patients in essence say to their physician, "You're the doctor, fix it," while often refusing to accept the physician's advice when the physician does indeed attempt to "fix it." Moreover, in this hiatus between the negotiation and compliance models, the maturity of the participants is rarely mentioned. It is as if one must choose between the relativism, if not indifference, of the negotiators and the absolutism of the compliance seekers.

Despite biomedicine's ideals, ambitions, technology, and pretensions, patients and families will do as they will and not as clinicians wish. Patient autonomy, freedom, pathology, and mere difference often come to be viewed and felt by physicians more as defiant affronts than as welcome opportunities or even as simple facts. Physicians often ask themselves and their consultants, "Why don't they comply?" rather than "What do they do?" and "What meanings, values, rules, strategies, unconscious conflicts, and economic constraints do they live with?" From the physician's viewpoint, the "problem" of compliance consists only of the patient's behavior (or misbehavior), not the physician's expectations or assumptions. Defined this way, compliance indicates that the practitioner's is the only legitimate point of view about the clinical relationship.

Physicians often depict compliance as an ongoing battle to outwit patients. Preoccupation with ever-new formulas and strategies for compliance (which physicians employ behavioral scientists to provide) may play out, prolong, and escalate the quest for control from which neither doctors nor patients can then extricate themselves. Because patients often serve as the proving ground for physicians' sense of competence at curing disease, physicians' personal stake in compliance can become enormous. Noncompliance portends defeat and the dreaded sense of failure that inverts the status of medical authority.

Clinicians may express their discomfort and frustration with noncompliance, chronic illness, and disablement through joking, avoidance, curtness, and overcompensation. The clinician who expects to be a successful healer may experience failure with incurable or terminally ill patients as a trauma, a narcissistic wound from which he or she seeks to recover. One means of diminishing self-recrimination for an inability to effect a cure is stigmatization of the patient. In his study ***Stigma***, Erving Goffman writes that the stigmatized individual is "reduced in our minds from a whole and usual person to a tainted, discounted person" (1963: 3). It is not the attribute, however, that is discrediting, but the system of relationships in which it is embedded. "A language of relationships, not attributes, is really needed" to account for stigmatization (1963: 3). Specifically, "a stigma . . . is really a special kind of relationship between attribute and stereotype" (1963: 4), an "undesired differentness" (1963: 5). The stigmatized person, however, is seen to possess and embody either a "discredited" or "discreditable" identity.

Stigmatization is a way of labeling a patient's personal identity in terms of one's own system of values, attitudes, and defenses. The clinician cannot undisguisedly say to the patient, "You are simply no good. You will never amount to anything. I thoroughly dislike you and all that you represent." But a practitioner can communicate this judgment to the patient through the impersonal medium of clinical language, thereby disqualifying the intent while conveying it. "If you don't try to succeed, you are a failure" translates clinically into "uncooperative, noncompliant patient." To the clinician, the patient who has given up on his or her disease is often a moral failure, just as from the clinician's and the patient's (and patient's family's) viewpoints clinical failure is a moral failure.

Psychiatrist Albert Vogel writes of the placebo's common use as a powerful (yet implicit) vehicle for stigmatizing the patient:

> Unfortunately, recent studies reveal that among house officers [interns] in a hospital (and likely among physicians in general) placebos are most commonly used when the physician is frustrated and angry with his patient, i.e., when in an adversarial relationship. Common examples occur when the physician is: trying to prove that the patient is not really sick or is faking; attempting to demonstrate that, contrary to the patient's belief, the illness in question is psychological not physical; feeling that the patient does not deserve analgesics or anti-anxiety agents, usually because of some disliked characteristic of the patient such as alcoholism, drug abuse, or noncontribution to society; trying to drive the patient away; punishing the patient; or aware that the patient will be upset, angry, or offended when he discovers that placebo has been used (1981: 8).

Stigmatization is often not limited to individual clinicians but is culturally shared. The patient who is applauded as a clinical success, and who likewise is approved as a moral success, mirrors to many physicians the external affirmation of their own defenses and ambitions. Conversely, the patient who is dismissed as a clinical failure, and who likewise is condemned as moral failure, represents to care-givers and to others a threat to their own defense system. In both cases, the patient is not experienced as a separate person but represents idealized and repudiated aspects respectively of the observers themselves who are assessing the patient's progress. As one PA said to me, "Most people working around stroke victims get turned off. They have to put up with the patient's constant dribbling from the mouth. Often the patient can't even talk. And often there's a complete loss of self-control. All of that is so foreign to them, they just can't take it." Losing control of one's bodily fluids and of one's feces; being cut off from talking, a form of communication heightened in American culture (as compared with, say, the expressive use of the eyes and of silence in Russian culture); being unable to control one's own muscles, limbs, and movements voluntarily; being utterly dependent on another to take care of one's needs—these are among the conflicts often reawakened in practitioners by stroke patients.

Many practitioners assume that patients with permanent spinal cord damage cannot have, will not have, and should not have the desire to maintain an active sexual life. But why the assumption? One PA suggested that the attribution to the patient needed to be translated into a self-defensive statement that would go something like, "The very thought of a person in your condition engaging in sexual activity is repulsive, disgusting to me." Sexuality carries with it cultural presuppositions about body integrity, beauty, motor coordination, self-control, and perception of power.

Geriatric patients present a special problem because according to the stereotype, to be old (say, older than sixty-five) *is* to be ill. Moreover, if one is old, one is also more likely to be ill. Aging, as Margaret Clark (1973) writes, is seen as a condition of inherent dependency, disease, decay, disengagement, and segregation. Aging is a vicious affront to the American insistence that the future is limitless, that youth is eternal. In the aged, the clinician sees what she or he attempts to deny will become her or his own condition. One way to create and sustain the delusion that aging is not a continuum is to parse it. Surely the young can say that the elderly have nothing to do with themselves, which translates into, "We don't want to have anything to do with them because we cannot bear to recognize themselves in us."

A fourth year medical student interviewed a sixty-five-year-old man prior to surgery. The patient inquired if when he recovered, he would be able to continue normal sexual activity with his wife. The student dismissingly quipped, "At your age, I wouldn't worry about it! A man your age wouldn't be much interested in that sort of thing anymore." This reassurance missed the point that the patient's abiding "interest" had prompted the question in the first place. Only "dirty old men," the saying goes, would maintain an interest in sex into their later years. What does "dirty" mean?: the Oedipal son's jealousy of the father's prerogative, together with the projection of his disavowed impulses onto the father.

The young drug addict presents a different problem. A chronic heroin addict may indeed be a master of manipulation, may seem to prey parasitically on the good intentions of the care-giver, may be psychopathically contemptuous of anyone else's rules, and may be impulsive. In the clinical setting, a struggle of wills is commonplace. Who will set the rules? When will they be broken? The stern, distant clinician ("bad father") insists on an inflexible set of standards; the gentle, protective clinician ("good mother") allows a rule here and there to be bent; and the addict manipulates one against another, just as the addict may have earlier triangulated with his or her parents (see Bowen 1978; Schwartzman 1975).

A practitioner who expects patient compliance finds patient deviousness instead. The clinician who expects to be in control of every medical situation finds his or her word and law challenged at every turn. The clinician who is accustomed to winning is now in a relationship in which she or he cannot win by being either good or bad because neither protective nor stern roles address the patient's underlying issues. The practitioner likely becomes a target for the addict's negative family identifications and "bad" ***inner objects*** (mental structures that echo parental wrath, abandonment, dread, as these are fused with one's own wishes, feelings, and fantasies). Not able to notice the schizoid emptiness, the paranoid terror, or the depressive despair behind frenetic acting out and clever calculation, the clinician may protect himself or herself via a clinically disguised righteous indignation.

The patient with chronic low back pain, whether or not there is visible spinal cord damage, is another condition ripe for stigmatization. This patient is typically regarded as "the low point in the [clinician's] day. Nobody looks forward to seeing him." This illness is not life threatening, and because in the biomedical view there is no real emergency and no cure, the clinician sees no possibility of gratification from treatment. The clinician continues to see the same patient, with the same condition, with the same complaint, with often the same attitude of chronic dissatisfaction. The patient may not comply with the clinician's order to rest in bed or undertake regular back exercises, for these would entail a change in the patient's lifestyle. The patient may also take his or her complaint against the world from the medical realm into the legal. Thus, practitioners are wary of the patient's potential litigiousness in quest of insatiable compensation when a "perfect back" cannot be made. The clinician-patient relationship is often adversarial from the outset.

Within medicine, the musculoskeletal is the least glamorous of the organ systems. It offers the fewest rewards in patient care. An angry and resentful patient is met with an angry and resentful clinical staff who "knows" what is coming. Consequently, low back patients are often circulated, or "dumped," from office to office, from clinic to clinic, or from one hospital service to another. The patient who "won't get better" because she or he "refuses treatment" is often labeled informally, if not diagnosed, as an "inadequate personality" or a "malingerer." Patients with chronic back pain threaten clinicians' very concept and self-concept of adequacy and become a convenient scapegoat and social casualty.

Here, neither identified patient, family of patient, health care system, nor culture can rightfully be blamed or exonerated. Rather, the portrait of stigmatization in chronic illness and disability is one of a systems pathology. Through stigmatization, the "normals" (from laypersons to medical practitioners who officially sanction normalcy) freely comment both on themselves and on the deviants. Likewise, those stigmatized comment reciprocally on the culture that labels them and on themselves by internalizing the judgment pronounced upon them. At one extreme, a chronically ill or disabled person may use the illness or disability in a self-punishing way for failing to live up to his or her own, parental, or cultural standards. At the other extreme, the patient may demand and succeed in exacting from clinical personnel and institutions what he or she could not secure from the natal family. The network of clinicians (and clinics) becomes the new family who will now be compelled to give—because medicine must care! On the other hand, largely through the agency of self-help groups based on illness or disablement identities, the stigma is reversed. As a result, many disabled people regard themselves as the real people, as special, and look scornfully at those whom they now disparage as "abies" (able-bodied persons).

Increases in neighborhood and regional localism, ethnic nativism, nationalism, divorce rates, medical malpractice suits, religious and political cults, practitioners' reluctance to make home visits, consumerism, and the proliferation of self-help groups all express a societal fragmentation rooted in regressive narcissistic self-preoccupation (see Kohut 1971; Kernberg 1975; Nelson 1977). Narcissistic isolation leads to intensified we-they dichotomies and stigmatization. In such an emotional climate, greater demands and dependency needs on the part of patients clash with the clinician's heightened concern about self-image, competence, mastery, autonomy, control—and liability. Both sides become increasingly antagonistic and judgmental. Further, this psychosocial trend is coming to characterize not only much of the United States but other Westernized and Westernizing societies as well.

The Cultural Context of Medical Moralism

Within biomedicine, issues such as compliance and social control are seldom explored as intrinsic to the practice of medicine. In fact, modern biomedicine takes suffering out of complex life and sets it within its own sanctioned province. But to segregate suffering from life and to relabel it *are* medicine's modern social roles. Foster and Anderson identify as one of the widespread functions of medical systems that of "sanctioning and supporting social and moral cultural norms. . . . Illness, seen as a penalty for disapproved conduct, is widespread in non-Western societies. Or, stated differently, the *threat* of illness as a consequence of socially unacceptable behavior plays a major role in many societies in maintaining the moral order" (Foster and Anderson 1978: 43).

That this statement contains an *aperçu* pertinent to biomedicine in contemporary America can be immediately recognized when we remember that such substances as ethanol, sodium salt, cholesterol, caffeine, animal fats, sucrose sugars, and tobacco (see Nolen 1987) and such "conditions" as obesity, lack of exercise, and casual sexual activity fall under the purview of social control—or at least the attempt at regulation—by biomedical physicians. In this view, failure to comply with highly abstemious regimes leads to disease, in which case both physician and society are absolved because, in the vernacular, such consequences are altogether the patient's own fault (see Becker 1987). In an article on health educators as the new puritans, Irma Kurtz describes the role of moralism in American biomedicine:

> Vaguely, we in Western society remember that once it was believed some sort of good came from restraint and moderation, but it has ceased to be a question of spiritual good. It is now the individual's physical good that is his or her utmost

> achievement. Health has become a religion. The body has become a sacred object. And the doctor has willy-nilly become a priest. Punishment for disobeying the doctor's orders is not delivered hereafter, but here and now. Punishment is not a bad conscience or a cursed soul, punishment is cancer, miscarriage, herpes or AIDS. That the doctor will probably recommend self-denial makes him a puritan. He is a militant fighter against refined sugar, promiscuous sex, and other implements of the new devil. The new devil doesn't give a damn for conscience or souls, he wants our livers and the muscle called heart (1987: 40).

Medical zeal has become religious fervor (Nolen 1987). In our era, medicine has been assigned, and eagerly accepts, the stewardship of the body at a time when, despite the resurgence of religious fundamentalism, people are less willing to think of their future only in terms of the fate of the soul. With unbridled fanaticism in intruding upon people's lives, medical moralism has—with the blessing of the wider society—redefined virtue and sin. Similarly, Marshall Becker, in "The Tyranny of Health Promotion," writes:

> the individual-responsibility approach has helped to establish "health" as the New Morality by which character and moral worth are judged. "Being ill" is redefined as "being guilty." The obese are stigmatized as "letting themselves go." Smokers "have no will power." Nonaerobicts are "lazy." . . . The as-yet unproselytized are treated as sinners. . . . Health promotion, as currently practiced, fosters a dehumanizing self-concern which substitutes personal health goals for more important, humane, societal goals. It is a new religion, in which we worship ourselves, attribute good health to our devoutness, and view illness as just punishment for those who have not yet seen the Way—a Weltanschauung that evokes Social Darwinism, the "Me" generation, and the 1980s (1986: 19–20).

American culture has tended to define and encompass as medical a wide variety of problems associated with the category of "control" (hypertension, alcoholism/drug abuse, anorexia nervosa, bulimia, diabetes). Such diagnosis often has the intention, if not always the effect, of relegating issues once associated with sin or "excess" to a morally neutral category of disease. Psychiatrist E. Mansell Pattison writes that contemporary Western culture has "subjectivized evil": "The problem of evil is a therapeutic problem, not a moral issue. Human values are persistently defined as health values. . . . Sin has been thoroughly transformed into sickness. There is no justice for evil, nor forgiveness of sins; rather there is therapy" (1984: 80).

No sooner, however, has the heavy judgment of sin and moralism been evicted through culture's front door than it silently reenters via a window or the back door. In a critique of the biomedical "disease" concept of alcoholism, Herbert Fingarette argues that

> instead of encouraging those concerned to see the drinking in the context of the person's way of life, and thus to discern what role or roles it may play for that person in coping with life, the logic of the disease concept does the contrary. It leads all concerned, including the drinker, to deny, to ignore, to discount what

> meaning that way of life may have. Seen as an involuntary symptom of a disease, the drinking is isolated from the rest of life, and viewed as the meaningless but destructive effect of a noxious condition, a "disease." The disease concept leads one logically, if tacitly, to the basic assumption that the alcoholic's way of life ought to be abandoned if at all possible—a devastating moral judgment on that life. . . . The drinker may be striving to express deep needs and genuine feelings—but how tempting to be freed of guilt and turmoil if only one will accept the bargain offered by the disease concept advocates! . . . Indoctrination with the disease doctrine gives the needed intellectual license and social encouragement to disavow the desire to drink, and thus to experience it as alien to self. Combined with the motive of evading inner conflict—the motive that is generic to self-deception—the proselytizing of the disease concept becomes a prime incentive to self-deception in the long-term heavy drinker (1985: 58–61, 61).

Moreover, the self-deceptive disavowal characterizes not only the drinker but the drinker's family, most of the medical and nonmedical treatment community, clinical educational institutions, law enforcement and lawmaking institutions, and the cultural group fantasy about alcoholism and chemical dependency in general. Were the disavowal only the lone drinker's defense, it would not work because it would be challenged. We must include virtually the entire contemporary American culture in Fingarette's clinical picture because what others are ill prepared to avow and explore in themselves they will be too frightened to recognize, confront, interpret, and empathize with in others. For instance, according to one widely used model of alcoholism, drug abuse, and treatment, all family members of alcoholics and drug addicts are labeled "co-dependents," thereby mystifying—by the appeal to concepts of substance, disease, and susceptibility—everyone's participation. Fingarette concludes that

> the irony is . . . that appeal to the drinker's own decision and self-discipline is made by those who insist that the alcoholic's drinking is the symptom of a disease, and hence is *not* voluntary conduct and not subject to personal self-control. This radical inconsistency between diagnosis and therapeutic expectations is typically ignored (1985: 62).

The demand that the alcoholic (or chemically dependent and co-dependent) voluntarily control an involuntary disease becomes an additional paradox induced by the treatment and legal community for the purpose of shoring up its own defenses (self-deceptions). Treatment becomes a way for the therapist to reassure himself or herself that *no one need candidly and painfully examine life*. Control becomes the only acceptable issue. Because doctrine and treatment symbolically and ritually reaffirm the splitting and repression in *all* participants' defensive organization, "alcoholics" and "addicts" remain permanently available as categories with which all widespread disavowed impulses, wishes, fantasies, and needs can be endowed. Anthropologist Dwight Heath (1985) directs our attention to the symbolism of alcohol, to the "dither about" drinking. He sees it as part of a more widespread, and ominous, clamoring for *external* controls on the part of a society that has difficulty internalizing superego functions (also see Stein 1985a).

John L. Falk suggests that contemporary scientific theories of drug dependence have the quality of myth:

> I'm afraid that many of our scientific notions about drug dependence are burdened with a heavy load of mythic, moral freight. . . .
>
> As each underclass begins to emerge in our society, as they become visible, they have attributed to them certain frightening characteristics. They are alleged to be aggressive, over-sexed and shamefully poor. This is typically the case for emerging foreign minorities, blacks, women, teenagers, and lately the aged or infirm. Each of these groups also gets some sort of substance dependence attributed to them as the mechanism of action which accounts for their ill-temper, hypersexuality, and poverty. Chinese and opium, Indians and alcohol, blacks and heroin or cocaine, teens and drugs, alcoholism in women, the homeless, and the aged. It's not that people don't have drug problems. What I question is that drugs are the major factor underlying their problems. And the problems that *are* attributed to these emerging groups are mostly not really their problems. These groups often function as wondrous screens on which to project our forbidden aggressive and sexual fantasies (1983: 390).

Alcoholism and other "chemical" addictions—both theories and treatments—express or manifest the mythic structure of contemporary society. They are a vital part of our contemporary folklore about ourselves rationalized in terms of the idiom to which we now confer highest status—science or medical science ("applied human biology"). One rationale for the medicalization of diffuse social problems is that it leads to more compassionate and objective treatment. Despite the ideology of therapeutic neutrality, in actual practice health and mental health often connote goodness, whereas disease and mental illness connote badness. Sin, good, and evil are smuggled in even as they are exorcized. Moral opprobrium persists in the form of physicians' (and staff's) attitudes toward categories of "difficult," "refractory" patients.

The broader social dynamic that persists is what William Ryan (1971) in another context labels "blaming the victim." Through such varied self-improvement and health maintenance–related activities as biofeedback, meditation, relaxation exercises, weight reduction, smoking cessation, jogging and other aerobic exercises, dietary change (less dairy and red meat products, more whole grains, bran, fruits, and vegetables), people are expected to take control of their own bodily destinies. Even if processes are medically or scientifically declared to be largely or entirely beyond conscious control or will, people are nevertheless held accountable should they fall from health or wellness. If they become sick, they have nothing or no one to blame but themselves. Righteous indignation masks widespread callousness toward those who have fallen ill. The "healthy" need to believe themselves to be an entirely different breed from the "sick."

Responsibility for health is both privatized and medicalized. Compassion and sense of responsibility toward those afflicted decreases, while social distance dramatically increases. Medical minimalism abandons the patient to his or her own devices and resources. It diminishes anxiety, guilt, and shame on the part of medical practitioners and educators because patients' fall from wellness or their inability to return quickly to productive health is their "fault."

Body Narcissism: The Wellness Movement and Core American Values

Recently, health, virtue, moralism, and nationalism have fused in the wellness movement. Scheper-Hughes and Lock locate the American wellness and fitness movement in the context of core American values and obsessions:

> In our own increasingly "healthiest" and body-conscious culture, the politically correct body for both sexes is the lean, strong, androgenous (sic), and physically "fit" form through which the core cultural values of autonomy, toughness, competitiveness, youth, and self-control are readily manifest (Pollitt 1982). Health is increasingly viewed in the United States as an achieved rather than an ascribed status, and each individual is expected to "work hard" at being strong, fit, and healthy. Conversely, ill health is no longer viewed as accidental, a mere quirk of nature, but rather is attributed to the individual's failure to live right, to eat well, to exercise, etc. We might ask what it is our society "wants" from this kind of body. DeMause (1984) has speculated that the fitness/toughness craze is a reflection of an international preparation for war. . . . Crawford (1980, 1985), however, has suggested that the fitness movement may reflect, instead, a pathetic and individualized (also wholly inadequate) defense against the threat of nuclear holocaust (1987: 25–26; also see Scheper-Hughes and Stein 1987).

As I argue (1982f, 1982g, 1982j), the view of wellness as preparation for war and as an inner attempt to control what externally cannot be controlled are not mutually exclusive. Externalization and internalization, projection and introjection, are phases of a cycle. The dread of death and the eruption of aggressive impulses intensify one another and thereby intensify both the panic and the wellness ritual one employs to try containing the panic.

On the face of it, nothing could appear more innocuous, even salubrious, than the wellness movement that arose in the United States in the late 1970s. Jogging, exercising, trimming down one's weight, renouncing indulgence in those popular vices so dangerous to health (nicotine, caffeine, ethanol, sodium salt, animal fats, sucrose, processed foods, to name but a few)—these are believed to improve respiration and cardiovascular circulation, reduce morbidity, and make for greater personal satisfaction. Professionals in public health and preventive medicine have for years promoted lifestyle change as a means of lowering both morbidity and mortality. Why, then, should wellness not be uncritically welcomed as an idea whose time has come?

Good nutrition and exercise are profoundly cultural notions. They are American prescriptions for a health in which the moral is closely allied with the medical. Education of the body has long been coupled with discipline of the spirit—one thinks, for instance, of the YMCA and YWCA movements, the Boy Scouts of America, Outward Bound, and the like. Physical fitness has always been a moral condition.

In the America of the early 1900s, warm breakfast foods, such as the favorite ham and eggs or oatmeal, were associated with sexual arousal. Social reformers such as Sylvester Graham, James Caleb Jackson, and John Harvey Kellogg (whose younger brother Keith founded the cold, dry breakfast cereal industry in the early twentieth century) endeavored to reduce the adult sexual drive and curb children's masturbation through dietary regulation. Historically grounded in humoral medicine in the Indo-European cultural tradition (such as the four temperaments; hot/cold, wet/dry dichotomies), reformist theory held that the fires of erotic arousal would diminish to controllable embers only if people ate those foods embodying virtues that opposed and counteracted sexual desire. Thus, many cold cereals that nutritionists and wellness zealots of today associate with dietary perdition were advanced a century or so ago as dietary salvation (Savitt 1982).

Moreover, in the nineteenth century as now, obsession with "health food" was not an isolated phenomenon. Rather, food was but one symbol within a pervasive temperance and reform movement that included the following emphases in its ethos: personal self-improvement; simplicity; romanticism of nature; widespread vegetarianism; rejection of the "harsh" remedies of regnant orthodox medicine; baths and water treatments (such as spas); vigorous exercise; cleanliness and purification of the body; proscription of all forms of intemperateness (indulgence in gourmet foods, alcohol, nonprocreative sex, stimulants such as coffee and tobacco); proper diet; fresh air; and a "great awakening" of religion, with the interweaving of religious, political, and health reform (Savitt 1982).

In *Crusaders for Fitness*, James C. Wharton (1982) draws parallels between the wellness movement of our time and this earlier era (also see Morantz 1983). He examines the personal hygiene movement in the United States between 1830 and 1920, a period of social ferment that has often been called the second great awakening. Among social reformers of this era, hygiene became the metaphor and vehicle for progress, optimism, and perfectionism. Hygienics was essentially a theory of balance. If only humankind would lead a hygienic life by forswearing temptations of the flesh and controlling their appetites, they could save themselves and help society attain the millennium. Prevention and treatment became forms of moral resocialization or acculturation. Medicine was enlisted as an agent of social control.

Through hygienics, science became a new vessel, so to speak, for failing religion. The language of medical science was conscripted into the service of ethical messianism. Canons of social virtue became canons of health. Conversely, the diagnosis of disease signified moral lapse or failure. Scientific denotations acquired heavily religious connotations. As the traditional religious framework became inadequate to explain the world and to satisfy emotional needs, health reform became the handmaiden of secular progressivism.

Our own era of social upheaval, doubt, and the quest for immutable verities and unfailing assurances might well be called a third great awakening. For patients, physicians, and populace alike, the union of medicine and ideology is as much a lure today as it ever was. The body remains a symbol—and often a battleground—of meanings and loyalties.

Insofar as we can characterize whole decades, one might say that in the 1960s and early 1970s many believed in salvation through sex. Since the late 1970s, many have come to believe in salvation from sex. Abstinence, a lean diet, and regular, vigorous exercise promise to keep the temptations of the flesh at bay. A current television commercial depicts a female marathon winner who had been an alcoholic running uphill; it concludes with the triumphant question, "Who says you can't run away from your problems?" Through society we collectively work out our need for inhibition, if not prohibition. Compulsive asceticism replaces the previous compulsive (and joyless) hedonism, just as obsessive indulgence had supplanted the earlier obsessive (and dour) puritanism.

The present era of wellness often uses the Vietnam War as an anguished external reference point. At first a trauma to be forgotten, it has become a trauma to be remembered if not brandished. The holding of American citizens hostage in Iran from November 1978 through January 1980 (after admission of the shah to the United States) was a later, secondary insult. Just as the shock of the Napoleonic conquests sparked nationalisms throughout Europe, and just as the sudden, unexpected end of World War I in 1918 became the great national trauma that Hitler promised to reverse, so today one hears of the need to "get tough." We have been steadily bracing ourselves for the good fight, one that can magically restore our self-respect, confidence, and purpose. Restaging or reversing the past, not mourning it, has become a national obsession.

Since the late 1970s, American society has witnessed a marked shift of emphasis from clinical or curative medicine to wellness or preventive medicine. With the publication in 1979 of the two volume set, *Healthy People*, the U.S. government gave its official imprimatur to this change in priority. The presidential election of 1980 elevated a spartan ethos to the status of the nationally representative. Such phrases as "belt tightening" and "trimming off excess fat" and President Ronald Reagan's now-famous trinity of "cut-slash-chop" well reflected the morally severe and economically stringent national mood. From workers' wages to federal overspending, from overeating to indulgent lifestyle, "inflation" was diagnosed as the disease. It followed unerringly that a stringent health was to be restored—from Reaganomics at the political level to personal "sacrifices" at the individual level.

The cultural climate of the 1980s has spawned vigorous political and religious fundamentalisms, nationalism, militarism, unbridled economic competitiveness and survivalism, increased provocation of external enemies (Libya, Nicaragua, Iran, the USSR), diminished sense of compassion and responsibility toward others in American society (including the elderly, the poor, the chronically ill, and the handicapped): in short, a renewed social Darwinism (Stein 1982f, 1982g, 1982j). "Back to basics" became a clarion call several years before economic hard times set in. A minimalist philosophy simplifies everything. Through nostalgia we are lifted from the frightful present to the reassuring past (Stein 1974b).

According to our widespread patently paranoid ambience, poisons abound everywhere, lurking in our national bloodstream to weaken and defeat us. In such a climate medical moralism, tidily and seductively mantled in the ideology of science, becomes as much a potential danger to the nation's health as religious and political fanaticism. Increasingly, to become ill is to be blamed for bringing the disease upon oneself. Righteous indignation masks and rationalizes widespread abandonment of and contempt for those who fall ill.

This is the regressive social climate in which the metaphor of health has come to dominate discourse about the body, the family, government, the nation, the national will, the environment, and the economy. Only the physically, mentally, and economically strong are worth bothering about. Others are permitted to languish or perish through neglect or are hastened out of sight and life by social policies that serve as collective externalized conscience. (Presidents, legislators, justices, and other elected public officials are "representatives" and "delegates" voted to embody and carry out group fantasies.) The recent proliferation of corporate, protocol-based hospital care (replacing individualized treatment with standardized care designed to get the patient quickly out of the hospital); of brief, short, focused, problem-oriented psychotherapies and family therapies; and of technological, technique-oriented treatments that bypass relationship and meaning in illness and therapy is symptomatic of the minimalistic climate in which scapegoating and victimization become forms of cultural therapy. G. Gayle Stephens courageously addresses this ambience in articles on the medical marketplace and on images of the physician (1984b, 1984c). William Carlyon (1984), Marshall Becker (1986, 1987), and William Nolen (1987) all identify symbolic issues in preventive medicine's zealotry.

The current fitness-wellness-health reform is also part of the culturewide anti-intellectual (or pseudointellectual) attitude that substitutes action for insight. The "therapeutic" goal is forgetting instead of remembering. If the acting out (and the justification of acting out) of aggressive impulses is a preponderant aim of the dominant group fantasy, it makes sinister sense that those projects and programs funded by the federal government, whose goal is the analysis and diminution of hostility, should be curtailed. This, indeed, is the case. In an address to the Pennsylvania Psychological Association on June 19, 1981, Clarence J. Martin reports that "at the National Institute of Mental Health, social research in rape, divorce, racism, sexism, family life, and aggression have been eliminated from all consideration for funds" (1981: 5). Moreover, in the Alcohol, Drug, and Mental Health Administration, research areas not to be supported include

> (1) Large scale social conditions or problems (e.g., poverty, unemployment, inadequate housing and slums, divorce, daycare arrangements, accidents, and criminal behavior); (2) animal ethology; (3) minority status and minority-majority relationships; (4) the structure and functioning of groups, institutions or societies; (5) social roles and career determinants of men and women; (6) decision-making models; (7) attitude formation; and (8) the legal or educational systems (1981: 8).

Social policy enacts group fantasy. The foregoing lists enumerate areas of life we do not wish to understand. Consequently, any motivated "mistakes" we make as a result of not knowing commit us to further action.

How one evaluates wellness (see Reed 1981; *U.S. News & World Report* 1982) depends upon where one looks, which is also to say, where one wishes to look and not to look. Nicholas Smith writes that "complex policy decisions are always set in social and cultural contexts which, more often than not, make objectivity difficult to obtain" (1981: 100). I would add that culture largely consists of consensual resistance to objectivity in order that "policy" be acted out with impunity.

Much of what has been written lauding wellness, has either narrowly isolated clinical variables (blood pressure, serum cholesterol, and so on) or has uncritically accepted psychiatrically naive self-reporting on miraculous reversals in well-being ascribed to the effects and ideology of wellness. Curiously, medical literature and popular literature omit discussion of the unconscious motivation that prompts sudden and dramatic changes in one's self-image, body image, and behavior. Often physicians, for unconscious reasons of their own, collude with patients' wishes and beliefs instead of helping patients to examine them. At this point medicine becomes part of the problem.

What, however, is the problem? Our bodies are never mere biological organ systems. They are meaning systems that attach to the body and pervade its functions. The result is often a spurious biology because meanings do not derive from the body but from fantasies about the body. If we have learned nothing else from Freud's legacy, we have surely learned this. Humankind is an inveterately symbolic animal who uses the body for symbolic purposes. One cannot discourse on the body and its uses without talking about the meaning the body has for the person who inhabits it.

Consider running, easily the most popular of exercise regimens. I would want to know what a person who regularly if not obligatorily runs is running for, perhaps running from, or running to. Surely running or jogging as a symbolic form or "symptom choice" can hardly be accidental. In a society that prizes personal freedom and mobility and in a world in which one can feel increasingly trapped if not paralyzed in life's options, running enables one to keep on the move, sustained only by one's own powers. One may be running from the past, from one's family, from the horror at the thought of one's own death. Running, in short, may well be a nativistic rite in which one attempts to intensify or revitalize the personal culture that one feels to be in decline (compare Wallace 1966). Running is culture before it is medicine. The same can be said for aerobic exercises, conducted in groups, often to the energizing pulse of music (see Cooper 1978). Although translated into the idiom of medicine, aerobics is nonetheless functionally the "dancing mania" of crisis cults in contemporary dress. These represent and enact shared fantasies about the body and lead to the implementation of medical means to achieve, and clinical ideologies to rationalize, fantasy goals.

Scheper-Hughes and Lock interpret the variously impulsive/compulsive eating disorders (see Chernin 1981) plaguing modern American society as enacting a central double bind of our culture:

> Crawford (1985) has interpreted the eating disorders and distortions in body image expressed in obsessional jogging, anorexia, and bulimia as a symbolic mediation of the contradictory demands of postindustrial society. The double-binding injunction to be self-controlled, fit, and productive workers, and to be at the same time self-indulgent, pleasure-seeking consumers is especially destructive to the self-image of the "modern," "liberated" American woman. Expected to be fun-loving and sensual, she must also remain thin, lovely, and self-disciplined. Since one cannot be hedonistic and controlled simultaneously, one can alternate phases of binge eating, drinking, and drugging with phases of jogging, purging, and vomiting (1987: 26).

J. D. Reed highlights the recurrent themes of time, aging, and anxiety about death that underlie the narcissistic pursuit of youthfulness through fitness. Reed provides ample evidence that through radical improvement of the body people strive to magically reverse time. "Paring it, preening it, pumping it up and pounding it down, the body national is being rejuvenated with a relentless impatience, slimmed with a fanatic dedication. . . . The country runs and runs, from fear of death and pollution and old age as well as longing for health, beauty and well-being" (1981: 95, 104).

"Health," "wellness," and "fitness" are cultural buzzwords, euphemisms for the darker realities that they mystify. From that viewpoint it is pointless to ask whether, say, jogging or any regular exercise regimen is inherently healthy or unhealthy. I am here inquiring into the meaning of behaviors as they are experienced through the ideology of wellness. When "obesity" or "fitness" runs rife with connotation, and biomedicine accepts those connotations as its own, we have removed ourselves from science, or, rather, we have superimposed upon science the weighty luggage of moralism, religion, and the widespread forbidden wish to indulge in excess. In short, the prevention of disease is not what healthy people and wellness are primarily about, the buzzwords notwithstanding.

Lest I be misunderstood, I do not favor the abolition of health education. Nor do I believe jogging to be intrinsically pathological. Preventive medicine is an essential, and neglected, way of approaching human health and illness. Programs in community medicine and schools of public health have historically been second-class citizens in a medical establishment, and wider culture, that more highly prizes curative, clinical medicine. When the jogging/fitness movement began in the late 1970s, many community medicine colleagues welcomed it as their vindication and championed it zealously. They responded with hostility to my attempts to understand its symbolism. In community medicine/family medicine conferences, discussions of patients' overeating or obesity frequently couch professionals' revulsion and supposed moral superiority in clinical language that barely disguises their condemnation. What I question is the subject matter of wellness, that is, what is being "prevented." More is being averted than the risk of heart disease, lung disease, stroke, diabetes, birth defects, and cancer among patients. For many practitioners and medical educators, as for their wide public, what is being prevented is also a deeply symbolic affliction that is represented by and focused into various disease entities and condemned lifestyles: the blurring of the boundary between what and who are moral and immoral, good and evil, alive and dead, worthwhile and worthless.

The obsessive preoccupation with health is one among many contemporary expressions of a narcissistic inward turning that follows a sense of frightened impotence to effect change in the world. One works overtime to maintain and improve one's body ("health status") because one feels so unable to affect the world. Wellness is offered as a cultural solution to our time of troubles, to our collectively emotional as well as economic depression.

Exercise and nutrition are the cultural vessels that carry the burden of rescuing the corporeal and national body from decay and decline and restoring it to potency and purpose. Wellness ideology not only treats complex human problems superficially (for example, running as a cure for depression) but diverts attention from pressing social concerns (regression, poverty, inflation, unemployment, nuclear war) by the self-preoccupation of each person with her or his individual well-being (see Cohen and Cohen 1978). Wellness is not merely superficial. It is a potentially dangerous displacement into medical language of widely shared unconscious conflicts. No longer able to redeem ourselves exclusively in the supernaturally derived dualisms of religion (good/evil, salvation/sin), we reembody the same issues in dualisms of medicine (health/disease).

We wage our ideological battles with our bodies—in the name of God, medicine (or both), and (now) nationalism. Wellness ideology mistakes and misplaces its subject: The principal referent of wellness is not the body but body narcissism. What we do to strengthen, improve, and restore the body consists of restitutive maneuvers that require prior regression in order to be felt necessary in the first place. It is to our group fantasies (deMause 1979), not to our biology in the strictly organic sense, that we must look in order to explain what we do with our bodies.

The medicalization of social Darwinism is culturally inseparable from its militarization in metaphor and deed alike. We as a nation have been bracing for war and may already have been psychologically at war since the early 1980s; there are trade wars, corporate wars, drug wars, wars against crime, wars against cancer and heart disease, war with smokers, and so on (see Stein 1985i, 1986a; deMause 1984). We do not have a congressionally declared war. Instead, we wage displaced wars within and outside the United States. If the function of scapegoating persists, then even if our current symbolic problems were to find resolution or the public were to become less interested in them, we would find others to brand with our malaise—most likely in the idiom of health, disease, and treatment.

Participation in clinical conferences and in clinical supervision persuades me that the doctrine of patient autonomy and patient responsibility is often invoked by physicians to keep the patient and the sense of guilt toward the patient at bay. It is as if people who cannot fend—and pay—for themselves have no place or right in this world. The poor, the elderly, the chronically ill, the psychosomatically afflicted, ethnic and racial minorities, homosexuals, and people with AIDS or genital herpes have all become social pariahs. Medicine is appointed the handmaiden and executor of social control. In short, it is difficult to treat—or educate clinicians to treat humanely—those upon whom we are waging war, those whom we would rather eliminate out of sight and out of mind—and out of conscience.

The Paradox of Biomedicine as Cultural Therapy

The age of DRGs, health maintenance organizations (HMOs), preferred provider organizations (PPOs), is one of bitter irony with respect to national health policies and choices. While cancer from smoking is a matter for public outcry, cancer from the global pall of nuclear radiation that would ensue from nuclear war merits mostly our stolid neglect. Our most devastating toxins turn out to be our most toxic subject. The connection between a culture and its medical ideology and institution could not be more perilous. Medicine serves the culture in which it is embedded. That medicine, together with its affiliated behavioral sciences, might be a critical agent of transformation is little discussed during these culture-conformistic times.

In his article "Medicalized Killing in Auschwitz," psychiatrist Robert Jay Lifton (1984) notes many disturbing parallels between the role of medicine in Nazi concentration camps and in contemporary American society. The medical technocracy of Auschwitz performed the "triage" in which inmates were selected for immediate death, for slave labor, or for medical experimentation. The identity pattern among SS doctors was founded upon, among other things, "the technicizing of everything," concern with efficiency rather than ethics, "psychic numbing, diffusion of responsibility, and 'derealization,'" the heart of which is "diminished capacity and inclination to feel" (1984: 28). Omnipotence and impotence were prominent in SS physicians' construction of meaning:

> SS doctors, in their literal life-death decisions, experienced a sense of omnipotence that could protect them from their own death anxiety in the Auschwitz environment. That sense of omnipotence, along with elements of sadism with which it can be closely associated, contributed to feelings of power and invulnerability that could also serve to suppress guilt and enhance numbing.
>
> Yet doctors could feel powerless, consider themselves pawns in the hands of a total institution (1984: 29).

Other defensive and adaptive mechanisms included the feeling among the medical victimizers "that they *themselves* were undergoing an ordeal" (1984: 30). They were attracted to order, to keeping "Auschwitz a coherent, functioning world," to maintaining the "orderly routine" (1984: 30). Lifton proposes the overall mechanism of "doubling" (similar to splitting) as a mechanism permitting clinicians to function as agents of death; it compartmentalizes "the prior 'ordinary self,' which for doctors includes important elements of the healer, and the 'Auschwitz self,' which includes all of the psychological maneuvers that help one avoid a conscious sense of oneself as a killer" (1984: 30). Finally, Lifton points to the "healing-killing paradox" (1984: 26) not only among SS camp doctors but among practitioners in all cultures:

> The distinction—the barrier—between healing and killing has always been more fragile than we wish to believe. . . . Whether the killing is done by mythological gods, by human medicine men, witch doctors, or shamans, specifically as religious ceremony (as in various forms of human sacrifice) or in connection with hunting or warfare, it is done in the name of a higher purpose—on behalf of a healing function for the tribe or people.
>
> In modern experience, the use of advanced technology radically alters whatever balance might have been maintained between healing and killing in the past. As the Nazis demonstrate, science in general, and biology in particular—however distorted or falsified—can be mobilized on behalf of a murderous claim to healing (1984: 31).

He concludes that "the elements contributing to mass murder, including extensive sadism and technized bureaucratic killing, were contained within an overall Nazi biomedical vision of mass murder as a healing process" (1984: 32).

Human history and the ethnographic record are littered with the human remains of those ethnomedically decreed to be "surplus men" (Rubenstein 1978) to their societies. "Voodoo death" by bone pointing or magical incantation, from Australia to Zambia to America (various forms of social Darwinism from McCarthyism in the 1950s to the wellness movement of the late 1970s and 1980s), is a widespread means employed in the preliterate and modern world of declaring an undesirable human being or class of human beings outside the moral community and as good as dead—with which curse the extruded and abandoned victim complies by dying. Among the Kubu of Sumatra merely to become febrile is reason enough to be left to die (Clark 1973). Among the northern Algonkians, to be accused of being possessed by the cannibalistic "Windigo monster" may result in one's execution, often by close kinsmen (Hay 1971). Such kinsmen may fear their own cannibalistic impulses, yet exercise their moral duty by killing the human windigo. Acting out continues as they often cannibalize their accused victim rather than risk being eaten themselves.

There is plenty of precedent in human history for scapegoating. In the past two centuries, nationalist movements have waged gruesome sacrificial campaigns against the unwanted—often first against the infirm. Invariably, the riddance of social undesirables occurs concurrently with the celebration of health, vitality, renewal, and raw aggressiveness. In the nineteenth century, such social reformers as Karl Fisher, Miroslav Tyrs, and Jindrich Fugner—the former, founder of the German Wandervögel; the latter two, founders of the Slavic Sokols, or Falcons—typified the romanticism of nature, youthful vitality, a turning away from the supposed sinfulness of decadent civilization, a return to the simplicity of the past, and abundant exercise (Kohn 1960). (Sokols are gymnastic societies devoted to character building and physical development, which organizations conducted mass gymnastic displays and were a major political force in many Slavic nationalistic movements in the latter nineteenth and early twentieth centuries.) Theirs was a program of wellness offered as a potent antidote to the sickness of imperial Europe. Body and spirit were to be made tempered and taut, life was to be renewed, and the evils responsible for decay were to be eliminated from the human body and from the body politic alike.

All nationalism's roads do not lead to National Socialism and Auschwitz. But in its regressive extremism, Nazism showed how the restoration and repair of the social body and that of the physical body became indistinguishable. The elimination of evil within—often in the metaphor of cancer—was a precondition to the attainment of inner unity, harmony, integrity, health, and renewed will. Health could be restored only by eradicating disease (those groups whose very existence symbolized decadence and death). The coupling of the euthanasia (and later extermination) program to eliminate undesirables and vestiges of the past with the *Lebensborn* program in which racially "pure" Aryan women attempted to breed the Germanic future in breeding centers was no accident (Kren and Rappoport 1980).

At this point in many comparisons an author will offer the gratuitous disclaimer that contemporary America is not Nazi Germany, that the purpose of the analogy is to illustrate a point in order to sound a warning. This disclaimer tends to make the Nazis and their era in German history far more ghoulish, bizarre, and exotic and far less human than they were. It radically separates "them" from "us" as if to say, "*They* do that sort of thing; *we* surely do not." At the same time it enables us to indulge our prurient interest (as we identify by projection with our image of them). After all, Nazism is a serious subject matter; surely we are studying *it*, not looking in a mirror of ourselves. But the lesson of Nazism is that they may well be us, and that nationalism everywhere declares categories of people discountable. Of our discounted groups, many even in medicine contend that they should not receive school lunches, job training, Food Stamps, free or subsidized medical treatment, resuscitation, suffrage, Social Security benefits, unemployment compensation, minimal wage, and so on. Those who are expendable are righteously identified as a threat to "public health," and their elimination promises recovery.

The danger is not that we will become the historical Nazis. That we might unconsciously identify with them and admire their hideous deeds is a separate matter. The fact of Nazism teaches that desperate people can do and have done anything to prevent the disintegration of the self, a selfhood that expands to incorporate the selfhood of the nation. That, at bottom, is what wellness as a cultural phenomenon is all about. Instead of facing the self and finding it flawed, vulnerable, frightened—human, all too human—we may well turn against some convenient others and attempt to solve our problems in them. Wellness and health are as much symptoms and symbols of our disease as they are therapy. The issue is whether we will have the courage to face our inner world or whether we will combat it outside ourselves by jousting lethally with phantoms of our inner night.

As a social movement, health and wellness are euphemisms of societal regression, metaphors of neo-Darwinian nationalism. So long as shared inner dramas are externalized into public spectacle, we shall persist in solving the wrong problem in the wrong place. At issue for the institution of medicine in the broadest sense is whether it wishes to promote additional symbolic modes of public self-deception or seeks instead to help its constituency (that is, patients and public alike) to understand just what it is they are acting out beneath the disguise of health. If wellness ideology and practice are at once the heir to and the contemporary form of the cycle of sin (indulgence) and abstinence, biomedical practitioners would do well to avoid taking sides in the fray but endeavor to understand both. By not encouraging patients toward either extreme, practitioners provide that stable anchor in reality that enables patients to understand emotional extremism and thereby lessen the need to find other symbolic means of discharging it (Stein 1982f, 1982g, 1982j). If then they exercise, restrict dietary intake, relinquish the consumption of cholesterol, ethanol, or caffeine-containing beverages and the like, their motivation for doing so will be for more bona fide health reasons uncontaminated by dimly understood emotional panics. Running, surely, can serve joy instead of dread.

In "The Transformation of Thought That the Nuclear Age Requires," Robert S. Wallerstein (1986) describes an inner awakening from unconsciousness that is as cogent to treating our official cultural out-of-control pathologies as it is insightful about nuclearism. The unconscious link between the two is that the United States as a nation has long psychologically prepared for war and has selected various categories of expendable, sacrificial people. To stop this metaphoric war already being waged, it will be necessary for us to reinternalize and feel as inside ourselves (not equivalent to "internal medicine") those pains, guilts, and anxieties that we have individually and collectively embodied in others and with which role they have complied for unconscious reasons of their own. Wallerstein writes that

> the "psychological transformation" required, as I see it, is the capacity at least in some people, and in enough of the key people who influence political policy and public opinion, to set aside our evolutionarily innate, powerfully sustaining, and automatically operating ego mechanisms of safety, of defense and adaptation, to be able to live with and in the face of what may be the almost unendurable levels of anxiety, actually of outright terror, that would be unleashed when confronting, *psychologically unprotected*, the frightful dimensions of our current plight (1986: 310).

The implications of this theory of medicalized social Darwinism are (1) that mainstream and "normal" society is as much a part of the problem of displaced moralism as are those officially designated as victims; (2) that an exclusive emphasis on pariah categories functions to divert attention from the larger national malaise; (3) that if the process of scapegoating is to diminish, we must understand why Americans seem to require scapegoats and why we are driven to conduct metaphoric war against them; (4) that if we wish to counsel, treat, or help patients, or teach practitioners how to do so, we cannot also be a part of the problem that needs their disease to distract us from ourselves; and (5) that we need to ask anew what kind of life is worth living and how or whether life can be worthwhile in a world without appointed moral casualties.

The privacy and confidentiality of clinical relationships are widely held beliefs and ideals in American society. Another assumption is that the physician (or the practitioner) is always or ought to be acting in the best interest of the patient (sometimes "family" substitutes for "patient"). As this chapter has shown, however, this is only one part of the story. Clinical judgment in behalf of the patient often blurs into if not conflicts with moralistic judgment in behalf of the society at which behest the physician is empowered and licensed to act. In this chapter I have thus shown that much clinical decisionmaking that is ostensibly and officially "for" the good of the patient is also "for" institutional and wider cultural groups. In the chapter that follows, I turn to the process of actual clinical decisionmaking in and by groups, in practice and training settings alike, and explore the consequences of these group dynamics for clinical judgment and patient care.

FOUR

THE INFLUENCE OF GROUP DYNAMICS ON CLINICAL THINKING AND PRACTICE

WHEN AMERICANS GET SICK, they say that they are going to "the" doctor or to "my" doctor—singular. Individual clinical judgment and action are prized and guarded. Although physicians are trained to consult with and refer to other practitioners, and more recently to work collaboratively in groups called health care "teams," they also expect and are expected to make independent clinical decisions. Such individuality safeguards the privacy and confidentiality of the physician-patient relationship and the physician's belief in his or her ability to master a clinical situation without being emotionally dependent upon others. To this belief system is further added the conviction that individual medical judgment is rational, scientific, professional, objective, and in the best interest of the patient. Widely shared, tenacious cultural images embody and express this belief from the physician's own premedical or preprofessional past as well as from society at large.

Throughout the years, many physician colleagues have invoked as their ego ideal the image of the Lone Ranger, the radio and television cowboy-lawman-rescuer hero of the 1940s and 1950s, who often single-handedly—albeit with the aid of his loyal American Indian partner, Tonto—restored order and justice from chaos. Similarly, among physicians and the public, the image of Super Doc, who can superhumanly cure all ills, is linked with Superman, hero of comic books, television, and movies since the 1930s. On an only slightly less grandiose mythical scale, physicians bear the burden of such popular-culture "medical" images as the kindly, always available, always wise Marcus Welby, M.D.; the young, brash Dr. Kildare; the decisive Dr. Joe Gannon of the series "Medical Center," which extolled the virtues of activism; Dr. Hawkeye Pierce of the series "M.A.S.H.," which portrayed the medical side of the Korean War; "Trapper John, M.D.," successor to "M.A.S.H."; and various characters in the daytime soap opera "General Hospital." These folklore images and their associated expectations have long been intrinsic to medical education and practice, something of a silent code of what a doctor as a "real man" (even if she by gender is a woman) is like.

Portions of Chapter 4 were adapted from information appearing in *New England Journal of Medicine.* James W. Mold and Howard F. Stein, "The Cascade Effect in the Clinical Care of Patients." *New England Journal of Medicine* 314(8) (Feb. 20, 1986): 512–514. Reprinted, with changes, by permission of *New England Journal of Medicine.*

This chapter paints a different portrait of medicine—one of physicians, and of clinical decisionmaking, in groups. Groups influence clinical functioning in a variety of ways: in the form of physicians and other practitioners actually working together and influencing one another; in the more subtle but equally powerful form of internalized group norms established by each professional, medical subspecialty; and in the form of federal and insurance corporation guidelines regulating reimbursement of medical expenses, an indication of societal tolerances and trends. If the Lone Ranger constitutes medicine's ideal and traditional self-portrait, group dynamics is the reality of medical education and practice. Any distinction between ideal and real, however, is made much more complicated by the fact that there are implicit as well as explicit values to consider.

For instance, although the "rugged individualist" physician is the most explicit ideal, in practice physicians often participate in what Michael Balint terms the "collusion of anonymity." "When the patient offers a puzzling problem to his medical attendant, who, in turn, is backed by a galaxy of specialists, certain events are almost unavoidable. Foremost among them is the 'collusion of anonymity.' ***Vital decisions are taken without anybody feeling fully responsible for them***" (1957: 76). Physicians and other health practitioners often deal with anxiety, guilt, shame, and uncertainty by ceding individual responsibility to the group "itself." One veteran rehabilitation physician remarked in a discussion about a medical team's response to an obnoxious, belligerent family member of an elderly patient who had suffered a stroke, "When you're a member of a medical team, you don't have to feel you're on your own. You can blend in the 'collusion of anonymity'—especially with patients you don't like. You don't have to take a stand. You just let the team take on all the responsibility." This group consensus-seeking helps physicians to escape pangs of anxiety and guilt that would come if more personal or solo responsibility for decisionmaking were taken. It may even permit the acting out of feelings and wishes that would otherwise be regarded as unprofessional and hence intolerable.

Moreover, since the onset of corporate medicine in the early 1980s, group pressures have increased regarding compliance with impersonal and depersonalizing institutional protocols. Physicians must accommodate DRGs. They must participate in, or compete with, increasingly larger and more bureaucratized group medical practices (corporate-owned hospitals, health maintenance organizations, prepaid physicians' organizations, and so on). They must anticipate careful scrutiny of hospital admissions and length of stay by physician peer review groups. Together these influences have made group-based clinical decisionmaking more of a reality if not a competing ideal than before (see Ritzer 1987; Ritzer and Walczak 1986, 1987).

By examining the group dynamics of authority and leadership, identification, role allocation, and "groupthink" (Janis 1982) and the unconscious "basic assumptions" (Bion 1959) by which groups are regulated, we discover some surprising answers to the question, "How do medical students, residents, and faculty decide which diagnoses, laboratory tests, procedures, medications, techniques, even curriculum items to select?" This chapter thus examines the influence of group psychology and group logic of choice itself in medicine. It explores emotional investments in the group and their consequences for decisionmaking and medical action. Further, I introduce "group dynamics" not as another new subject to vie for time in the already densely crowded curriculum of medical education but as an ordinary, inexpugnable fact intrinsic to all medical subjects in which groups are involved in thinking and acting together.

The Team Concept in Biomedicine

One specific institutional, cultural, and historical form taken by groups in biomedicine is the team. The abundance of terms associated with medical teams attests to the popularity of the concept as well as a tendency toward reification and personification: team meetings, team spirit, teamwork, team building, team player (= loyal), team leader, team morale, team approach, crisis team, mental health team, outreach team, health care team, coronary care unit team, and so forth. From numerous discussions with physician colleagues (especially with Alvah Cass, M.D. [1988], whose insights inform the following paragraphs) and from an examination of pertinent literature, the following picture of the medical team concept and function emerges.

Ideally, medical teams are formal or ad hoc small group organizations of persons from several medical professions (physicians, nurses, medical assistants, physical therapists, clinical psychologists: as on a rehabilitation medicine team) who combine their skills and knowledge in the service of patient care. The team is a means of achieving a clinical goal, of striving toward cooperation among its constituent members, and of expressing leadership. Teams developed in medicine in response to several circumstances: (1) greater role specialization in health care, beginning with the physician/nurse dyad; (2) the "hospitalization" of America since the late 1800s; (3) the increased treatment of multiple diseases in one person; and (4) the shift from the predominance of acute illness (such as infectious disease) to chronic illness.

Until the 1940s, hospitals were largely places in which one could have a dignified death. Since then, hospitals have become associated with the aura of the miraculous cure. Based greatly on scientific and technological innovations spawned by World War II, the medicine of the 1950s witnessed a technological explosion. For a number of decades prior to this, the hospital team consisted only of physicians, nurses, nutrition specialists, and cooks. With the technological explosion and greater professionalization came greater specialization and the concomitant need to coordinate the increasingly fragmented system of functions.

Role specialization and professionalization, fueled both by increased medical technology and by societal demand, led to greater numbers of different people doing differing tasks or functions in medicine, which led in turn to the type of coordination for which the team concept was the cultural response. Milton Roemer, for instance, recently writes of the increase in numbers of nurses:

> The 1910 U.S. Census reported little more than half as many trained nurses as physicians and surgeons. Even with the addition of nurses (untrained) and midwives, the total nursing personnel in 1910 numbered less than 1.5 times the number of physicians and surgeons. By 1980, there were almost 2.5 times as many registered

> nurses as physicians. Counting all levels of nursing (registered nurses, licensed practical nurses, nurses aides, orderlies, and attendants) there were 6.8 times as many nursing personnel as physicians. Considering only registered nurses, they increased from 55 per 100,000 population in 1910 to 502 per 100,000 in 1980 (1986: 69).

Nancy Aries and Louanne Kennedy, following Eli Ginsberg (1983: 483), note that "in 1900, 1 out of 3 health workers was a physician. Now only 1 out of 16 health workers is a physician." In much of the medical literature on teams, "the medical model of physician control remains dominant" (Aries and Kennedy 1986: 205), and the physician is the "'Captain of the Team'" (Fuchs 1974, quoted in Aries and Kennedy 1986: 204). At the same time, as exemplified by the professionalization of numerous health workers, "the epitome of the professional is the autonomous individual practitioner" (1986: 204). According to Spiegel (1971), the conflict between hierarchical and individualistic values is both rife and endemic in American history. This conflict is played out in medical team relations and in the larger social process of which its members are a part. Aries and Kennedy note that "physicians . . . are the central figures in defining the limits of health and disease and the scope of medical practice" (1986: 196). Later, they argue that

> health workers have two options before them to increase their power and autonomy within the medical care system. One choice is to seek professional status similar to that held by physicians. This has typically been the choice of higher status health workers such as nurses. The second choice is to unionize. In this case workers seek power through their unity with other workers regardless of position within the medical care hierarchy. . . . The strategy of professionalization, however, has largely failed to accomplish the goal which the allied health workers had set for themselves. It has not given them the control over their work or the recognition and status in the health care hierarchy they sought (1986: 204).

The complex role, status, task, and attitude issues become implicit if not explicit agendas of the team.

Much of the team literature consists of lists of team members and their formal roles or responsibilities. For instance, in a discussion of the "home health care team," Mary Dete (1987: 66) lists the following members: physician, registered nurse, health care aide, homemaker, physical therapist, occupational therapist, speech therapist, medical social worker, dietician, pharmacist, durable medical equipment dealer, and volunteers. Dete further writes that "similar to the hospital team, the home care team utilizes one another's skills for problem-solving and for ventilation of frustration when the patient's gains are not forthcoming or when the patient and care partner are not compliant or are passively resistive to the physician's plan of care" (1987: 67).

So culturally ingrained is the segmental approach to medical care, to thinking about the health care system, and to teaching medicine that it is no easy matter for the clinical scholar or researcher to find such "obvious" terms (cultural categories) as "team" or "health care team" in the indexes of many a textbook! On the other hand, entries for discrete professions (physical therapist, dietician, cardiologist, home health care nurse) are abundant. A segmental, rather than a systems or holistic, view of the team concept still widely prevails. The complexity of teams follows the burgeoning of new health professionals: for example, PAs in the late 1960s and health care technicians in the 1970s. Earlier simple teams, such as the doctor/nurse dyad, have given way to complex teams, such as stroke teams (physicians of several specialties, speech pathologists, nurses, occupational therapists, physical therapists), oncology teams (physicians, residents, nurses, physical therapists, social services, chaplain, and patient advocates), and coronary care unit teams (cardiologists, residents, nurses, respiratory and physical therapists).

Since the 1970s, centralization via the hospitals has given way to decentralization and increased outpatient, community-based teams, corresponding to the "dehospitalization" of America as a means of lowering medical care costs. An abundance of community outreach teams and home health care teams, especially for the elderly and for postsurgical patients, has been spawned since the emergence of corporate medicine. A common issue in the dynamics of any health care team is the interplay, if not conflict, between "vertical" (hierarchical) and "horizontal" (whether individualistic or consensual) organization (see Spiegel 1971 for an excellent discussion of this tension throughout American culture). Often, "team leaders" welcome diverse "input" from all team members but then make a final, binding decision to be executed by the group. A more subtle variation on this theme is the leader's careful orchestration of group process so that vertical organization appears to be more democratic. On the other hand, in hospitals in which physicians are more the passers-through and nurses the permanent inhabitants, nurses often make decisions in patient management (such as ordering and starting medications) and notify their physician leaders later.

Further complicating team dynamics is the fact that team members come to and participate in the *culture of the team* with often different if not divergent *professional cultures*—with their specific values, priorities, concepts, procedures, loyalties, and perceived statuses. In the day-to-day world of team functioning, it is difficult to know with certainty which members are the "independent practitioners," the "dependent practitioners," and the "supporting staff" (Jonas 1986: 56; Freidson 1970a). There is likewise often a distinction (stated in action rather than recorded in an organizational chart or protocol) between the official "chain of command," or hierarchy, and the actual process of decisionmaking and influence. Health care teams exemplify what Anthony Wallace (1961) labels the "organization of diversity" concept of culture. Precisely because of the professional diversity within the team, and the chronic possibility of conflict and schism, football terms—"quarterbacking," appealing to members to be loyal "team players" with a shared "game plan" so that all can reach the "goal line" together—abound in health care teams to foster if not coerce some superordinate image of unity. Nevertheless, a stable team with face-to-face meetings develops interactions and a distinctive *small group culture* of its own, which is to say, some claim to uniqueness and boundaries that form distinctions between "itself" and others. Within the team boundaries and beyond them, its members play out the group dynamics identified in this chapter.

Medical Specialties: Us Versus Them

In a wide variety of case conferences I have attended in many medical disciplines, the official and ostensible goal of patient care is often superseded by a specific group dynamic through which the medical specialty strives to reassure itself of its professional identity and status by contrasting itself (concepts, models, techniques) with competing medical specialties. At a family medicine clinical case conference presided over by a family physician and family therapist, the official, explicit agenda was the diagnosis and treatment of a patient and her family. This was used by the presenters for an implicit agenda that included the inculcation of the distinction between what is "us" and what is "them."

Early in the conference, the presenters said, "We were afraid that the anorexic patient and her husband would go to a psychiatrist rather than come back to us." Later in the conference, while discussing the patient's inability to swallow and her fear of swallowing, the family therapist instructed the group of assembled family medicine faculty and residents: "You want to avoid saying to the patient 'this is psychological,' but rather humanize it." At one point during the conference, the family physician presenter looked toward me and said, "I know that Howard [the writer] is probably thinking along psychoanalytic lines about her trouble swallowing, but . . ." At that point I briefly interrupted, remarking that I had said nothing but that he was doing fine to mention it himself as his own thought.

He continued by contrasting a psychoanalytic line of thought they did *not* want to follow and the family interactional line of thought they staunchly advocated. This teaching exercise had as its implicit agenda the shoring up of boundaries between what was admissible data within their concept of family medicine (family therapy, "humanizing") and what was to be excluded (psychiatry, "psychologizing," and possibly "Howard"). In this group process, I was explicitly associated with the negative group identity, that is, as an example of how not to think or treat.

Diagnosis and patient care can become the battleground, so to speak, for expressing interprofessional boundary conflicts and for shoring up professional group identities. The official, explicit agenda of the preceding case conference was to understand the particular case, to formulate a correct diagnosis, and to offer an improved treatment plan. The unofficial, implicit agenda was to reaffirm the rightness, internal goodness, and security, if not superiority, of the conference group and of the professional discipline. At conferences dealing with pregnancy and delivery, and with children's diseases, family medicine faculty, interns, and residents frequently contrast their field's humane treatment of patients with obstetrics' mechanical impersonality and family medicine's concern for the whole person and the whole family with pediatrics' ostensible narrow focus on disease or the child. The teaching of specific surgical, prescribing, counseling, or family therapy skills often has the implicit agenda of affirming the group's professional identity and its members' sense of belonging. "This *is* what *we* do" is often conveyed by means of contrast—often with ridicule and contempt—with "That is *not* what we do" or "That is what *they* do."

At a case conference, a physician presented a case of a woman in her early forties suffering from dysfunctional uterine bleeding (DUB). The group consisted of approximately thirty resident and faculty physicians and nonphysician behavioral science faculty. The woman had experienced some six months of irregular menstrual periods after having had years of regular periods. She was increasingly concerned about her husband's safety as a longtime police officer. She found herself worrying that he would die in the line of duty.

The presenting (family medicine) physician used this case as an occasion to distinguish between family medicine, which attempts to treat the "whole person," and obstetrics, which had treated the woman in the past, as more organ or disease oriented, and as more mechanical. His explicit case presentation was that of a woman with DUB. His implicit purpose was to make a boundary-creating and boundary-maintaining rhetorical distinction between us and them. Those on the inside were ascribed good qualities, and those on the outside were ascribed bad qualities. (I discuss this process in interethnic and international relations; see Stein 1987b.)

Later, during the discussion portion of the conference, a lively disagreement erupted about the extent to which the woman's ostensible depression played a role in her menstrual dysfunction. One participant argued that the group might be looking too hard for psychosocial explanations (depression, neurosis, stress) for the patient's malady, whereas we should instead take her physical complaints more seriously. She raised the issue of possible sexism: namely, that male physicians often dismiss patients' menstrual problems as "just" neurotic. Her position was endorsed by a female physician in the group.

Male participants, on the other hand, arguing for the complexity of DUB, propounded what they viewed as a more biopsychosocial, integrative approach. They argued that although one can *recognize* a hierarchy of levels in any medical problem, one can justifiably *choose* to address only one at a time (for instance, the physical pain or the unpredictable bleeding). Instead of reaching clinical consensus, however, group discussion ended with two positions or subgroups within the larger group—male versus female, us versus them—in which diagnosis and treatment were caught.

I commented briefly on the group process and subtle polarization itself. I said that sometimes it becomes more difficult to listen to the patient and family and address their issues when we inadvertently use the patient to fill our own unconscious or political agendas. We then "treat" the patient, family, or disease for our problems and anxieties instead of those afflicting the patient. It is easy to inadvertently define medical problems in terms of formulas that are shadows of ideological positions. When we do so, the patient—the official focus of the problem to be solved—becomes a medium through which the group consensus or conflict expresses itself. What I wish to generalize from this conference is that the conference dynamics themselves are always part of the clinical subject matter and decision-making process. They are as important a factor as are the disease, patient, and family upon whom clinicians and clinical teachers direct attention.

In case conferences, grand rounds, tumor boards, utilization review committees, quality assurance committees, and the like, ideas that produce anxiety are more safely identified and placed outside the boundary of the professionally acceptable. The message at these groups can become in essence, "You don't have to or shouldn't think about these anxiety-evoking things. In fact it's not only OK but mandatory that you keep within the limits that reduce all our anxiety." As a result, the presenters' scotomata (blind spots) become the residents' and faculty's blind spots, now rationalized and shored up with physician and group authority and acted upon by the group with diminished anxiety and guilt.

The creation and validation of the group's belief system often become the primary function of the group. Although patient or family diagnosis and intervention (care) may serve the stability of the group, the primary focus of attention and anxiety may be the clinical group itself. Stated differently, groups are always trying (unconsciously) to conduct therapy for themselves, and they employ official processes such as clinical assessment, diagnosis, treatment, and prognosis as an extension of that therapy. Unconscious group processes can occur parallel to the "work" agenda, or groups can use that work agenda as their vehicle for symbolic realization of their aims. (The reader interested in pursuing issues of group definition by opposition is referred to Spicer 1971; Stein 1980d, 1986b, 1987b; Stein and Hill 1977.)

The ordering of certain tests or procedures may be used as a group ritual to affirm the rightness and sanctity of professional group boundaries. Then, in essence, the group is saying, "What is good for us must be good for the patient." I have often heard a senior resident or veteran physician (of a number of specialties) adamantly say, "I do it the way I was trained in (1) internal medicine, (2) the city, (3) the medical center, or (4) Dr. X's service." The authority behind one's choice may thus derive from multiple unconscious sources of motivation, not simply from scientific considerations (see Katz 1984a).

The question of what is good for the patient may inadvertently become secondary to what confirms the integrity of the group's identity. Stated differently, patient diagnosis and treatment may become a means to achieve group identity resolution by retaining the sense of goodness inside the group and expelling any badness outside. An underlying group task that cannot, or may not, be acknowledged, except perhaps through metaphor, may overtake the official agenda of "getting the job done." The unconscious group agenda may become the affirmation of the rightness and integrity of the group itself via the official content or agenda (patient care, curriculum, and so on).

Clinical Decisionmaking: The Emotional Limitations of Groups

A sizable literature has accumulated on the dynamics of dyadic doctor-patient relationships, doctor-family relationships, and the culture or social organization of Western medicine (Balint 1957; Bowen 1978; Fox 1959; Freud 1912; Gerber and Sluzki 1978; Katz 1984a; Stein 1982h, 1983b; 1985g; Stein and Apprey 1985; Parsons 1951). Virtually absent, however, are comparable studies of the middle ground, so to speak, of local, relatively small biomedical groups in which clinical decisionmaking occurs. Yet, the group dynamics of clinical decisionmaking, although little investigated, deserve to become part of the forefront of thinking about biomedicine and medical and residency education because they have significant consequences for the process of diagnosis and patient care. I use the phrase "clinical decisionmaking" in the widest possible sense to include diagnosis-treatment-referral of individual patients and families, medical case conferences, grand rounds presentations (lecture or case-review format), curriculum committee meetings, tumor conferences, quality assurance meetings, medical faculty meetings, physician-nurse hospital staffings, and so forth.

When listening to group dynamics in clinical decisionmaking, one identifies, in Wilfred Bion's words, "the emotional states which find an outlet in mass action of the group in behavior that seems to have coherence if it is considered to be the outcome of a basic assumption" (1955: 476). That is, "emotionally the group acts as if it had certain basic assumptions about its aims" (1955: 476). The purposes served by thought, decisionmaking, and action in groups cannot be automatically assumed by taking decision trees, organizational charts, or official tasks at face value (see La Barre 1951). In his distinction between the pragmatic, reality, task-oriented level of group functioning that he labels "work" and the symbolic, unconsciously driven level of group functioning that he labels "basic assumptions," Bion (1955, 1959) affirms that both are concurrent.

> I do not believe that we are dealing with two different kinds of group, in the sense of two different aggregates of individuals, but rather with two different categories of mental activity co-existing in the same individuals. In work group activity time is intrinsic: in basic assumption activity it has no place. . . . [Moreover], the more the group corresponds with the basic assumption group the less it makes any rational use of verbal communication (1955: 463, 473).

I do not question that medical groups perform genuine work group activity that benefits patients. But such rational, purposive learning often serves the deeper purpose of fulfilling the group's basic assumption activity. Stated differently, patient care, curriculum content, and administrative policy choices can all readily become means toward fulfilling unconscious ends. Collectively as well as individually, physicians and other practitioners can use diagnosis and patient care as forums if not battlegrounds for quelling their own unvoiced anxieties (see Katz 1984a; Mold and Stein 1986; Stein 1985g).

At a family medicine case conference attended by some thirty faculty, interns, residents, medical students, and behavioral scientists, the presenting physician discussed the topic of amenorrhea (suppression of menstruation). He was uncomfortable in discussing women's bleeding. When reviewing an overhead on amenorrhea and coming to a paragraph on menstruation, he said only, "You can read that. . . . I don't say those words," followed by anxious group laughter. His discomfort was expressed by his total control of the conference agenda, by his highly technical language, and by his inability to be psychosocially sensitive to the patient's situation while professing the need to do so. There was much group laughter when the resident stated that the patient had profuse galactorrhea from breast self-stimulation.

The resident made a number of parapraxes (unconscious "slips"); he referred to "my flow (chart)" (group laughter) and while discussing the logic of karyotyping (an examination of chromosomal structure) said, "feminization in my case" (a double entendre; the audience burst into laughter). The "slips" attest to the momentary and anxiety-evoking transgression of the boundary between physician and patient, and between male and female. Instead of saying "flow chart" (which is a clinical decisionmaking schematic), he omitted "chart," thereby symbolically becoming a male physician with a menstrual flow. The laughter-inducing "feminization in my case" derives from the dangerous ambiguity over whether the patient was female or whether he was, or feared that he in some unknown respects might be female.

Anxiety about gender identity permeated discussion of the case by speaker and audience—"If there's no secondary sexual features at age sixteen, do a workup. . . . If there's no breast tissue . . . you might find out it's a he" (audience laughter). An epidemiologist in the group tried to remind participants that "rare" does not automatically mean "pathological," but the presenter and group's patent discomfort with ambiguities in sexual identity did not permit this to be truly heard. Although amenorrhea was the official, explicit conference topic, the implicit topic was males' fear of being or becoming female. The presenter and group's subjective involvement in the topic were disguised and channeled through ostensibly scientific algorithms (decision trees) that were consciously designed to improve decisionmaking (and implicitly designed to deal with the anxieties about menstruation and male/female difference).

Although official biomedicine radically dichotomizes objectivity and subjectivity, hard science and soft social science, real medicine (organic medicine) and background information, group process at medical conferences large and small is heavily influenced by unconscious agendas that the officially espoused work agenda implements. Joseph and Anne-Marie Sandler note that shared members' needs are expressed and reflected in group process (such as clinical meetings):

> Members of a group will "negotiate" with one another in terms of the responses which each one needs and in terms of the responses which are demanded of him. The members of the group may even make unconscious "deals" or "transactions" in terms of the responses involved so that each gains as much object-related wish-fulfillment as possible in return for concessions to other members of the group (1978: 291).

Group dynamics can unwittingly appropriate any subject or topic, while participants ardently believe they are above such subjectivity. As the following example illustrates, group members can suddenly become fascinated with the patient's "exotic" or different culture as a means of deflecting attention from their sense of uneasiness about how they have managed the case (Stein 1985c).

At the beginning of one case conference, a medical student presented the following summary: An eighty-year-old Native American male was admitted to a large midwestern urban hospital from the emergency room, having been brought to the hospital by his son following a three-day history of fever (104°F), weakness, chills, malaise, decreased appetite, and questionable hematuria. An elderly house painter still active in his work, the patient had been completing a job with his son just before being brought to the hospital. Although he had several daughters who lived throughout the urban area, his son and daughter-in-law had taken responsibility for his health care.

During an earlier hospitalization, the patient had been diagnosed as having septic arthritis and had surgical drainage of the right knee, with cultures of fluid positive for *Staphylococcus aureus*. He had also experienced difficulty with urination and had been diagnosed as having benign prostatic hypertrophy with obstructive uropathy (difficulty urinating due to an enlarged prostate). A transurethral resection of the prostate (a surgical procedure used to remove part of the prostate) had been performed. During this previous twenty-one-day hospital stay, intravenous oxacillin (an antibiotic) had been administered every four hours, and treatment had continued for five subsequent home care days under the supervision of a visiting nurse. Following physician instructions prior to discharge the patient's son and daughter-in-law had devotedly administered his intravenous oxacillin treatments. While at home, he developed complications as manifested in the presenting three-day history of fever. The son brought him to the hospital for a second time. During this second admission a different physician was team leader overseeing his care. The patient was put on intravenous Keflin (another antibiotic) and had good response to therapy. He was subsequently diagnosed by liver function tests as having oxacillin-induced hepatitis.

Near the end of the hospitalization for the oxacillin-induced hepatitis, the second physician team leader planned a meeting of patient, son, daughter-in-law, and nursing staff. He was concerned that because the patient had become sicker while at home, the family might feel a sense of guilt or disappointment in the care the patient had received. At that point in the conference discussion, this physician expressed puzzlement about why a *son* rather than a daughter would take such responsibility and be so reverential toward the father. He speculated that this might be due to the patient's Native American culture. He turned to me, a faculty behavioral scientist/medical anthropologist, and asked if I would say some things about this patient's culture and its salience to this case.

The shift in topic felt abrupt to me. I felt uneasy and replied that we knew absolutely nothing about the specifics of the patient's culture or cultures. I asked the conference participants to imagine, for example, what kinds of valid and clinically apt generalizations we could make by knowing only that the patient was European. Although we could say a few things, they would mostly be cultural platitudes so broad as to tell us nothing about this particular patient and his family configuration. "Were there not," I asked, "many males of various European backgrounds in the conference room who might take devoted care of their father even if there are sisters in the family?" I said that I could continue with a line of questions to the presenting medical student, team leaders, and team members, all of which might elucidate more about this patient's culture.

I said that I felt that something clinically more pertinent was going on *in the group* and that it would be tangential to spend much time then gathering data about the patient's culture. "Why," I asked, "are we suddenly now so interested in the patient's culture?" I continued, noting that often a fascination with a patient's culture or family is a way of displacing attention from unresolved emotional business in the clinical group. I drew their attention to the topic and process of the group's "free associations" during the nearly half-hour preceding the second team leader's question to me. I speculated aloud whether—especially in the light of the amount of time the conference participants had devoted to discussing medications—members of the teams felt and wanted to discuss any lingering guilt.

At this point, the team leader for the first hospitalization declared adamantly that he did not feel guilt about the management or outcome of the case. But during the remaining fifteen or so minutes of the conference, members of both teams sorted through their feelings. They discussed their sense of responsibility, the sense of unfairness felt by the second team with their illusory "success" for making the patient feel better (because the first team had not done anything medically wrong). We discussed the inevitability of fortuitous as well as calamitous mistakes in medical practice, and so on (compare Katz 1984a). Because the patient's family was under financial stress, conference participants felt lucky and relieved that a new medication (intravenous Ancef®, a brand of sterile cefazolin sodium, an antibiotic), prescribed following the most recent hospitalization, was far less expensive than oxacillin.

I felt that the conference was "back on track" in dealing with the clinically pertinent subject—the culture of the medical group and the delineation of clinical responsibility. The patient's culture (specifically, the issue of who in a family was responsible for the father's care) would have been for the moment a clinically spurious topic. I might add that in this instance, I refused to accept the assigned conference role of cultural anthropologist who talks about "culturally different" people. Rather, I paid close attention to the unconscious or at least implicit intention of the delegation process (see Stierlin 1974) instead of paying attention to the content (and its association with my role) alone. Instead of colluding with group members to distract them from their own uneasiness, I redirected them to their group issue, that is, back to their own culture. At this time, as in others, I have found that I can be clinically useful—if also for a time resented or dismissed as impertinent—when I urge and help them to examine their own culture.

Psychiatrist Casper Schmidt writes that

> the capacity for effective working-through of emotional conflicts within groups is restricted. Bion [1961] has shown how groups have great difficulty in performing real work, and how insidious and predominant are those emotional positions which he called basic assumptions (where fantasy solutions hold sway over realistic ones). The commonest pathway for the discharge of dammed-up group tension, historically speaking, is recourse to action (1984: 40).

In medicine as in other institutions, reality and technical know-how may be manipulated to serve shared fantasy ends. While striving and purporting to conduct "patient care," medical conferences also frequently, although inadvertently, use the process of assessment, diagnosis, treatment, and prognostication to "treat" their own anxieties.

At one case conference, a resident hurriedly discussed a patient who had had a recent myocardial infarction, and devoted the remainder of the conference to a biomedical diagnostic workup complete with a virtuoso review of the EKG reading. This was a conference at which discussion of multiple levels of biopsychosocial factors was part of the official agenda. While diagnosis occupied center stage, prognosis was tabled. I was puzzled by the virtual group taboo on discussing personal and familial aspects of the MI. As a relative newcomer to these conferences, I felt reluctant to make a comment at the time and remained silent.

Afterward, several colleagues and I discussed the group process of the conference. The group felt to me to have been in something like a trance: as if it could talk only about EKGs. The very denial that characterizes patients with MIs, and that makes it difficult for physicians to diagnose MIs in patients, also makes it difficult for a roomful of physicians and medical educators to discuss mortality and risk-ridden achievement drivenness, anxiety about time, and hostility. Significantly, early in the presentation the presenting physician had rushed through an enumeration of risk factors in MIs.

After reflecting on this conference experience I concluded that the doctor-patient relationship can become contaminated by physicians' unconscious need to protect themselves from the uncanny sense that they share—or could easily share—the disease or predisposition that afflicts the patient. Clinical conferences frequently confirm participants' defenses, as all present protect themselves from the scourge of dread, decay, and death evoked by the identified patient. To help the patient, practitioners must first know how the patient moves or influences them and then how they unwittingly use scientific validation from medical colleagues and the professionalism of diagnostic workups to keep personal issues at bay. Doctor-patient and doctor-patient-family relationships can be therapeutic only insofar as physicians can avoid using doctor-colleague-staff relationships as a bulwark against painful self-knowledge and against clinical knowledge of the patient and family (see Stein 1985g; Stein and Apprey 1985).

R. H. Hook writes that "Freud discovered that the latent content, the *real* meaning of the dream, can best be understood as a reflection of wishes or ideas which can only be tolerated when expressed in a suitably disguised form" (1979: 269). One can transpose this observation into a statement about group functioning as well. In medical decisionmaking groups, the latent wishes or ideas can be tolerated only when expressed in the subtly disguised form of the official, ostensible agenda or task and acceptable metaphors and similes. The formal agenda thus may represent group wishes or fantasies while at the same time diminishing anxiety and guilt by disguising or displacing attention from them (also see Boyer 1979).

The following events took place at a regular weekly medical corporate meeting on physician-patient and physician-corporation relationships. Beforehand, rumblings among some junior physicians suggested there was a major conflict with administration. The chief executive officer (CEO), a male authority figure in the group, was present when the meeting began. A female facilitator began the session by asking whether the group wanted to talk about any administrative issues before we started in with a difficult case. There were no takers.

One of the junior physicians then presented a passionate account of a recent encounter he had had with a woman and her baby during a "well baby" visit. The physician said he had been forty-five minutes late for the appointment (an accepted circumstance of scheduling at this clinic), and he had apologized to the patient. He said that in response to his questions, she had said she felt depressed. She also had said that she had to be somewhere else soon and could not stay for a long appointment. The physician felt frustrated because he had wanted to explore her depression and its etiology more, but the patient had left before he could do so. He said he had asked her whether she was taking drugs—he suspected cocaine—and she had replied, "No."

As the conference continued, the presenting physician, and then many of the participants, including the CEO, became convinced that the woman had been on cocaine. The CEO, who smokes cigarettes, suggested deception to elicit admissions of addiction and gave this example of a strategy to persuade patients to quit smoking: "You listen to their chest with the stethoscope, and even when you can't hear any unusual sounds, act and talk as if you do, to pull their bluff, saying, for example, 'It sounds pretty bad. You must smoke pretty heavy,' to get them to admit their addiction and be frightened into quitting smoking."

The presenting junior physician and many in the group often referred to the baby as a "victim" of the mother's probable neglect and abuse. Many group members aggressively pushed the presenter to do more to rescue the baby from the bad, victimizing mother. I briefly commented on how we might have jumped to conclusions about the mother's "addiction" because we had so few facts. The group continued unanimously, however, as if it were an indisputable *fact* that a bad mother was endangering the life of her innocent infant. (The group had identified with the victim-child fantasy.) The group consensus was that the woman should be persuaded to return to the clinic soon and to admit that she was on drugs.

Much of this case and subsequent discussion concerned the physicians' need to gain control of their practice, of the patient, and of the patient's addiction. Attempts to discuss difficulties in controlling patients, or the reality that clinicians do not control their patients' lives, were to no avail. The group almost single-mindedly branded the woman as bad and in need of treatment (punishment?) in order to ensure protection for her helpless child. The presenting physician became the perceived instrument of the group will.

Shortly thereafter the physicians began to discuss their own mistrust and resentment about their ambiguous role in the medical corporation. The CEO had left prior to this part of the discussion. The group talked resentfully about the recent firing by the CEO of a senior physician in the corporation and about their hope that he could be reinstated. They clearly felt that he (the senior physician) had been victimized by some sinister administration plot of which they had not been informed. The facilitator and I both tried to help the group to distinguish between what the CEO was actually doing to them and what they imagined him to be doing to them. The group rejected this distinction because they felt persecuted and exploited by him.

After the group had dispersed, the facilitator and I continued to discuss the entire process. We concluded that the initial "crazy" case and overdetermined response had really been a metaphor for the group issues that later emerged. The case showed how *concrete* a group metaphor or fantasy could be. At least for the time being, it was impermeable to challenge.

Early in the session the junior and senior physicians in the group had talked about the need to "deceive" patients in order to force them to admit their bad habits or addictions and in order to frighten them into changing. The junior physicians later used the same word—"deceived"—to describe how they felt at the hands of their CEO. There was thus a progression in the mental representation within the group from (1) an unconscious identification with the fantasized (CEO) aggressor, which then turned into an active desire to rescue an infant with whom they had also projectively identified, to (2) a subsequent conscious perception of themselves as victims of the leader's presumed aggression, deception, manipulation, and betrayal of trust. The final issue brought up by the group was the recent dismissal from the corporation of a well-liked senior physician. Further group discussion suggested that group members identified with the victim (as this latter physician was perceived) and were unable to mourn his loss.

The recent history of the corporate group itself may have unconsciously governed the selection (symptom choice) of the initial case example by the junior physician. Shared group history likewise may have accounted for the continuous reiteration of the themes of victimization and deception throughout the two-hour discussion, regardless of the official subject matter. The group, however, was unwilling to accept any suggestion of a thematic link among the various segments of the marathon meeting.

In recent years a number of writers (Diamond 1984, 1988; Fornari 1974; Kets deVries 1984; Mack 1986c; Mitscherlich and Mitscherlich 1967; Montville in press; Stein 1987b; Volkan 1979) have explored organizational and international conflict from the framework of psychoanalytic object relations theory. This framework attempts to integrate biological drive theory, early experiences in family life, and the structuring of internal mental representations of these relationships. A frequent theme among these writers is the role of mourning in achieving liberation from the past and thus in diminishing the need to repeat the traumatic past and cling to its inner representations. In the face of loss—individual or group, personal or institutional, of actual persons or abstractions of the self such as land or leaders or ambitions—aggression is often mobilized (1) to lessen the pain and anguish, (2) to deny that the loss has occurred and is therefore irreversible, (3) to reclaim or revive the dead object, and (4) to exact vengeance upon the real or imagined cause of the separation or loss (Klein 1946). Personal and group defenses, unconsciously designed to be self-protective, are ultimately self-defeating. They interfere with perception of the world and with memory in order to exclude the unpleasurable (A. Freud 1965: 104–105). These defenses further distort judgment and interfere with realistic decisionmaking. Mourning achieves the opposite of these; it facilitates genuine change rather than the changelessness—and timelessness—of historical repetition (Nedelmann 1986).

In group decisionmaking, participants may often seek consensus—that is, sensing together, unanimity of vision—in order not to have to "sense" separately, independently. In medical decisionmaking groups, as in others, the borrowing of authority (from the leader, from mutual identification among participants) and emotional consensus often lead to distortion of the subject matter under scientific scrutiny. Even though medical professionals pride themselves on independence of judgment, group decisionmaking often becomes a way of ceding and suspending critical, individual judgment in favor of merger with the group.

Leadership and Group Dynamics

In "Group Psychology and the Analysis of the Ego" (1921), Freud notes that groups are organized by the emotional ties people have to one another and to the leader. (Freud emphasizes conflict-ridden father/son and fraternal relationships at the level of the Oedipus complex; later writers more closely examine the influences on group psychology of early—"pre-Oedipal"—mother/child relations and of inner, affect-laden images of oneself and others.) Often in groups the individual ego ideal is replaced by an external or group ideal that is usually embodied by the group leader. Individual judgment is ceded over to the leader. Kets deVries (1984) has edited a volume that contains psychoanalytic studies in management and that shows how unconscious management style and group dynamics affect decisionmaking. Leadership, for example, is often perceived in terms of splitting. In medical training settings, the physician director may be seen by his/her colleagues, residents, employees, and students as wise, fair, decisive, kindly, thoughtful—in short, as a good mother or father figure. Contrariwise, the administrative director may be perceived by the same group as aloof, manipulative, unavailable, inconsiderate, coldly calculating, rejecting—in short, as a bad mother or father figure. (Similar splits in the armed services are well known.)

In his study of American civilian and military policymaking groups, Irving Janis (1982) reveals that beneath the surface picture lies a deeper agenda, which he calls "groupthink." In this frame of mind, group participants secure morale and diminished anxiety at the price of critical thinking. Loyalty and commitment to the group and to its leader are purchased at the price of reality testing. Among the characteristics of "groupthink" are the illusion of invulnerability, the assumption that one's group's position is moral, stereotyping about one's own group and outgroups, group pressure on dissent from policy, self-censorship to avoid deviating from consensus by voicing misgivings about policy, the illusion of unanimity (the unwarranted assumption that silence = assent), the search for policy validation only within the group, and the emergence within the group of "mindguard[s]" who "protect" the leader from adverse information that might shatter consensus.

Janis's valuable and popular descriptive social psychological work in *Groupthink* (1982) nonetheless lacks the specificity and depth of psychodynamic approaches to group process in organizations. To the degree that unconscious agendas fail to be brought to conscious awareness for greater access and control in work groups, organizations fail to "develop" in the sense of maturing and evolving. Instead they continue to repeat old patterns or "mistakes" (Kets deVries 1984). Conversely, as groups become better able to develop insight into these powerful underlying factors, they increase their ability to be liberated from the tenacious pull of the past and to explore genuinely new alternatives. An example will illustrate this process.

Some years ago I served as consultant to a medical firm that I shall call Medical Consortium (MC), a group of practitioners that was a subsidiary of Corporate Health Planners (CHP). Around the time of my arrival, the senior executive physician (CEO) of MC had just resigned from the position he had held for eight consecutive years. The resignation came close upon the heels of a routine organizational reevaluation of all senior executives in which virtually universal disaffection had been expressed by junior personnel.

His resignation was followed by an immense sigh of relief among the personnel of MC. Several of the junior physicians used the expression "fresh air" to describe the good feeling and their hopefulness toward a future with the firm in which they would exert more control. A day or so later, however, several began to voice concern about how they would function once the momentary good feelings began to abate. "It is all well and good to feel good about ourselves and the freedom we have, but what are we going to do? Where are we going to go with it?" one pointedly asked.

As discussions continued, individually and in small groups, many group members began to realize that they had been participants in their unhappy relationship with their former boss, not entirely victims of it. They came slowly to realize that they had projected or allocated their aggressive impulses to the leader, whom they had then accused of being heavy-handed and treating them like children. They gradually recognized how much they in fact had needed their ("counter-Oedipal") old boss to do the "dirty work" of politicking, making hard choices, setting administrative priorities, and "being a son of a bitch" (in the words of one) in order that they could feel more clean and pure. They began to feel less triumph over his departure and more uneasiness about taking upon or into themselves aspects of the authority they had disliked in him. They remained far from eager to take over a leadership role, let alone to compete with one another.

There commenced a grieving process, one that seemed to supersede the exuberance and relief—a mourning for the loss of innocence, for the realization that they were far less pure in motive than they had hitherto thought. The mending of good and bad parts of themselves had only begun; a few days could not undo the psychic work of eight years. When I left the week-long consultation, I felt that I had resisted taking sides with them against their boss, or with him against them, but had instead helped them to understand what he had represented to them. I was hopeful that their organization would not stagnate, dissipate, or repeat its former pattern.

I am persuaded that this genre of example is more rule than exception in such mundane activities of group decisionmaking as determining curriculum content in medical education, deciding upon medical diagnosis and treatment plan(s) during the course of medical case conferences, arriving at group consensus during medical grand rounds lectures and discussions, and allocating funds and determining group priorities during the course of medical faculty meetings. Although slogans and dominant self-images such as "hard data," "cost effectiveness," and "rational man," represent the party line about the nature of participation in medical (and other) organizations, the fact remains that group decisionmaking is influenced if not driven by powerful unconscious agendas. If unrecognized and not worked through by the group, such issues will be ultimately destructive even though at the time they might feel exhilarating.

The Mirror Image of Families in Groups

Elliott Jaques (1955) observes that in corporate consultations organizational groups unwittingly use group relationships and roles as a defense against shared persecutory and depressive anxiety. Howard Stein and Daniel Fox (1985) show

how the metaphor of the "family" affects interpersonal relations and decisionmaking in medical and nonmedical environments. John Kafka and Joyce McDonald (1965), and before them Warren Brodey, Marjorie Hayden, and Othilda Krug (1957), discover that conflictual relationships among health care and administrative group members often are a recreation or reenactment, via identification, of relationships in the family of the patient. Kafka and McDonald, for instance, write that

> in one situation where the father was ignored by the mother and patient, the administrator seldom met with the social worker and therapist. Furthermore, we have noted that a family in which the internal power structure is being tested by the family members may also test the power structure of the hospital staff in a parallel way. For instance, a family, in which the father's power was being questioned, repeatedly tested whether or not the Medical Director of the hospital would or would not overrule the decision of the unit administrator. Members of the hospital's administrative hierarchy were informed of this family pattern. The resulting approach interrupted the family's long-established pattern of moving the patient after brief hospitalization from one institution to another (1965: 174–175).

If this parallelism is not analyzed by group members, but is instead acted out, the patient's and family's problem may be perpetuated. Here, the group response becomes a metaphor for understanding or misunderstanding the patient and family.

In a similar vein S. H. Foulkes (1948), D. Wilfred Abse (1974), and Vamık Volkan and David Hawkins (1971, 1972) observe that when teaching a group of psychiatric residents about psychopathology, the group by identification reenacts aspects of the patient's symptoms or family history. In a discussion of this literature, Volkan (1984) remarks that

> whenever the residents met regularly to review the psychotherapy of a patient being treated by a member of their group, aspects of the patient's psychopathology, behavior pattern, or family history were reenacted in the teaching group in what is called the parallel (or echo) phenomenon. It is as though the group itself brings facets of the patient's situation "to life" in order to identify with his problems and respond to them empathically (1984: 3–4).

The dynamics of Balint groups, like those of medical case conferences, medical grand rounds, hospital staffings, and the like, often recapitulate the unhappy relationship between physician and patient. In discussing the use of small groups in medical training, R. Gosling, D. Miller, D. Woodhouse, and P. Turquet point out that "sometimes it is possible to notice how the doctor is identified with his patient and starts to impersonate him in the [Balint] seminar, and gets the other members to respond to him as if he were the patient. . . . For example, a doctor says 'no' to all the suggestions and remarks made to him by his colleagues in the seminar" (1967: 16, 37).

In this example, the presenting physician is consciously aware that he is frustrated, perhaps even angry, with his "difficult" patient. The physician is not aware, however, that he has unconsciously identified with the patient and has begun to act like the patient in the group. The other medical group members, identifying with the frustrated presenting physician who is trying to be helpful to the patient, in turn become the counterplayers. For their part in the "symmetrical" spiral (Bateson 1972), group members make numerous suggestions and offer more and more advice. The group thus reenacts (acts out) the drama of the physician-patient relationship.

Practitioner-patient, presenter-group, and other clinical relationships also embody and play out early family relationships and parts of participants' mental structure. DeMause (1974a), for instance, identifies two widespread parental reactions to their children: "projective care," in which the adult uses the child "as a vehicle for projection of the contents of his own unconscious" (1974a: 6)—for example, giving one's infant the indulgent care one craves for oneself; and "reversal reactions," in which the adult uses the child "as a substitute for an adult figure important in his own childhood" (1974a: 6)—for example, seeing in one's infant a tyrannical, willful mother or father, the child "becoming" one's parent. DeMause notes a "continuous shift between projection and reversal, between the child as devil and as adult, [producing] a 'double image,'" (1974a: 21), one that deMause documents as "a precondition for battering" (1974a: 21). In clinical relationships and groups, various members can unwittingly be endowed with, and accept, such roles as hero, villain, fool, caretaker, or dependent.

Otto Kernberg (1965) identifies two types of practitioner countertransference: "concordant" and "complementary" identifications with patients (these processes occur in groups as well). In *concordant identification*, the practitioner identifies with the corresponding part of the patient's mental structure: for example, the therapist's superego (conscience) with that of the patient. In *complementary identification*, the practitioner identifies with the patient's transference objects—that is, with those people (more correctly, their mental representations) who have been emotionally important in the patient's past. In complementary identification, the practitioner feels what it was like to be various aspects of the patient's parenting figures, a process similar to what deMause terms "reversal."

Ideally, the Balint group leader, or another insightful member, recognizes and comments on these processes rather than participates in their repetition and escalation. If he or she offers an interpretation, the group may attempt to understand rather than perpetuate the fruitless cycle (both in the group and in the physician-patient relationship). Ideally, through understanding their own reaction to the patient, group members widen their repertory of future responses. A clinical group's emotional response during the process of data-gathering, diagnosing, and decisionmaking about treatment can thus contribute to or diminish members' abilities to understand and treat the patient. Similarly, how a group answers the question, "Where is the symptom located?" not only influences how the group intervenes but likewise reveals (often implicit) constraints upon its intervention.

Many years ago, I served as a guest case discussant for a consultation psychiatry team at a large urban hospital. The patient, Gracie Jordan, was a forty-five-year-old black female with unrespectable carcinoma of the lungs and a previous surgical removal of a brain tumor. Following a recent regimen of radiotherapy, she thought she was cured. She attributed her recovery to the radiation acting in concert with her and her family's prayers and faith. After a brief remission of symptoms, she began to experience shoulder and neck pain and was increasingly unable to use her legs to get about.

Her family had been informed that she had approximately two more months to live, but they asked that she not be told of the seriousness of her illness. They feared that she might not be able to accept it. Although she knew that she had "had" cancer, she believed that it had gone away. Her family asked that she be told that she would get better. The family's prescription coincided with her own wish.

The attending psychiatrist advanced a psychiatric diagnosis of hypomania (a mildly agitated state). The patient's hypomaniac activity and denial protected her family—her mother and sisters—from becoming depressed. This appeared to be her function or delegated role in the family's emotional economy. So far, then, the team had discussed mostly the patient and patient's family and the cultural setting. The psychiatrist then wanted to know more about how the patient perceived her situation, what she thought the future held for her, and what she thought was the effect of her illness upon the family. He planned to broach these questions in a hospital interview.

We walked onto the patient's ward, then entered her dark room. The somber ward had the unmistakable aroma of cleanliness. Ms. Jordan's room was the very last at the end of a long corridor. Of the four beds in her room, hers was the one in the farthest corner. As is true of the placement of many terminally ill patients, the psychogeography (Stein 1987b) of the ward, and of interaction between staff members and patients on the ward, communicated a powerful symbolic message: She was literally at the end of the road.

The hospital interview proceeded like an unsuccessful assault upon a medieval bastion. To say the least, this woman was well defended, despite the psychiatrist's insistently confrontive interview style. Her answers to a barrage of questions about her knowledge of the illness, her assessment of the future, and the implications of her illness for her family revealed her resolve not to consider her situation dire. For her, cancer was entirely a matter of the past tense. A steadfast smile accompanied her words. Although she anxiously clutched the bed railing on four separate occasions during the twenty-minute interview, in her words she adamantly refused to accept what was taking place in her life. She already "knew" what she could not tolerate to know. Tomorrow, we learned, she would be discharged. She had requested to return home to take care of her mother. Her sense of responsibility to her family was too great for her to allow for the possibility that cancer had metastasized to her legs.

At the conference's end, the psychiatrist asked, "What should we do now?" Almost as different voices entering a Bach fugue, everyone urged that the family be convened as a whole, which would be a "first" during the patient's long course of treatment. In the family conference, at least, the anguish that had necessitated the network of secret alliances could be addressed. For, so long as clinicians dealt with the family exclusively as subunits (each protecting the other), the family would indefinitely postpone coming to terms with death.

The presiding psychiatrist wondered aloud, "Why had this patient been presented for consultation?" Aware that they were dealing with both chronic disease and chronic mental illness, medical hospital staff members (oncology, internal medicine, nursing) had been uncomfortable in dealing with the latter. Consequently, they had rid themselves of this discomfort by relegating (turfing) this aspect of the patient to the consultation psychiatry team. It quickly became clear to the consultation psychiatry team that it would be premature to explain everything in terms of the patient's individual psychodynamics, family process, and ethnicity alone. Somehow, the medical system, too, had been involved.

Like Ms. Jordan's family, the hospital staff had shored up its denial through silence, thereby buttressing the patient's denial (while the dread secret seeped out via her placement in the hospital). Staff members, too, became sustained through her. With its own strategy, the family had anxiously engaged the collusion of the medical system, and the health care system had complied for reasons of its own that corresponded to the family's own rationalizations and the patient's own denial. Death anxiety had spread like a quiet panic: from family to hospital staff to psychiatric team. Each transfer had been an appeal for social control that had never quite sufficed.

In this case consultation the patient, her family, her support network of religion and its ideology, the medical system, and finally the wider cultural system had unwittingly colluded in shortcircuiting the process of grieving. Because the symptom had been widely shared, it had been difficult to recognize it as a problem. In fact, it was a solution. Genuinely therapeutic interaction with the family could begin to take place only because, at least in one segment of the health care system, the mutual vow of silence had been broken first among team members, which in turn had permitted the taboo to be examined. Stated somewhat differently, ad hoc "group therapy" within the consultation team preceded and facilitated whatever family therapy might subsequently occur. The case was thus not only about Ms. Jordan but about what she represented to all involved (E. Becker 1973; Brain 1977).

Treatment often becomes a personal and group defense by the practitioner(s) against what the patient is experiencing. Only as we could recognize and accept our group defense against death and dying could we then address that process in the patient and family, rather than fend it off. Change in the family was thus possible via prior change in the team. Team members discovered that the boundary of the symptom had encompassed the team itself, that the team had unwittingly contributed to the homeostatic process that had kept the grief buried. This suggests that medicine's dictum, "First do no harm," might be reframed in group systems terms to read, "First do not collude."

Groups as Human Bodies: A Focus of Anxiety

Not only do groups recapitulate family dynamics (their own, those of the patient), but members of groups also imagine their group and other groups to be *human bodies* that protect and menace one another. Groups can thus describe themselves as being born, mating, giving birth, having adolescence, aging, dying, being male or female. In the group process of medical committees (academic, corporate, hospital, clinic), I often hear, "We've got to . . . present a united front . . . protect the rear . . . guard our flanks . . . protect both our fronts . . . launch a frontal assault . . . conduct a two-front war. . . . They're bleeding us to death. . . . Make sure the enemy doesn't get a chance to come in the back door." These metaphorical statements convey what Bion (1959) terms "basic assumptions" about what it feels like to be a member of a group (see also deMause 1977: 11).

Of course, whatever else a clinical department or medical conference is, it is not a human body with a protective or vulnerable "front" and "back" (or "top" and "bottom"). But when in groups, under the influence of powerful fantasies and shared sense of endangerment, we quickly come to feel, think, and act as if our group had become a single human organism whose front and back are menaced and must at all costs be protected (see Stein 1980d). Metaphors are useful halfway houses for expressing thought and feeling. Nevertheless, in group medical decisionmaking as in other "corporate" activities, participants often fail to examine the truth value of these expressions and hold them to be true, absolute, and necessary. Stated differently, the group is indeed conveying a symbolized truth (a compromise formation that both reveals and conceals the shared unconscious wish and object), but the truth is displaced and projected from its real source. The group is trying to solve an enshrouded problem in the wrong place. Metaphors may take on the group psychological function of defenses that resist the type of knowledge that would release what is being defended against. The formidably most important group agenda may unwittingly become the defense of the group body, not the project all had originally and rationally gathered to undertake.

In Chapter 1, I briefly discussed one groups' unofficial splitting of role and status identity issues between two floors on which medical faculty offices were located. An erotically tinged ethos pervaded relations between the two floors. One male non-M.D. faculty member adamantly declared, "In medicine there are only two kinds of people, two roles: You're either a doctor [which is to say, male] or you're a nurse [which is to say, female]. Either you screw or you get screwed." The perception of group structure as bifurcated into gendered bodies (subdivisions) contributed to the intensity of this group's frequent upheavals, attempts at role reversal (acculturation if not assimilation, acceptance, "passing") by nonphysicians, and attempts at disassociation from nonphysicians by physicians.

Group fantasy may thus dramatically set the tone for minute particulars of day-to-day decisions and group interactions. It may serve as the larger, overriding metaagenda that is at once implemented in ordinary decisionmaking activities and reaffirmed by those activities. It is the often unstated reference point without which decisions and group actions would not occur in their specific form or feel "right" to those participating. In an article on organizational diagnosis of communities, and political units, Tobias Brocher writes that "[in groups] it is possible to destroy or divert individual insight and to prevent reality perceptions by creating social dependency needs, thereby forcing the individual into primary process operations through collective regression in the interest of collective unconscious drive needs and satisfaction" (1984: 374).

Decisionmaking in medical groups is often founded on the paradox that although strict objectivity is the official rule, participants unwittingly appropriate reality (secondary process) to fantasy ends (primary process). In this dream-scaped wonderland of primary process, there are no negatives, time and space are distorted or are altogether irrelevant, omnipotence of thought and wish-fulfilling fantasies reign unfettered, the part may represent the whole, and a thing may be represented by its opposite. Ultimately, ideas and wishes may be displaced and condensed into symbolism (Freud 1900b).

Cascades in Medicine: Group Action as Acting Out

The topic I chose for a behavioral science seminar was physicians' difficult and painful decisions involving death and dying among elderly nursing home and hospitalized patients. Around the table sat perhaps a dozen doctors, nurses, and medical assistants. The presenting physician began:

> I'm having trouble with my elderly patients. When I think I've worked things out with a patient and his family, I get fooled. The patient agrees to die at home, but then the family calls me when they're afraid he's dying. It's OK for the patient to get worse at home, but not to *die* at home. Or, even when Hospice is involved, the family sometimes still calls the ambulance. Before things take a turn for the worse, everybody accepts that the patient is dying. But when things look like they're going down the tubes, the family suddenly wants more aggressive treatment. Then my phone rings off the wall. What am I supposed to do? They're supposed to die, and then they bother me when the time comes for them to die.

A second physician talked about the grief cycle: "Sometimes a prolonged death lasts six months. You never know exactly when death is going to happen."

A third resident, fidgeting nervously at the table, interrupted, "I like to put out fires, not watch them burn. If you're going to die, then die. But I don't like to be morbid or to hang around morbid people. My attitude is: We're going to whip this. We're going to give it everything we've got."

The second resident said diffidently, "How do you know 'We're going to whip this' in a particular case? How do you know whether to do a Code Blue? And when you start one, how do you know to keep going or not? There's a fine line between what's terminal and what is not. And how do you know which side of the line the patient's on?"

A fourth resident—who always had a tender social conscience and the reputation for being a rabble-rouser—added:

> You've got to take into account the legal implications of "doing nothing" in the hospital. What you call "dying" might look like to others that you're a patient-killer. We talk glibly about "supportive care," but we can't predict how aggressive treatment will turn out until we try. Not to treat an infection is mercy killing medicolegally. Treatment is all or nothing. When you elect to do nothing, like not feeding a patient, you are walking the line of malpractice. You've got to look at it two ways, the humane or personal way, and the medicolegal. We spend more time covering our rears than practicing good medicine. The first rule if you want to avoid the medicolegal route is to make sure a dying person, at home or in the nursing home, is not brought to the hospital in the first place. Because once you're in the hospital, a different set of rules applies. Everything starts to go on automatic.

The presenting resident wondered aloud, "They say we're not supposed to play God. But when I treat elderly patients, I assess the quality of life and make decisions based on that. I've played God before, and I will continue to play God, because that's my role. I think it's dishonest for us not to own up to that fact."

A nurse who was active in a local Hospice group introduced a distinction:

> I think that part of physicians' discomfort is that hospitals are places where people are supposed to be fixed. Hospice offers an alternative. With Hospice, my patients are supposed to die. We talk about it, and they know it. We acknowledge that the person is going to die and that there is going to be no treatment for it. I wish it were that simple, because down the road when the patient starts bleeding out or coughing up blood at home, the family might throw their earlier agreement out the window and call an ambulance. But at least in Hospice, people are *talking* about dying. Here in town, Hospice has gotten very few patients because the doctors refuse to tell their patients that they're dying. To give a referral to Hospice the physician first has to face the fact and tell the patient that he's terminal. But there's still a pall of silence because to most physicians, death is not an acceptable medical outcome.

Kernberg poignantly notes that

> understanding organizations in depth can be painful; at times, such awareness does not improve the effectiveness of staff members; but understanding always makes it possible to gain a more realistic, even if painful, grasp of what the future probably will be. The parallel to the painful learning about aspects of one's unconscious in the psychoanalytic situation is implicit: there are similar pathological defenses against becoming aware of reality in the place where one works (1984: 44).

I am not arguing that official content under consideration by any group (differential diagnosis, treatment plan, curriculum choice, leadership choice) is of little real consequence for the group. Rather, I am arguing that this content is often the foil, vehicle, or symbol of other, deeper agendas that are rarely directly addressed. Instead, such agendas are acted out ***in the name or guise of that content***. Group dynamics are really about all levels simultaneously, although groups act as if the only acknowledgeable reality is the official topic of the content under consideration. There are ominous consequences for group morale, medical education, and patient care when participants remain unaware of all the parameters (levels of agenda) involved. Medical group fantasies have real outcomes.

In a study of "the double-bind between [kidney] dialysis patients and their health practitioners," Linda Alexander argues that "case conferences, staff meetings, patient forums and exchanges are all presently characterized by detailed itemizations of persons' proclivities, symptoms and character, rather than by consideration of the interactive structures that occur in clinical environments" (1981: 323). As a result, a group labeling process may occur. Diagnosis by group makes sterotyping easier than when diagnosis is performed alone because one can borrow and justify "license" from the group (more technically, from one's inner image of the group). In an overview of "the social labeling perspective on illness," Nancy Waxler remarks that "illness labels are created in social negotiations between several parties, including professionals and the troubled individual, and they occur within institutional and social contexts that play an important part in the negotiation. Ideologies and organizational procedures as well as the relative power and interests of the negotiating parties contribute to the label of illness" (1981: 296). Later she argues that "even the information from hospital or clinic records that we tend to think of as 'hard' data can also be conceived as the product of social processing. Labeling theory suggests that facts such as diagnosis, length of stay, prognosis, may tell us much more about the social characteristics of selected patients and the workings of the treatment system than about a biomedical process" (1981: 302). For example, case conference participants can quickly stereotype an elderly patient as suffering from a chronic illness condition (to be old equals to be chronically sick), when in fact the patient had only recently become acutely ill (Stein 1985g: 21–23). Physicians can "transfer" powerful, aversive past medical experiences inappropriately onto current ones (Stein 1986c).

As I noted earlier, hospital tumor boards or oncology conferences often proceed according to a formula in which the patient is initially identified sequentially by age, race, marital status, and gender. The ensuing discussion of cancer staging and treatment proceeds as if there were no person, only a disease. Such group-sanctioned defenses as depersonalization and rationalization are employed to keep the painful feelings of identification, fragmentation, and decay "off limits" to the discourse (Stein 1985g; Stein and Apprey 1985). Group anxiety, however, can trigger a cascade of action more designed to quell the clinicians' anxiety than to actually help the patient (Mold and Stein 1986; Stein and Mold 1988).

In biology, cascade refers to a process that, once started, proceeds stepwise to its full, seemingly inexorable, conclusion. Cascade events, whether at a molecular level or in clinical patient care, sometimes serve a very useful purpose. Consider the clotting cascade, in which a small tear in a blood vessel leads to a chain of events that results in closure of that tear, or consider the series of events that occurs when a patient arrives at the emergency room pulseless and without respirations. But, the danger of a cascade is that it can be inappropriately triggered (as, for example, in disseminated intravascular coagulation, that is, excessive blood clotting); once triggered, it is virtually impossible to stop.

Processes that occur in molecular systems often have correlates in larger systems. The cascade effect as a clinical group dynamic generally consists of an initiating factor or factors, followed by a series of events that seem to be a direct result of previous events, often catalyzed by some characteristic of the system—usually anxiety. This chain of events often proceeds with increasing momentum, so that the further it progresses, the more difficult it is to stop. Participants in the process are often unaware that it is a cascade effect, and they frequently fail to recognize its cause. The following case (adopted from Mold and Stein 1986) exemplifies the cascade effect as it occurs in the clinical care of patients.

A fifty-nine-year-old man was admitted to the surgical service of the University Medical Center for elective repair of an inguinal hernia (in the groin area). He had a history of coronary artery disease with mild stable angina pectoris (episodic heart pain) and had undergone coronary arteriography (a procedure using dye to visualize the coronary arteries) nine years earlier that showed mild to moderate coronary artery disease with no area of stenosis (narrowing) greater than 75 percent. He also had a history of chronic obstructive pulmonary disease and reflux esophagitis (lung disease and involuntary regurgitation). His family physician had evaluated him for a variety of chest complaints and had decided that his coronary artery disease was stable.

On the patient's admission to the surgical service, however, a cardiology consultation was obtained because of the vague chest complaints and the history of coronary artery disease. The cardiologist suggested delaying surgery until an exercise-tolerance test could be performed. Unfortunately, the patient had to wait six hours at the heart station for the exercise-tolerance test. During that time he became anxious, agitated, and angry and had some mild chest discomfort. Because of the discomfort, the test was not done, and the patient was transferred to the telemetry unit because of the possibility that he was having preinfarction angina (chest pain that may precede a heart attack).

The situation went from bad to worse. The patient became more anxious and agitated, and he had more chest pain, as well as electrocardiographic changes (in the electrical activity of the heart). He was transferred to the coronary care unit, where he was given intravenous nitroglycerin and oral calcium-channel blockers. There was no elevation of cardiac enzymes in his plasma. He eventually underwent coronary arteriography, which showed a slight improvement since his previous arteriogram nine years earlier. His primary care physician was left to try reassuring the patient that all the tests and precautions had been necessary and that the results indicated he was not in any danger. At that point, the hernia repair could not be performed because of a full operating room schedule, and it had to be rescheduled for two weeks later. The patient eventually underwent hernia repair without complications.

Physicians taking care of this patient after his transfer to the telemetry unit felt powerless to stop what seemed to be a succession of problems, each one building on and worse than the previous ones. The chain of events seemed to be fueled by the patient's anxiety and by the "anxiety" of the health care system, which could not accept the small risk of a potentially life-threatening condition. Although the series of precautions and interventions can certainly be justified medically, the fact remains that this patient entered the hospital in stable condition, and it is unlikely that his condition would have coincidentally become unstable enough to require the testing and interventions that he eventually received.

Physicians' anxiety, which through identification may reverberate throughout the entire health care system, often fuels clinical cascades (Bowen 1978; Devereux 1967; Katz 1984a; Stein 1985d, 1985g; Stein and Apprey 1985). It can be operative at several steps in the process. First, physicians who are anxious about a patient's problem may be tempted to do something, anything, decisive in order to diminish their own anxiety. Second, when physicians feel incapable of managing their anxiety because they think they do not know enough, they often turn to a consultant who, they hope, will gain control of the situation. The anxiety of the referring physician and of the patient may in turn be transmitted (by identification) to the consultant, who begins with more anxiety than if he or she had seen the patient initially. Physicians may project onto patients their own sense of being out of control and intensify their efforts to control the patient.

Third, physicians (as well as other practitioners) attempt to diminish anxiety by creating and adhering steadfastly to prescribed formal institutionally codified response sequences for medical situations and diagnoses. In an effort to decrease anxiety, physicians and/or other health care personnel (nurses, psychologists, drug and alcohol counselors) and administrators may set up protocols through which all patients with ostensibly similar problems (presenting complaints, diagnostic category) are treated identically. Although this procedural simplification often "works" well, it ignores individual differences, situational differences, and the desires of patients. In treating the protocol rather than the patient (or treating the patient as refracted by the protocol), all participants to the medical encounter become standardized and dehumanized. Bureaucratic standardization of treatment through case management protocols is at least in part designed to alleviate the anxiety of uncertainty, complexity, and personalization that invariably arises in clinical practice. In a sense, by ascribing responsibility to the protocol, physicians do not have to think and feel as much about choices and their consequences as they would were the buffer not there. Through a cycle of projection and internalization, personal responsibility—reality-testing ego functions as well as superego functions—is ceded to institutions (see Parin 1988; Jaques 1955, 1976; Diamond 1984, 1988; Diamond and Allcorn 1986).

Early in the twentieth century, Frederick Winslow Taylor (1911) advocated rigidly hierarchical principles of scientific management and conducted careful time-and-motion studies of industrial workers to make them more productive and efficient. This bureaucratic or organizational philosophy emphasized the accomplishment of the task, rather than the person per se, who was paid only to do the task. Since the advent of Taylorism, the regimented, bureaucratized language and ethos of "management" and "efficiency" have pervaded American society. Its most recent permutation has been the school of thought introduced by Peter Drucker (1954) in his influential book, *The Practice of Management*. Leadership, followership, and participation in work groups are formalized in the technique called management by objectives. One powerful offshoot of this style in educational (including medical) circles has been the molding of curricula into a format of goals and objectives, which transforms teaching and learning into a disspirited assembly line. Robert F. Mager's *Preparing Instructional Objectives* (1962) is the cultural locus classicus of this pedagogical genre (see Gardner 1977).

In a cross-cultural study of organizational management, Geert Hofstede observes that "in the United States, MBO has been used to spread a pragmatic results orientation throughout the organization. It has been considerably more successful where results are objectively measurable than where they can only be interpreted subjectively" 1980: 58). MBO emphasizes "the idea of replacing the arbitrary authority of the boss with the impersonal authority of mutually agreed-upon objectives" (1980: 58). These "objectives become the subordinates' 'superego'" (1980: 58). "MBO presupposes a depersonalized authority in the form of internalized objectives" (1980: 59). Hofstede characterizes MBO management style as "fact based"; "'fast decisions [are] based on clear responsibilities' rather than the use of informal, personal contacts and the concern for consensus" (1980: 59). The learning, teaching, and clinical practice style of fact-based management has diffused culturally throughout biomedicine.

Impersonal clinical management protocols (both outpatient and hospital) specify medical objectives, how they are to be achieved, and the outcomes that are to be expected. From the first day of medical school, medical students, interns, and residents are told by their basic and clinical science teachers how many and varied are the "facts" that they must amass during their medical education, how many of these facts will be obsolete before they complete their medical education, and how great the need is for continual reading in order to "keep up with the new facts that are being generated." The cultural language of narrowly contextualized facts is inseparable from the managerial norms that govern group behavior throughout biomedical institutions. The physician-as-technician who "manages" patients is in turn "managed by" and an extension of clinical and administrative protocols that dictate precisely what constitutes relevant (and reimbursable) facts. Likewise, since the early 1980s the corporate ethos has promoted (marketed) medicine as "managed health care systems." Patients, like facts, are to be managed quickly, technically, efficiently, impersonally.

Protocols are thus potent *initiators* of stress-reducing cascades. They are based on the assumption that a given disease-entity should be treated the same way in all patients. The era of corporate medicine has intensified and proliferated this diffusion of responsibility through corporate medical protocols that lead even more than in the past to narrow treatment of the diagnosis rather than the patient. Since the late 1970s, legal pressure has been added to the physician's internal drive to render good care as factors in medical practice. To protect themselves from the prospect of a malpractice lawsuit or from too zealous peer review, physicians often practice increasingly defensive medicine, which results in cascades to reduce the threat and confer the sense of security. In the onrush of anxiety-reducing cascades, medicine violates Sir William Osler's plea that it is more important to know what kind of patient has the disease than what kind of disease the patient has.

Not all medical decisionmaking results in virtually unstoppable cascades. During the course of clinical decisionmaking, however, as physician anxiety increases, physicians utilize the following recurrent, often cascade-producing, decision patterns (identified by Stein and Mold [1988]) to reduce that anxiety:

1. Inadequate collection of the patient's medical, personal, familial, occupational, and culturally based historical data, which would place the symptoms into the context of the patient's lived world
2. Excessive lab testing (which is often designed to save the time the physician spends with the patient—only to displace time and cost elsewhere)
3. Overinterpretation of lab results or overconcern about positive lab test results, thereby making lab testing more magically oracular and less scientific
4. Excessive prescribing of medication (often as a way of feeling that one is "doing something" and of conveying this to the patient)
5. Premature consultation, together with transfer of the physician's anxiety onto the consultant (with the attendant demand to "do something that I cannot do")
6. Too frequent scheduling of medically oriented follow-up appointments, resulting in the medicalization of all of the patient's problems

7. Overhospitalization of patients (probably less of a problem since DRGs)
8. Misinterpretation of the patient's historical data and of the patient's behavior based on biases that result from physician countertransference

The question remains whether action cascades in medicine can be stopped before they start or once set in motion. There are plenty of grounds for pessimism. As I argue elsewhere, much of American culture, and the biomedicine that serves it, inculcates and rewards, rather than tries to analyze or stop, cascades. If it is true that "the first mistake is the worst mistake" (Ober 1987), it is likewise true that to make such "mistakes" is individually and collectively built into medicine—largely out of the fear of making mistakes. Cascades can be interrupted or their initiation avoided only as practitioners and medical educators begin to ask what the drivenness to act and to control is about rather than simply acting upon it.

There is no easy, immediate way that an entire cultural way of thinking, feeling, and doing can be revised. Nevertheless, in medical school, internship, and residency training, greater attention could be paid to the dynamics of physician-patient-family-colleague-staff relationships and to the group dynamics of clinical and administrative decisionmakers. Furthermore, practitioner and residency Balint groups (Balint 1974; Gazda et al. 1984; Scheingold 1988) in which physician-patient, practitioner, and group relationships are explored could be instituted in all medical training. Finally, the considerable literature on the doctor-patient relationship and on the topic of countertransference could be more widely utilized in clinical curricula.

Medical as well as nonmedical decisionmakers must examine their own individual and group emotional investments and cultural meanings in order to diminish the distortion these invariably impose on the best laid plans (see Devereux 1967; LaBarre 1978). Subjective involvements tend to remain an unanalyzed case within the case, so to speak, and they profoundly influence the kind of work the group undertakes. The value of devoting attention to group dynamics within medical meetings of all types is that as participants are able, in a nonjudgmental setting, to identify underlying conflicts, fantasies, wishes, fears, assumptions, participants will have greater access to and control over them. The process of the work group would be facilitated and liberated rather than contaminated.

Every time yet another curriculum component is suggested for medical or residency education, an outcry can be heard from already swamped students and residents: "Don't we get enough thrown at us already? How will this new item help us be better physicians? Won't it detract from the really important topics we're already studying?" What justifies devoting attention in medicine to group dynamics? Nothing less than the fact that given our out-of-awareness subjective investment in our groups and in the topics we discuss, such attention serves as a corrective to our tendency to distort the very topic under consideration. We are always in groups. In medicine, as in all realms of human activity, our problem is not what we know, but what we prefer to think must be true when, for unconscious reasons, we overextend our theories, impose on the subject matter what in fact belongs to ourselves, and then proceed to treat the screen of our projections as if the image belonged to it.

This perspective can be extrapolated beyond medicine to all corporate (group) decisionmaking to suggest that those hidden agendas that are collectively brought to work groups be routinely addressed. This effort would help organizations to truly develop and not merely enact the defensive chimera of change. Medical groups, like other organizational groups, often select and focus on seemingly palpable problems in order to divert attention from the fact that one is always part of the problem one studies and in which one endeavors to intervene. The ability to reinternalize and examine what one (or one's group), for defensive reasons, has displaced and projected away from oneself is the starting point for bona fide development in biomedical and all other groups.

The chapter that follows extensively documents one such egregious failure of internalization within the institution of biomedicine. While heated discussions about health care financing, coverage, and reimbursement rage in corporate medicine, in Congress, in insurance companies, and in industry, and between practitioners and a host of third-party payors, there remains a pall of silence between practitioner and patient around the issue of payment for services rendered. Physicians may literally touch some of the most intimate parts of their patients' lives. But money is enshrouded in taboo and delegated to a cadre, indeed an industry, of business office and collective agency henchmen whose role is to be the "heavy" in the drama of medical care. To the many dualisms that haunt medicine—Cartesian mind/body, patient/practitioner, internal/external, hard/soft—is now added the division of labor between those who engage in patient care and those who receive, solicit, or attempt to exact appropriate payment.

FIVE

Money and Medicine: An Identity Problem

This chapter identifies the dynamics and consequences of a curious taboo in official American health culture: namely, a prohibition upon allowing physicians to appear concerned with financial matters within the physician role. From a content analysis of advertisements in the *American Journal of Nursing* and the *Journal of the American Medical Association*, Krantzler writes that

> in advertisements depicting physicians, the white [lab] coat and stethoscope have predominated as identifying symbols. [Nevertheless,] these symbols have undergone some changes in the past two decades. While in 1965 the white coat and stethoscope clearly predominated as physician identifiers, their use decreased in 1982 with a rise in the depiction of physicians in street clothes (suits or dresses). When drugs are advertised, the physician is more likely to wear a white coat and stethoscope; when business-related concerns are advertised, these are less likely to appear. This symbolically suggests the separation of healing from earning money, part of the ideal image of medicine (1986: 935).

What I shall describe as a taboo represents an irreconcilable conflict between "caring" values and "business" values in medicine. This conflict has defied solution within the culture of medicine despite continuing attempts to resolve it.

At first glance, the very existence of this taboo seems implausible. Soaring health care costs and their containment are hotly debated public policy issues. Hospital utilization review boards vigilantly oversee inpatient medical care. Lectures, seminars, and practica in "practice management" have become standard fare in medical curricula. Small placards on which appear a message indicating the physician's willingness to discuss fees with patients are frequently posted in physicians' offices. Behavioral scientists employed in medical education settings emphasize the dire necessity of practitioners' knowing the patient's current and past life situation, including financial concerns, as a guide to intelligent patient care as well as a

Portions of Chapter 5 were published in Howard F. Stein, "The Money Taboo in American Medicine." *Medical Anthropology* 7(4)(Fall 1983): 1–15. Reprinted, with changes, by permission of Gordon and Breach Science Publishers S.A.

means of improving the overall clinical relationship. These facts do not disconfirm the existence of the taboo. They both coexist with it and intensify it.

American medicine characterizes itself according to many diverse, even competing images: a biomedical science, a form of service, a high-technology trade, a helping profession, an intellectual pursuit, and a clinical practice. That medicine is also a business is at once an obvious fact and an identity that medicine has sought to minimize. As with every form of employment, medicine is a means of earning a living. Physicians and society alike, however, scorn this way of putting it.

An examination of the folklore of finances, profit expectations, earnings, and lifestyle within the culture of medicine reveals many contradictions and much ambivalence. Society accuses medicine of gluttony, of an insatiable appetite for wealth. The public expects physicians to lead lives of self-sacrifice yet likewise expects physicians to flaunt their income in expansive homes and expensive automobiles. In their turn, physicians seek to earn a comfortable living following decades of self-denial during their education, yet minimize if not disavow the importance of recompense in their lives. Societally, it is as though medicine should be rewarded and punished for its monetary interests. Medicine must simultaneously live up to the ideal of utter selflessness while pursuing luxury and ease. Because anything less than ascetic self-abnegation (à la St. Francis of Assisi) earns a fall from public grace, even devoted doctors who spend their lives "on call" may serve as objects of savage gossip. One veteran family physician, who had for decades devoted himself to his patients, bitterly revealed his sense of caution and betrayal from his interactions with patients. He counseled his family practice residents: "Don't expect a word of gratitude from your patients. And don't get the idea that you're indispensable when they tell you that they wouldn't know what to do without you. Because when you die you'll still be warm in the ground when they're already running over your grave after another doctor to take care of them."

Medicine must labor overtime to disavow those sins of avarice and gluttony from which it cannot escape accusation and condemnation. One form this disavowal takes is the virtual embarrassment at incorporating any financial considerations into the content of medical education. Several generations of medical practitioners and residents have lamented and complained to me that nowhere in their training did they receive instruction on how to organize a billing system for their practice, let alone learn about the complexities of the "alphabet soup" (HMO, PPO, PRO) of corporate medicine. Physicians describe and experience the financial aspect of medicine frequently in terms of what Erikson describes as the "negative identity" (1968), that repudiated yet alluring portion of the ego identity that one is admonished *not* to be. The myth of the old country doctor who was always available and who lived only for others haunts medicine in nostalgia-bound American society.

Caught in the unrelenting double bind of societal ambivalence regarding financial gain and/or regulation of income in medicine, the very profession that stands accused of being consumed with interest in money must behave as though uninterested in anything monetary while pursuing the good life. Only the Albert Schweitzers and Marcus Welbys who renounce the world for the souls and bodies of their patients gain exemption from stinging societal denunciation and envy. Otherwise stated, physicians constitute a category of society's loyal deviants who must conform to the ascetic ideal *and* violate it. Historically, in American medicine, money has long had a bad name. It is not my intention to polish money's tarnished image or to cleanse its soiled reputation. Rather, my goal is to inquire into a taboo that continues to divide medicine into irreconcilable sacred (helping) and profane (business) realms.

During the course of my work as an applied medical anthropologist in medical education, I have repeatedly been caught in the factional conflict between caring and business within medicine. Convinced that the clinical relationship is the keystone of all clinical work, I noted that discussions of the patient's economic situation were virtually absent from doctor-patient interactions, even when they affected the patient's ability to purchase prescribed medication, for instance. I regarded the financial picture to be a vital, if neglected, dimension of the patient's history and current life situation. Moreover, I felt that an inclusion of a discussion of physician's fees (or clinic fees), laboratory costs, and hospital costs within the clinical relationship would enhance both the patient's trust and the patient's likelihood of feeling responsible to the physician to pay the bill. This, admittedly, was an outsider's perspective.

My first seminars on this subject, however, led to a rude awakening: Often one learns the most sacred rules only by first innocently violating them! I found myself severely rebuked or met with embarrassed silence when I raised the issue of discussing fees or outstanding bills with patients. It was as though patients' ability to pay was simultaneously assumed and could not be examined by the physician. This was one intimacy that, for some reason, was declared to be off limits by physicians themselves. One family practice resident adamantly argued, "It's nobody's business what the doctor and patient talk about in the privacy of the examining room. The doctor-patient relationship is a special relationship in which you're trying to help another person. To bring up the subject of fees or collection would make them wonder whether you had some ulterior motive and not exclusively the patient's interest at heart."

Although I continue to broach the subject in annual seminars, the topic is never welcomed. Somehow, it does not belong. Confidentiality, privacy, and beneficence, three of the most exalted virtues of medicine, confer upon the clinical relationship the dual qualities of exclusiveness and sanctity, not to mention a certain unreality. The introduction of money matters into medicine proper constitutes a violation of the sacred by the profane, the clean by the dirty.

Front Versus Back: Identity Splitting in Medicine

During several years' involvement in residency training, I gleaned the presence of a chronic but low grade conflict between medical and administrative staff about paperwork. Physicians wish to devote their full effort to patient care, unencumbered by "administrative detail." "It is not our problem," they often insist with respect to "accounting" matters. In part, this is precisely why they employ receptionists, transcriptionists, bookkeepers, accountants, and business managers. Yet even though the latter group is recruited for the purpose of assuming the burden of financial arrangements, its members have difficulty gaining the cooperation of the physicians.

Nevertheless, a persistent effort has taken place to improve communication between the receptionist-business sector and the medical sector of the clinics with which I am familiar. Attempts have been made to modify various forms to enable the resident physician to feel less burdened by paperwork: to come to agreement upon lists of patients whose charts are incomplete, others whose accounts are delinquent, and still others who are not to be seen at the clinic because of their steadfast refusal to pay for services received. A recurring focus of this ongoing conflict has been the patient "charge ticket" that specifies type of visit, procedures, and tests and that the physician is to fill out upon completion of each patient encounter and hand to the patient to take to the front desk at the clinic. This charge ticket has been redesigned several times. Its use requires constant reclarification. Common agreement on its purpose and utility has been virtually impossible to achieve. (I add in passing that another symbol and focus of these clinics' chronic illness is the hapless laboratory slip that specifies what tests are to be ordered, their results, and so on. Bad feelings intermittently erupt between nurses or medical assistants, ["the girls," as they are called in "the back"] and the laboratory technician[s] as to who should take the responsibility for filling out the slips, especially when the clinic is busy. Each considers it an imposition by the other, a feeling fueled by the perception that the lab is not an authentic part of "the back.")

At times, I attempted to interrupt the chronic misunderstanding and mutual recriminations between the business, or administrative, sector and the medical, or healing, sector by bringing the two groups together into joint seminars. They usually seated themselves at opposite ends, or on opposing sides, of a large conference table! I found myself identified, however, as siding with administration for having raised financial matters publicly. Although physicians assumed that financial arrangements and expectations were present, they preferred that such matters remain implicit. Business agendas were not to be discussed. Emoluments of the profession (trade) must remain a silent matter, despite the public outcry about health care costs. To address it publicly, then, was to violate the privacy and exclusivity of the doctor-patient relationship. One primary care physician said, "At the MEC [minor emergency clinic], after I put the stitches in, I go hide. [Gesturing with a wave of the hand:] Bye! I don't like the fees we have to charge. They can tell them [the patient] the bad news up front [at the reception/business desk]."

My "discovery," therefore, was simply that there was a widely recognized problem that somehow could not be resolved despite everyone's earnest efforts. The administrative sector could not understand why every effort to simplify the paperwork and make it more efficient was greeted by the physicians with such uniform contempt and seeming subterfuge. After all, the administrators complained, they were only trying to help make life easier for the physicians; they were only doing their jobs. For their part, the physicians felt that no problem existed because their responsibility lay only with treating patients' sicknesses. In fact, they felt that the administrative sector was creating unnecessary obstacles for them, placing barriers between themselves and the patient, "contaminating" patient care. They felt that administration was asking them to do what the administrators themselves should have been doing outside of the physician-patient interaction.

Attending faculty physicians tended to support this latter view. Their own interest—be it during grand rounds, hospital rounds, or patient consultation—centered upon honing the resident's differential diagnosis of disease, assessing and improving the resident's clinical judgment with respect to ordering tests and procedures (with occasional consideration for cost effectiveness), and putting the finishing touches on the resident's biomedical techniques of patient management. Attending faculty physicians tended to be as uneasy in directly dealing with financial matters as were the trainees. It thus became impossible to solve a problem that only one party to the dispute defined and perceived as a *shared* problem.

At issue in this problem was a discrepancy between competing value orientations (Kluckhohn and Strodtbeck 1961), specifically, between ideal and operant values (Spiegel 1971), between espousable and inexpressable values within medicine and between the medical and management sectors of medicine. The conflict between medical-associated values of caring and business-associated values of profit management was here compartmentalized into the institutionalized division of labor between the medical and business sectors. Staff, residents, and faculty alike spatially divided the clinic into two distinct realms: the front and the back. (Other medical institutions, such as hospitals, vertically bifurcate between upstairs and downstairs or compartmentalize functions in different buildings, some separated by miles.) The physicians in these clinics had "resolved" the problem of ambivalence regarding management of finances within medicine by allocating the unacceptable part of it to administration.

The front of the clinics under discussion referred to the reception area and the business office located adjacent to it or closely associated with its functions. The receptionists and clinic administration worked in this area. Among the chief responsibilities of those working in this area were to request, collect, or arrange terms of payment from a patient upon the conclusion of the encounter with the physician. The back referred to the corridors and rooms in which the resident physicians, nurses, medical technologists, and faculty worked. It included the nursing station(s), which served as a protective barrier for the physicians, who were thereby able to work with minimal outside interference.

The nursing station with its attendants was a perpetual "liminal" (Turner 1969) or transitional region, neither front nor back, one that bordered upon two adjacent yet mutually exclusive roles. The function of the station was to conserve the sanctity of space and time in the examining rooms, which were, as many have put it, the "Holy of Holies." All that was medically nonessential (that is, nonurgent from the medical viewpoint) did not get conveyed through this barrier (except perhaps for incoming phone calls from physicians' families and other doctors). Through the nursing station, the separation of and commerce between front and back were regulated. Likewise, the front was somewhat of a liminal area mediating between the clinic and the outside world. From the perspective of the back, it was the primary function of the front and the nursing station(s) to police and mediate the flow of information and patients into and out of the sacred space.

Whereas patient care was the principal activity of the back, financial matters constituted a preeminent concern of the front (others included scheduling patients, transcribing medical tapes, answering telephones, sorting mail). Emphasizing the importance of their role in the clinic operation, members of the front repeatedly invoked such adages as "Quality service at a fair price"; "You only get what you pay for"; "The one who doesn't charge doesn't get respect [from his or her patients]"; "The more you charge, the more you're respected."

Resident physicians, on the other hand, maintained that "money is not our problem. We need to see lots of patients regardless of their ability to pay. We need the patients for our training." Physicians often interpreted clinic staff's requests for payment following an office visit as an expression of hostility toward the patient. They would often intercede in the patient's behalf, an act that employees at the front interpreted as "interfering" with their jobs. In the angry words of one business manager:

> It is the receptionists' job to ask initially for payment when patients leave the doctor's office. When they do their job, they are accused by the doctors and nurses of being "ugly." They say we're "hassling" the patients. If I hear the word "hassle" one more time, I'm going to explode. You can't win. If you do what you're expected to do, you get accused of being inconsiderate of patients. You're in a bind. The doctors make the girls up front to look like they're money-hungry. For instance, one doctor will say to a patient. "If you pay just a little each month, they won't be mean to you," or "they won't hassle you" or "get on your case." "Getting ugly" is my term, one I got from living in the South. It means hostility. But there's nothing especially hostile about asking a patient to pay for a service they've just received.

At an earlier case conference, one physician characterized the staff in the clinic reception/business office as "the bad guys" who are hired to deal with money matters. On such occasions, I combine gentle confrontation with interpretation to try helping physicians to recognize that they are able to be the "good guys" only if another group is willing to serve (and be paid to serve) as the "bad guys." In fact, such virtuousness and superiority are purchased and sustained at the price of chronically diminished clinic and institutional morale. Occasionally, defenses such as splitting and projection diminish in an individual resident, and the role internalization of "bad" topics that had been exclusively allocated to other staff occurs. For the most part, however, the need for the splitting and projection and the institutional-cultural rewards for them carry the day.

Front and back representatives came to hold reciprocal or mirror images of themselves and the other. Both saw themselves as conscientiously doing their job and perceived the other as violating the rules and undermining their own best efforts. Each saw the other as making unfair demands on their time, energy, and sense of responsibility. Each branded the other as "greedy." Each likewise felt that if only the other would give in a little, everyone would be "one big happy family" again. These mirror images served as what Wynne (1965) calls "traded dissociations." They kept the conflictual relationship going and in turn prevented resolution.

The medical division of labor is ostensibly founded upon culture-specific "scientific" management principles. But it is as much based upon what Stierlin (1972, 1973, 1974, 1976) refers to as the "delegation" of a disavowed portion of one's personality to another, appointing that other to act as unconscious proxy of the first. This other is sent out, entrusted with a mission (Stierlin 1972). Indeed, accepted management norms almost successfully disguise at the same time as they implement this delegation. Through the division of labor between care and business, medicine can deny and project the profit motive onto the ulterior and therefore unsavory motives of the business office and collection agency at the same time that medicine pursues these motives ***through*** others who identify with what is projected onto them, adapting to their roles in addition to having been drawn (recruited) to them. (For studies of these dynamics in international relations, see GAP Committee on International Relations and Stein 1987; Stein 1987b; Volkan 1988.)

Physician and patient commonly negotiate a dyadic alliance that triangulates a third member or unit to bear the burden of potential conflict within the dyad. The business office, receptionists, collection agents may serve as the target or container of unacceptable or bad parts that cannot be integrated into the doctor-patient relationship (such as tallying up the amount of money owed and collecting it) without threatening to disrupt it. The physician-patient relationship can preserve the preambivalent, good, nurturant constancy only so long as the bad is allocated to others, who thereby become "their" attributes. The current torrent of medical malpractice lawsuits serves to further heighten physicians' fear lest patients avenge themselves should physicians fail to fulfill the image that the good doctor requires. The practice of defensive medicine has thus led to further attempts to expel outside the doctor-patient relationship anything that would tarnish the aura of beneficence.

Seen in this light, receptionists, bookkeepers, administrative managers, and collection agencies all serve as psychological extensions of part-functions that cannot be assimilated into the physician's own concept of the physician role. Such a division of labor can be an interpersonally and institutionally implemented compromise formation in which one can simultaneously pursue capitalistic (profit) interests while repudiating them. The intolerable flaw of imperfect compassion and altruism that physicians often criticize in their administrative staff is one they have allocated to personnel in the reception and business sector of the clinic or hospital or practice. In turn, this sector acts out these financial interests in their (the doctors') behalf by performing assigned tasks with great industry.

Conflicting Priorities Within Medicine

In this same clinical setting, considerable difference of opinion existed between front and back factions as to whom the clinic was designed for and what constituted responsibility or accountability. Did the clinic exist for the sake of residents, staff, patients, and educators or for some wider mission or target population? What merited greatest emphasis: service to patients, training for residents, income production for the office? There was little consensus on these answers.

The following event illustrates the ordinariness of priority conflicts as ingrained within a variety of personnel in medicine. It occurred at a community-based primary care residency training setting that was an affiliate of an urban-based tertiary care medical center and school of medicine. An administrator of the community program (clinic) asked me to give him an ethnographic consultation on a problem. Earlier that day, the director of the clinic laboratory had come dejectedly to the administrator's office saying that medical assistants in the back (the patient care part of the clinic) were refusing to draw blood during periods of high patient volume. The lab was responsible for most of the workups for the outpatient population that the clinic served. The lab director reported that there was no way that she could do all the phlebotomy and run all the tests for all the clinic physicians.

The larger context of the problem, it should be noted, was a profoundly depressed local and state economy; a reduced medical, clerical, and business office staff due to repeated cutbacks mandated by the medical school administration; and the presence of a full complement of residents in need of patients and support staff for their training. For more than fifteen years, various receptionists, medical assistants, nurses, and even residents had eagerly pitched in during times of heavy patient load. They had learned and performed others' roles. Such generalist role adaptations had been a source of increased group camaraderie and of chagrin by division heads, who were often appalled that helpers simply jumped in and improvised ways to perform tasks instead of following clinic protocol.

Shorthanded, in the transition zone between the busy "flu" (winter) and "allergy" (spring) seasons, the clinic had recently had heavy personnel turnover, and each division head was busily training new personnel. In such an atmosphere, a more specialist role mode had settled in. The head nurse in the back had refused permission for her medical assistants to perform laboratory-related functions. She felt that there was enough for them to do already in the back. The laboratory director then felt abandoned and "in the middle," with heavy clinic demands yet little support for her efforts. Complicating matters further, the lab director was one of the few-remaining "old-timers." She began to feel virtually demoted rather than rewarded for her loyalty to the clinic's teaching and patient care efforts.

Moreover, in later months, several residents had complained at clinic meetings and at case conferences that educational activities were being sacrificed for an increasing quantity of patients who were "mysteriously" appearing on their schedules. In fact, one source of acrimony conveyed by resident physicians was their sense of having no control over their own schedules. Residents wondered how they could take time to visit with their patients or to learn about various rare diseases or management if they were allotted so little time per patient. When could they study up or consult with faculty physicians?

The clinic administrator sought my perspective because I had the reputation of being holistically "all over the place," with wide geographic range of the clinic. My first comment was that everyone was trying to give 200 percent under extenuating circumstances. Further, although I did not see this as primarily a conflict of "personalities," all employees' self-esteem was bound up with their ability to perform their role successfully and to be recognized as contributing to the program. I suggested that he talk with the nurse, medical assistants, and laboratory director together, eliciting and encouraging them to compare their own expectations and expectations of the others. In this way their recriminations might diminish by greater face-to-face understanding of each other's situation.

But I further suggested that we widen the scope of the problem so that it was not limited to the medical assistants versus the laboratory. I said that in my opinion, part of the reason that the laboratory director was asking for help from the medical assistants, while the nursing department was declining such requests, was that both departments were feeling overwhelmed by the need to take care of so large a volume of patients. Such a perspective, even if only partially correct, required that we ask about the premises underlying the performance of the receptionists and business office (who often likewise substituted for each other in various roles, including time-consuming telephone answering).

Employees in the front had long prided themselves on doing their utmost to increase patient volume and keep the physicians' schedules full. During annual program orientations for new residents, medical and administrative directors routinely emphasized that all personnel, regardless of role, were as much participants in teaching functions as those officially hired as instructors. Quickly, however, that function receded in importance in comparison with the more preeminent one of maintaining patient flow. Perhaps of all staff personnel, the duties of the receptionists were the least formally integrated into residency training and most resembled the front office of a private, group, or corporate practice. I said that in a sense, the receptionists in the front were doing too well at the job they thought they should be doing. Not only their income, but their self-esteem as well, depended on how well they were performing their role.

The conflict between the laboratory and the back was thus a symptom of the wider medical culture conflict between the front and the back. More subtly, it was also a conflict between the educational function (in which, I urged, the receptionists should be given a more explicit, visible, recognized role) and that of patient care tied to clinic income generation and hence survival. Finally, I added, the place where I would begin was not with the laboratory and the back, or even with the front and the back. Rather I recommended that the administrator first have a soul- (and role-) searching discussion with the clinical director, who was locally responsible for setting medical policy for the program.

Staff (medical and administrative), residents, and faculty concurred that the clinic and the training program were created to train resident physicians to practice medicine. In the strictly educational sense, all participants involved in the clinic program—patients included—were there for or in behalf of the residents. In the strictly clinical sense, however, everyone was there to serve the patient population. In yet another sense—one only rarely made explicit and then mostly by administrative staff—the residents were there also in behalf of the clinic; education, service, and income were to be balanced in a quid pro quo. That is, the clinic was a service facility in which patient-generated income partially sustained the educational facility.

Residents' and medical faculty values could be arranged in a hierarchy (following Kluckhohn and Strodtbeck 1961; Spiegel 1971) according to which professional education occupied a first order (highest) position, patient contact occupied a second order position, and production of income for the clinic or training program occupied a third order position (if indeed it was present at all). Business was clearly subordinated to educational and clinical values. Moreover, patient contact was a means to a career end. Seen from the short term, patient care was an instrumental rather than final value. In this perspective, of course, patient contact and education were often indistinguishable. (Occasionally, especially during high patient volume times, even this was an area rife with conflict. Interns and residents complained that the front was "movin' 'em out" [as in a cattle drive!] so fast and filling the clinic schedule so completely that the residents had no time to read, to conduct literature searches, and so on.)

Administrative staff (managers, bookkeepers, receptionists, secretaries) did not rank order these value orientations. Instead, they tended to balance the three delicately as co-equals (education, service, business). They tended to see residents and faculty doctors alike as idealistic, but by contrast perceived themselves as practical and realistic. Whereas physicians tended to measure success almost exclusively in terms of thoroughness of clinical workup, accuracy of diagnosis, patient satisfaction, compliance with prescribed regimen, return visits, and recovery, administrative staff was equally concerned with cost effectiveness.

Administration's attempt to balance its three co-equal priorities also assured a constant tension among them—and a constant need to reresolve them. On the one hand, staff members prided themselves in their compassion ("No one will be turned away just because they are unable to pay"). On the other hand, they vigorously pursued delinquent accounts by turning them over to collection agents. They maintained an active, updated list of patients whose accounts had been officially closed by the clinic and who therefore would not be seen at the clinic.

These patients nonetheless managed to "get by" the receptionists and were seen by resident physicians who were unaware of or oblivious to the ban. One receptionist complained to me, "Some doctors have patients come in through the back door to circumvent the front entirely." Precisely because administration attempted to satisfy inherently incompatible values simultaneously, the administrative staff could appear inconsistent, contradictory, even capricious. Resident and faculty physicians, however, felt that they themselves appeared consistent because their values and priorities were so clearly rank ordered. They faulted administration for "creating" problems because, in their own scheme, the problems did not exist.

Glaring exceptions notwithstanding, physicians generously offered their knowledge, advice, wisdom, availability, and time. The physician who devoted his or her life to *giving* felt acutely uncomfortable talking with patients about *receiving* (let alone demanding) payment for services rendered. Residents expressed embarrassment at the thought of bringing up money matters to a patient or family who may be down and out, perhaps financially as much as physically or emotionally. Reciprocity for clinical services rendered was simultaneously assumed and unmentionable.

Administrative staff often retorted sharply to this sentiment with a stern word of warning: "Just wait until they're out in private practice in the cold, cruel world. Then they'll learn the value of a dollar. That'll change their minds quicker than anything else. You can't eat or feed your family on good will alone." This lesson in reality, so to speak, was the administrative staff's *fantasy* about stark economic reality that administrators conveyed in the language of perception and prophecy that promised to vindicate the staff's own values. It was also the staff's psychologically delegated function to be "cold" and "cruel," from which role staff members recoiled even as they executed it. They were *recruited* for roles that they were subsequently accused of executing too zealously. They rationalized their behavior by projecting the necessity for it upon the external world, just as the physicians rationalized their own behavior by projecting their darker sides into roles they created for their administrative staffs. Through externalization, both front and back could feel good, vindicated, about what they did. Each was the other's evil double or disavowed counterpart.

In my experience, the chronic conflict between business and patient care sectors of medical training and community practice institutions alike accounts for many of the brush fires that seemingly erupt spontaneously—and this between persons who at other times harbor boundless goodwill toward one another. This conflict can be viewed as something of an enduring institutional, if not cultural, structure that becomes manifested in or channeled into various and diverse forms. A psychodynamic view of this chronic irresolution suggests that a shared unconscious story or agenda ***generates***, ***sustains***, and ***assures*** the ***displacement of attention*** onto superficial (in the sense of surface, but not in the sense of inconsequential) issues.

To illustrate this, let me briefly return to the metaphor of brush fires. On various occasions, disputes arise about the medical charge ticket, what information is to be charted in the medical record, who is responsible for filling out laboratory slips, procedures to be followed when patients telephone their doctors, the determination of what fees to charge the patient, the pursuit of delinquent accounts, and the like. These are temporarily solved, subside, and flare up again. These various brush fires constitute the surface picture, the focus of firefighting activities.

For the most part, however, among members of this biomedical culture, the focus is consistently mistaken to be the cause or source. Although clinical charge tickets, lab slips, and patient scheduling are bona fide realities, they bear the burden of a shared unconscious division of labor between the medical and business sectors. This constitutes the underlying picture, the arsonists, as it were, who are responsible for setting particular fires and keeping them well tended. It is the fantasy structure of the group that keeps the underbrush ready to be enflamed. Such implicit patterns are responsible for the form taken by many surface cultural features, although the specific content of these forms does not necessarily reduce to these underlying patterns. Stated differently, the conflict between front and back did not create the need for charge tickets or scheduling rules. But through a kind of psychodynamic functionalism, these items of cultural content serve as frequent media through which the unconscious fires continue to burn, where the flames are allowed to be seen and the heat felt.

Many psychiatry, family medicine, and occupational medicine interns and residents vow that their private practices, partnerships, HMOs, and hospitals will be nothing like their training environments. In their training environment they object to the feeling (never stated directly to them) that teaching-learning activities take second place to seeing patients in as great a volume as possible. Brief, technology-intensive visits also tend to prevail because "time is money," thereby diminishing familiarity with the patient's story and a more personal relationship with the patient. Training environments tend to be dominated by high-dollar, income-generating procedures. Yet, early in practice, these physicians tend to repeat the clinical routines and implicit priorities of the training environments they so detested. Although they have more autonomy and authority than they previously had as interns and residents, they are for the most part unable to escape those scarcely articulatable conflicts between business- and patient care–related values. In fact, such conflicts are as much institutionalized into physicians' mental structures and choices as they are property of medical bureaucracies.

From having worked with psychiatrists and family physicians for sixteen years, I found that the discrepancy between the ideals, expectations, and conflicts of the training period and those of subsequent private or group practice was not nearly so great as either residents or management tended to believe. Reality did not simply transmogrify every physician from idealist to mercenary, nor did a greater degree of autonomy lead each formerly harried practitioner to devote more emphasis to the doctor-patient relationship. Some physicians privately railed against welfare and condemned patients who exploited their dedication by failing to pay. Yet, to these same patients they nonetheless gave of themselves generously. Others justified their avarice by appeals to external conditions of the medical marketplace. Many physicians outside academic medicine continued to be troubled by the conflict between giving and receiving. Problems described in this clinical training setting permeate the wider practice community and culture of medicine as well. Even such buzzwords as "accountability," "responsibility," and "efficiency" have different frames of reference within the medicine and business systems. The conflict between these two value subsystems is institutionalized into the very social organization and practice of medicine.

The Sacred Shrine of the Bottom Line

Since the early 1980s, no discussion about values, standards, choices, even ethics in medicine can elude mention of the bottom line. If it is not the new societal summum bonum, the highest good, it is at least the image of final appeal, the argument stopper. Anthropomorphized, it ranks with the ancient mythological characters of fate and necessity. The bottom line is one of the central organizing, obligatory, if also egregiously oversimplifying official stories, clichés, and shibboleths of our time. (For a discussion of money as symbol of anxiety, see Ebel 1980.) Since the late 1970s, and especially the early 1980s, no story is imaginable—or, rather, tolerable—that is not "reframed" or sanctified by it. It is a kind of metastory, or underlying folklore motif, that supersedes, qualifies, or disqualifies all others. Its severe judgment renders some clinical stories legitimate and others illegitimate.

The corporate-industrial metaphors commit biomedicine to fateful choices and destinies. When these metaphors, crystallizations of standardizing stories, become imperative, they become the measure by which reality will and must be assessed. Alternative ways of looking, hearing, feeling, and acting become tantamount to heresy. In such a symbolism-dominated climate, the pursuit and practice of science, of scientifically grounded medicine, and of humane patient care often become insuperably difficult, just as the appeal to such standards in medical professionalism often becomes little more than sham.

In narrating the story of the cut-slash-chop era of the bottom line, I do not claim that the prior fee-for-service era was some golden age of biopsychosocial integration in clinical teaching and practice or of copious compassion for underserved populations. But at least "quality," "care," and "whole person" were part of the lexicon and, to some degree, part of the institution of medicine. Stephens observes that "the industrialization and privatization of medicine are no reforms at all, but the mere extension of a narrowly conceived Scientism into the organization and management of medical practice" (1988b: 187). The institutionalization of corporate medicine—with the cultural blessings of survivalism, social Darwinism, competitivism, minimalism, nuclearism, militarism, and nationalism—has carried the mechanization process many steps further (see Eisenberg 1988: 208–209).

John E. Mack, M.D., writes:

> We tend to treat economics as if it were separate from political power. Yet as political science professor Robert Heilbroner points out, power is "inextricable from economics" (Heilbroner 1988). Heilbroner further suggests that the blindness of economists themselves to the importance of power and ideology—treating business activity as if it occurred in a political vacuum—has limited and distorted our understanding of the social nature of economic behavior (1988: 10).

Kormos observes that

> perhaps more than anything else, one hears that medicine is essentially and simply in a financial crisis (Halenar 1979, Havighurst [and Hackbarth] 1979, Klarman 1977). . . . The question this line of thinking does not answer is why 8% or, for that matter, 10% or even 16% of GNP [Gross National Product] would so obviously be an unacceptably high level of expense for medical care (1984: 324).

Regardless of where the crisis truly lies, a social consensus has formed around the belief that medicine is itself in a crisis that must be remedied by austere means. Kormos concludes about the future of the physician's professionalism that

> obviously the professionalism of the doctor should be sufficient guarantee that his practice will remain of the highest calibre at all times. But what if this professionalism itself is undermined by a gradually increasing regimentation, subtly suggesting that proper medical practice is really more a matter of obeying norms than of exercising judgment? There remains an inherent contradiction between the industrial doctrine of strictly controlled production methods and the physician's obligation to exercise his best judgment at all times (1984: 336).

Admittedly, it is easier now for the entire disavowed component of clinical reality concerned with the assessment and collection of fees to be delegated to third parties ranging from business offices of clinics, hospitals, and health maintenance organizations to insurance companies. In the biweekly newspaper *Family*

Practice News a front-page story, "Family Physician Finds HMO Is His Kind of Practice Arrangement" (Delmar 1987: 1, 46), offers *continuity* to the split between health care service and business functions, together with their associated meanings, that likewise characterized the prior (more individual and group practice–oriented) medicine.

> It's been about 6 years since Dr. Bruce Blumenthal graduated from his residency training program, but it wasn't until recently that he found the kind of practice arrangement that makes him happy: It's one that enables him to practice family medicine without the worries of a businessman.
>
> Dr. Blumenthal found it in an HMO. . . . Now someone else worries about the hiring, the firing, the accounts, the furniture, and even about drumming up enough patients to keep the practice going.
>
> "I am very happy being outside of the business end of things," Dr. Blumenthal said in an interview with FAMILY PRACTICE NEWS at his HMO office (Delmar 1987: 1, 46).

There are a number of paradoxes in this quotation and in the cultural genre of similar ideas I have heard from physicians in recent years. To begin with, the arrangement described here fragments patient care far more than had occurred previously. There is less opportunity for the physician to engage in staff/clinic development and morale building, because the staff is not the physician's "own." Similarly, the furniture in the waiting area, or the amount of space in the examination room, can very much set the tone for the practice climate; yet in the new era, such matters are usually beyond the physician's control.

A play area with toys can be used not only to keep children "occupied" while their parents are waiting or seeing the doctor; it can often double for play therapy. Practices with a large elderly population can benefit from having waiting room chairs that are moveable, rather than fixed. This would allow patients who have a difficult time hearing one another or turning their bodies to adjust the chairs for this significant social occasion. Finally, examination rooms need to be spacious in order to accommodate the presence of family members (or friends) in addition to the patient (who usually is seated on the examination table).

The physician who is primarily the employee of a medical corporation has less authority in the design of the practice environment (or in making policy, hiring staff, and so forth) than physicians in an earlier era had. Yet, these domains, which are germane to patient care and satisfaction, are increasingly relegated to the administrative or business office. Stated differently, what the physician himself or herself, and what the medical corporation itself, defines as within the purview of patient care is narrowing dramatically. This trend appears to be occurring in part by physicians' preference and in part by acquiescence to (if not identification with) the local and national corporate administrative structure (see Deal and Kennedy 1982; Parin 1988).

A medical administrator colleague who had long felt that he had to subordinate his ideas and wishes to the dictates of hospital and clinic physician-superiors triumphantly said to me when the first DRGs were instituted in 1982, "I look forward to the day when we administrators will tell physicians what diagnoses they can and cannot do." Increasingly, the medical domain is shrinking, while the business domain is expanding. There is additional irony to the physician's belief that by joining an HMO he would extricate himself from "the business end of things"—HMOs and other medical corporations came into being to promote cost containment and profitmaking. The business end of things is increasingly integral to clinical decisionmaking and patient care, even as physicians strive all the harder to assign business functions to others. The more inroads that business has upon practice, the more physicians must deny that such inroads have occurred and must widen or deepen the split that has long been there. If anything, the incursion of business concerns into medical practice has intensified the need to delegate to others the distasteful role of exacting payment for medical care. Donald A. Bloch, M.D., writes that

> Control over access to health care is the way in which the burden of costs is allocated and benefits distributed. It is difficult for most of us to get a handle on the subject of health-care economics, and when we do so as professionals, it is in the narrow sense of trying to influence hospital privileges (access, again), or licensing, or reimbursement, or third-party payer procedures. But out of these moment-to-moment decisions emerges a big picture, a picture that is fateful for our personal and professional lives. . . . Deliberately or inadvertently, health-care consumers and providers are set against each other; each of a multiplicity of competing interests advances its own narrow view of self-interest. Survival in a system so created requires inordinate time spent on record-keeping and paperwork, so that the energy demands of simply negotiating the system are formidable. Practice strategies develop in a context that contributes to the problem by maximizing the economic return from more and more fractionated and particularized approaches to clinical work. A sure recipe for disaster. In Pogo's timeless words, "We have met the enemy and he is us" (1987b: 403).

The image of the bottom line enhances the cultural value and the reimbursability of technologically mediated tests and interventions and likewise sanctions the brief, depersonalized clinical relationships that accompany them. The business metaphor concomitantly downplays the cultural value and severely limits the reimbursability of careful listening, commitment, intimacy, and the taking of time with one's patient. Here societywide conflict, if not shift in values, is culturally defined and displaced onto medicine as if cost containment (economics) were the entire issue.

In a courageous challenge to the sanctity of bottom line as the dogma of final appeal, David Himmelstein, Steffie Woolhandler et al. offer a physicians' proposal for a national health program for the United States. They begin with a verdict that has been little heard publicly during the last decade:

> Our health care system is failing. It denies access to many in need and is expensive, inefficient, and increasingly bureaucratic. The pressures of cost control, competition, and profit threaten the traditional tenets of medical practice. For patients, the misfortune of illness is often amplified by the fear of financial ruin. For physicians, the gratifications of healing often give way to anger and alienation. Patchwork reforms succeed only in exchanging old problems for new ones (1989: 102).

If a thorough and honest debate about corporate medicine, and about standards for setting health policy, is to occur, the bureaucratization of medicine must not become the new scapegoat. Until the cultural meaning of the bottom line is understood, until the perennial split between health providers and administration is addressed and healed, and until the symbolic burden of money in medical care is appreciated, even the next wave of American health care reforms—no matter how consciously high-minded they are—will flounder and will "succeed only in exchanging old problems for new ones."

Aggression: The Phantom in Medical Finance

Medicine remains an income-producing profession that must disavow that it benefits or profits from others' ailments—both from the illness itself and from the experience of regression that leads to some degree of dependency attendant upon asking another for help. With nervous laughter, physicians wonder what would become of them were they too successful in eradicating disease or too equal a partner in treatment. Medicine goes to considerable lengths to create and sustain the illusion that emoluments do not exist.

Many of the younger generations of doctors are not as torn between medicine and money as I have suggested. Many are business-people first and doctors second. Their secretaries and other administrative staff are tailor-picked to reflect their stern financial priorities, making it impossible for welfare patients even to get an appointment. This new attitude within medicine does not vitiate my argument; rather, it attests to the tenacity of the taboo in the very aggressiveness, almost indifference, with which it is violated. Likewise, the sheer obtuseness or bravado with which many physicians now flaunt the business side of medicine has an unmistakable protest quality to it. The refusal to be guilty is, nonetheless, a way of dealing with one's guilt feelings.

The following statement represents a sentiment that I have heard many physicians articulate since the early 1980s. Even the most conscientious physicians have expressed frustrations in finding adequate solutions to the problems of money management in medicine.

> When I started out in medical school, there was an acute doctor shortage. Now they say there's an oversupply of physicians. Patients have gone to the ER for every little thing, and doctors have kept patients hospitalized far longer than they should have. We've had it coming for years. If we can't police ourselves, somebody will lay down the law on us—and it'll be far worse than if we had done it ourselves long ago. Families and communities have got to learn to take care of their own. Medicine isn't a charity; it's a profession like any other. But there's going to be a lot of suffering because of these changes, especially among older folks and the poor.
>
> I'm beginning to wonder whether we're not becoming agents of financial institutions rather than advocates of patients. I don't hear much anymore about quality of care. Just get the patients in and out of the hospital as fast as possible. I hate to think that we're treating lab results instead of patients. Then we have to resort to sleazy ways to circumvent the system in order to treat patients with the care they need—

like running additional tests to find some laboratory abnormality that'll justify our keeping them in the hospital or admitting them.

It's a whole new world that we're entering in the middle 1980s. Less and less compassion. All we hear about at conferences is the dollar. Instead of talking about patients, they talk about "consumers." Health care is supposed to be some kind of "product," and I'm constantly being notified of seminars and journals and books that promise to tell me how to "market" my practice. We've got to attract patients, but I get uneasy about the big sell. How do you build trust with patients and with a community in such a hyped, contentious climate? And you're torn in several directions at once. The patient sues you if you don't diagnose right, but the government doesn't want you to do all those tests that would eliminate or confirm the diagnosis. I see more paperwork these days than I see patients. And this is supposed to be less government. It's harder and harder to walk into an exam room and try to help patients when all this other weighs on your mind.

Against this background, one begins to understand the only apparent contradiction between physicians' idealism as expressed in their dedication to patient care and their resistance to medical prepayment plans that would guarantee them but also limit them to fixed salaries. The flaw in their idealism is their forbidden aggression. They cannot openly elicit recompense for their services but must rely on others to perform such tasks. These support people are in turn scorned precisely because their function must be disavowed even as it is required. Yet in many physicians' views, socialized medicine or a national health care policy is a threat to the free enterprise system that would allow them fulfillment as cultural Americans. Their idealism and free-enterprise medicine are entirely compatible so long as physicians do not directly pursue capitalistic self-interest within the clinical context. Corporate medicine offers financial incentives to practitioners who are cost effective, while sanctioning or weeding out those who are not. By merging self-interest with the economic success of the organization, physicians can be aggressive on behalf of the corporation without feeling that they are placing personal gain above patients' best interest.

That fantasies and wishes dealing with aggression, and defenses against them, heavily underlie health care personnel's reluctance to deal with financial issues directly with patients is illustrated by the following example (also see Paul 1978, 1988, for a discussion of aggression and human nature). The setting is a clinical department's meeting convened to discuss turning delinquent patient accounts over to outside collection agencies. The meeting was attended by about twenty physicians, administrative/financial staff, and myself. On the formal agenda, presented by the business manager, were six sequential items: (1) when patient accounts are to be considered delinquent; (2) first collection letter; (3) notification of physician; (4) final collection letter; (5) when delinquent accounts are turned and patient is notified; and (6) withdrawal from patient care, plus attached sample letters. At first, most of the discussion was legalistic, polite, euphemistic. Questions arose as to how much time to allow patients before they are contacted because many businesses would not allow ninety days to pass before a bill was turned over to a collection agency.

Early in the meeting two physicians briefly raised the question as to whether patients and their families would understand such phrases as "Your account with us is becoming delinquent"; "Your account will be subject to further collection efforts"; "Your account has been turned to our agency for collections." These two physicians' inquiries into the language of the letters—"Will our patients understand these letters?"—were not picked up on by the group, which returned to legalistic and leniency issues. Ten or fifteen minutes later, I again brought up the issue of possible disparities between what we were trying to convey in the letters and what patients and their families actually read. I took the linguistic issue further, noting that *we* as a group were trying to be nice about a subject that was inherently not nice: asking people to pay money, especially asking people who had not shown a willingness to pay. As a result, I wondered aloud, were we clouding the issue by being too euphemistic or abstract?

Suddenly, aggressive wishes and fantasies were unleashed in the group. One participating physician seriously suggested that instead of writing, "Your account with us is becoming delinquent," we should write, "You owe us money." Another added, "Pay up, or we'll break both your legs." The group broke into laughter. Several members of the group criticized the phrase "subject to further collection efforts" as being too euphemistic, too passive, that we could state the issue more straightforwardly. Shortly thereafter, one physician suggested that we draw a picture of a gun pointed at a person's head, together with a picture of a wallet, as a means of being concrete about our wishes. He added, "Get Godzilla with a baseball bat, saying, 'Fork over your money or else.'"

From numerous discussions such as these, I have realized that the splitting between the clinical and business sectors of medicine, the use of euphemism and legalism in communication about money, and the avoidance of direct conversation with patients about the costs of medical care and what they owe all serve the function of repression and displacement of aggression. The medical practitioner becomes the repository of the good, the libidinal, while the business office implements the bad, the aggressive. Role and personnel splits prevent physicians' aggression from getting out of control. At the same time, the less it can be integrated into the professional self of the practitioner, the more monstrous it becomes.

In this system of splitting, each participant within the clinic setting is trying hard to do his or her job well, unaware of the emotional division of labor beneath the official job description. So long as physicians are presumed to be selfish, are expected to be selfless, and solve their dilemma by hiring others to be responsible for them, the conflict *cannot* resolve. All efforts at conflict resolution that do not address these unconscious issues in the division of labor are condemned to failure, not because the participants lack goodwill but because they fail to recognize where the problems are located and what sort they are. Stated differently, the problem cannot be solved so long as the participants adhere to shared psychocultural premises about medicine's identity. In order for the conflict to be solved, what is taboo must be addressed openly. Yet it is of the very nature of a taboo to obscure its subject matter (wish) by displacing it into symbol and ritual. Sadly, given the premises that the taboo sustains, putative solutions are but a restatement of the problem. Only as medicine can cease to be "sacred" and business "profane" can the problem be truly resolved.

Finance in Medicine: The Elusive "Big Picture"

The dynamics of the money taboo presented here would seem to give credence to the proposition that problems defy resolution when they are incompletely posed—that is, when efforts to solve them occur at a level that does not encompass the entire scope of the problem. More than cognitive, perceptual, and logical Aristotelian processes are involved, however. For problems that *cannot* be solved are usually those that *must not*, for affective reasons, be addressed. Certainly, in the present case, a problem that must not even be discussed is hardly amenable to resolution! More often than we would like to acknowledge, techniques of problem-solving and clinical methods of treatment are rituals mainly designed to alleviate anxiety by preventing the full scope (breadth and depth alike) of the problem from arising to conscious awareness.

Thus conceived, ritual "solutions" are shared defensive maneuvers unconsciously designed to reassure participants that they are doing something about the problem as they perceive and define it while mystifying its more terrifying sources. Ritual solutions are compromise formations that simultaneously reveal and conceal. They are a shared form of resistance to insight into the full problem, a means of avoiding it. Such solutions assure the persistence of the problem because in the structure of the unconscious the problem itself represents a kind of solution. So long as individual, family, institution, and society collude in their efforts to solve problems in this manner, even with all the effort and goodwill in the world, they will nonetheless further entrench themselves while firmly believing that they are at last digging themselves free. This leads, I believe, to the inescapable conclusion that just as "ritual makes explicit the social structure" (Leach 1954: 15), so likewise does unresolved conflict that takes the form of insuperable "social problems" keep implicit the unconscious structure of the society while acting it out.

I have in recent years arranged for an annual seminar to be offered to the resident groups by a financial counselor. These seminars consist in part of a series of exercises in value clarification and rank ordering priorities, together with an enumeration of representative types of financial planning (insurance, property, stocks, bonds, extended family resources). My intention in organizing these seminars is to help the residents to think about their own life goals, the time frameworks in which these goals are located, and the means or options available to achieve these goals. Guiding this diversion from patient care is my hope that in taking the resident physicians' life situations and futures seriously, I also prepare them to take that of their patients likewise more seriously.

Resident and faculty physicians alike express gratitude for the availability of these presentations and are attentive and inquisitive during the seminars. They diffidently acknowledge their naivete and inexperience in financial planning. The residents' location in their individual, familial, and occupational life cycles only partly explains their overall obliviousness to financial matters. In my own experience, as in that of the financial counselor whose clientele includes physicians of all ages, physicians in general are not predisposed to careful long-term financial planning for themselves or for their families.

The overarching framework for physicians' perception of time is that of the patient's course of illness and its management, which is to say, short term, the immediate future. Physicians' lives are embedded in a daily cyclic schedule of office visits, hospital rounds, chart reviews, procedures, and meetings. To use a personal example, one of the most exasperating facets of my clinical teaching and supervision is that even though my behavioral science conferences and Balint groups are well publicized on official schedules, most residents, interns, and faculty consistently do not consult them to organize their time. Although patient care qualifies as a formidable justification for a physician's absence, this smokescreen does not tell the whole story. Physicians tend not to think of time in terms of the hour of the day (except at night!). Rather, they tend to think of it patient by patient, exam room by exam room, until no more patients remain to be seen. Physicians only rarely consider life outside this rather rigid framework, which thus makes long-range planning somewhat foreign and mysterious and likewise tends to leave the physician vulnerable despite short-term financial security.

Physicians also assume that this cycle of activities—and therefore its financial rewards—will continue indefinitely. "The future" is envisioned to look remarkably like the present, which is to say that the distant reality of physical decline and death *in the physician* is averted through an almost exclusive involvement within the preserve of immediate cure through patient care. "I'm too busy to think of those kinds of things" is an oft heard retort to administration's entreaties that the physician deal with patients' financial matters and is likewise a commonplace reply to attempts to help physicians in their own financial planning. Whatever its partial truth, it is a shared rationalization, the *purpose* of which is to keep at bay the ultimate motivations for keeping busy. Taken as a whole, the ritual side of medicine is an elaborate attempt to bring vulnerability, frailty, and death magically under human dominion. Uneasiness about money reflects uncertainty about the extent of one's control, goodness, and, finally, immortality. Linear time is inexorable; it cannot be reversed. Neither physician nor patient can be "cured" of time's affliction (see Becker 1973; Brain 1977; Shapiro 1988, 1989).

Thus, not only is money an embarrassing subject for physicians (wherein a sense of shame and humility can partly mollify patients' envy), and one that arouses guilt (for fear that one is exploiting the vulnerable); at a deeper level, conscious consideration of money issues threatens to undermine the physician's use of medical practice as a massive defense against biological time. Anthropomorphized, time is a formidable adversary, a menace who lurks behind every symptom, diagnosis, and treatment plan. If souls cannot be saved, perhaps at least bodies might be salvageable from death. Biomedicine is in part a battle to postpone, if not defeat, death. The physician-patient relationship is likewise often used by the physician to mirror the physician's elusive self-ideal of untempered goodness and perfection. This ideal is one born of childhood need and now reenacted as the physician strives to bask in the adulation that comes from clinical success and patient satisfaction. Yet timeless love and perfection are imperfectly mirrored by a refractory clinical reality. With inevitable ambivalence, error, and loss, inexorable time further intrudes upon every effort to arrest it.

The pursuit of medical cure is the pursuit of control as well as the conscious effort to assist a suffering human being. Through the patient, the physician pursues the struggle for control over death. Part of the aversion physicians have to dealing too closely with money are the imperfection and mortality that money elicits (symbolizes) in time. If "time is money," then money is also time. It is little wonder that physicians prefer not to hear about, or to deal with, money in conjunction with patient care. It is likewise little wonder that receptionists and business offices feel saddled with an oppressive burden in handling doctors' financial affairs. For ultimately, in trading in time and money, administrative personnel are trading in unconscious matters deeply aversive to their employers and to themselves as well.

The single conspicuous exception to this taboo upon incorporating financial matters into the intimacy of the doctor-patient relationship is psychoanalysis. The sheer amount of time, and money, often spent in psychoanalysis devoted to scrutinizing the patient's resentment at paying high fees to the therapist is by now proverbial. Money neurosis is likewise the subject of unabating humor within this profession. That money is such an emotion-laden issue in the clinical relationship, and that money is used as manifest content of the patient's transference, helps us to understand the ***prohibition*** against including it within the doctor-patient relationship in medicine.

There is yet a further layer to the badness associated with money. Nearly a century of psychoanalytic, clinical, historical, literary, and religious research has suggested that money is symbolically bound up with feces, the holding on and letting go of aggression, the transformation of pleasure into duty, secrecy, guilt, and anxiety (Freud 1908). One of the most thoroughgoing analyses of the cultural history of the symbolic equation money = feces is offered by Norman O. Brown in ***Life Against Death*** (1959). Similarly, in an exhaustive analysis of German culture through folklore, Dundes explores the emotional links among feces, death, money, and aggression. He poignantly shows (1984: 119–142) how "the image of the Jew in Germany is very closely tied to feces" (1984: 119) and how the Nazi extermination program was created to "cleanse" Germany of those who embodied Germans' own "dirt"—a dynamic of splitting that is to a less murderous degree played out in the American medical/administrative role polarization discussed earlier in this chapter.

DeMause notes that

> ever since Freud pointed out the anal origins of money, it has been common knowledge that money unconsciously represents shit and reflects our ambivalent attitude toward our body products. The rich are "filthy with money," "so rich they stink," bank officials are ***Dukatenscheisser*** [money shitters], and debtors are "up to their necks in shit." As we used to say in the U.S. Army, "on payday, the eagle shits." This language reaches all the way back to the beginnings of money in early civilizations. The Aztecs called it "the shit of the gods," while the Babylonians called it "the shit of hell" (Bornemann 1976). The valued and the devalued have always been acknowledged to be combined in money (1988: 3).

DeMause continues by discussing the guilt associated with possessing and accumulating wealth and the ways that people try to divest themselves of this guilt.

In a similarly breathtaking sweep of the psychohistory of money, Henry Ebel observes that

> whole societies now participate, from top to near-bottom, in the fecal accumulative fantasies that power the entire process; and the process is then perceived as "going out of control." In addition, of course, the flight into gold in a period like our own can be seen as a direct psychological regression. Thus, fecal imagery having to do with the "poisoning" of our planet by radiation and chemicals coincides with direct appeals to the hoarding impulse, as represented by the quantities of gold coins and bullion now finding their way into safe-deposit boxes throughout the world (1980: 229).

Our own era, which demands stringent measures of cost containment in public and private areas alike, is also one redolent with greed, rampant competitivism, corporate takeovers, and panicky capital accumulation. In one sense, there is a dichotomy between "good shit" (gold, money, property) and "bad shit" (pollution, industrial and nuclear waste). Yet, as is exemplified by the discussion of biomedicine in this chapter, no sooner is some shit good than it quickly becomes tainted and must be handed off to and handled by others, who in turn are perceived as somehow dirty, aggressive, bad, greedy, hostile, all disavowed anal retentive/expulsive features of clinicians deposited in business staff as "poison containers" (deMause 1988). The pleasure of frenzied wealth accumulation is made more acceptable, devoid of guilt and shame, when others are delegated the onerous (dirty, execrable) task of doing the actual accumulation in one's behalf.

The most sacred color of biomedicine, and of Western Judeo-Christian religion, is white, color of purity, cleanliness. It is associated with the physician's lab coat and the nurse's uniform, with cure and salvation (see Brain 1977). Black, even dark brown, is associated with dirt, feces, evil, "lower" as opposed to "higher" thoughts, feelings, and kinds of people. Joel Kovel's book, *White Racism* (1971) grimly documents the psychohistory of American whites' perceptions and treatment of blacks, whose social role was to embody whites' disavowed anal aggressiveness and other "impure" impulses.

It is to some degree a paradox that physicians, exposed constantly to their patients' flowing blood, excrement, vomitus, nakedness, and body parts, should be so timid about dealing more directly and self-assuredly with money, which is "merely" a symbol rather than the real thing. It is, however, less of a paradox when one realizes that of all the physical examinations and procedures physicians perform, those associated with the rectum and colon are most disdained and are associated with the most raunchy humor. Faculty physicians, performing chart audits of interns and residents, constantly question why "rectal, deferred" is written in the patient's chart when a complete physical exam was supposedly being performed. In medicine, as throughout American culture, both one's own "shit" and other people's "shit" are the hardest to take, so severely repressed if not split off is the pleasure with which accumulation, holding, and elimination are emotionally charged. Patients, practitioners, staff, and society are all participants in a danse macabre of embodying and trying desperately to disembody their own and others' shit.

In their medical education, physicians are rarely trained to deal with the demandingness and aggressiveness of patients—except to try satisfying them or curing them by doing "more." Even less are they prepared to experience let alone put to use their own disavowed aggressiveness as it threatens to erupt in unwelcomed countertransference. Thus, what cannot be uttered in biomedicine must therefore be relegated to auxiliary staff members. The administrative staff (and billing offices and collection agencies) become the disavowed and reembodied aggressiveness of the physicians whom the staff serves. As Freud (1900a) discovered, where there is no wish, there is no need for prohibition. What is split off and repressed does not remain inactive. It wends its way into such compromises between impulse and prohibition as dreams, religion, folklore, art, and leadership. As this chapter has shown, taboo and its discontents can also be the foundation of a division of labor.

Thus far in this book I have explored the values, metaphors, social roles, group process, and taboos that are facets of the cultural organization of biomedicine. No culture, however, is organized by the interplay of these parts alone. Although the biomedical culture I have thus far portrayed is dynamic rather than static, important sources of its dynamism have not yet been considered. Decades ago, in his 1950 Marett Lecture, Edward E. Evans-Pritchard (1962) eloquently argued for the centrality of a historical perspective in anthropology. He noted that a purely synchronic approach was insufficient to explain either the existence or persistence of a sociocultural system, a point that Kroeber (1948) repeatedly made as well. Evans-Pritchard wrote that "a term like 'structure' can only be meaningful when used as an historical expression to denote a set of relations known to have endured over a considerable period of time" (1962: 181). Earlier chapters have already considered cultural-historical forces that contribute to the shape of American biomedicine. The next chapter closely examines the rigorous educational cycle by which a layperson is prepared to be and is transformed into a doctor. This chapter on formal, institutionalized professional training is then followed by an exploration of the role early childhood development, family relationships, and unconscious structure play in setting the stage for the choice of a medical career—in short, the ontological precursors of medical identities. I hope to show that many of the roots of biomedical culture history can be found in individual and group psychohistory.

SIX

Socialization and The Process of Becoming a Physician

THIS CHAPTER EXPLORES the rite of passage, the socialization process (Turner 1967, 1969; Van Gennep 1908), by which medical students, interns, and residents become doctors. (Much of the discussion can be transposed to describe the process by which a person becomes any type of biomedical practitioner.) The chapter examines the interplay between the "outer" and "inner" experiences of the initiates and of their clinical teachers or preceptors. Clinical teaching/supervision, facilitating Balint groups (see Balint 1957), and counseling interns, residents, and faculty physicians have helped me to perceive unconscious issues and transformations in personality structure during the course of medical training.

From a technical, cursory viewpoint, medical school, internship, and residency are places and processes during which one learns the knowledge, skills, and sacred lore—first in theory, then in apprenticeship—of doctoring. The seven or more years of biomedical curriculum set the stage for the young physician to meet the legal and clinical regulatory standards for medical professional certification and governmental licensure. These, however, are but a part—and from the cultural viewpoint a small part—of the educational task within medicine.

The central task of medical education is the transformation of a lay or "civilian" person into the role and status of a physician. The acquisition of specific intellectual knowledge, clinical methods, and skills are all part of, and subsidiary to, this ritual transformation into a member of the medical profession. Orientations or assumptions intrinsic to the culture of biomedicine strongly inform the lessons that medicine wishes to teach through any selection of medical curricula. Such metamessages account for what it *feels* like to become a physician. This chapter describes the process through which—in the language of physicians—medicine becomes one's "identity," "life," "jealous mistress," "profession," "guild," and "fraternity"—something one is, not only what one does.

The process of going through medical school, internship, and residency does not create young physicians' values, attitudes, expectations, and beliefs ex nihilo. Scores on nationally standardized examinations, interviews with medical schools' admissions committee members, and previous academic preparation in "premed" college curricula (chemistry, biochemistry, biology, microbiology, physics, engineering) are used as powerful screening tools. These select and admit to medical school candidates whose characteristics are most congruent with those of the

TABLE 6.1
RECIPROCAL SELECTION PROCESS

Early Family Environment	Personal Career Decision-making	Institutional Selection	Professional Preparation	Practitioner Role Identification
Family role, childhood experiences, unconscious structure	Self-selection for healer role, personal role, premed curriculum in colleges	Medical recruitment by institutions, congruence w/ admissions committee and institutional ethos	Medical socialization for practitioner role; medical school, internship/residency	Practitioner role; affirmation by patients, peers; social role in institution and community

admitting medical institution and its clinical cultural ethos. Medicine selects to intensify through formal education those characteristics most like "its" own, which promise continuity to medical culture. In a sense, medical training teaches candidates what they are most receptive and eager to learn because medicine has first selected them for this aptitude. There is thus considerable continuity between the applicant's family role, mental structure, and institutional "character" fit—the latter of which prepares the medical student and resident for the practitioner role, the eventual social role of physician. See Table 6.1 for an overview of this initial selection process.

In his anthropological study of religion, Anthony F. C. Wallace describes a "ritual learning" process (1966: 239–242) that also occurs in secular settings such as medical education. Philip Bock summarizes this process as "the rapid reorganization of experience under conditions of stress, resulting in far-reaching cognitive and emotional changes" (1988: 190). Following recruitment into medical school, one undergoes a process of "conversion" from a layperson to a medical professional. More is involved than the acquisition of knowledge and technique. One's view of oneself and of the world is restructured during this ritual process.

The educational rituals of medical school, internship, and residency have as one of their major functions the creation of boundaries. Good identities and feelings are cultivated, kept inside oneself, and become associated with being inside the safe boundaries of biomedicine, if not within the specific borders of one's chosen medical specialty. Bad feelings are translocated outside. In writing of the function of ritual, Volkan begins with

> Erikson's [1977] idea that ritualization deflects onto outsiders our feelings of unworthiness. This is especially true in adolescence, when the various rituals of confirmation act as "a second birth" (p. 83) by integrating all childhood identifications into a wider view of the world. At the same time they crystallize as ideologically foreign all those belief systems, wishes, and images that have become undesirable (1987: 915).

In medical school, one learns ways *not* to be, think, and feel and how to replace these with prescribed ways of being, thinking, and feeling commensurate with the clinical role and status one eventually hopes to assume. The "stress" of medical school, or of any other ritual, is *intrinsic* to the emotional climate of learning in which one's very self is to be restructured.

The ritual learning process is a five-stage sequence that Wallace characterizes as invoking the "law of dissociation."

> This is the principle that any given set of cognitive and affective elements can be restructured more rapidly and more extensively the more of the perceptual cues from the environment associated with miscellaneous previous learning of other matters are excluded from conscious awareness, and the more of those new cues which are immediately relevant to the elements to be reorganized are presented. How permanent such a new cognitive synthesis will prove to be depends, presumably, in part on the maintenance of the dissociation (by such devices as actual isolation from prior contacts and the continued presentation of the selected matrix of new cues, including direct suggestions) and in part on reinforcement in the conventional learning sense (1966: 239–240).

The five stages of ritual learning proposed by Wallace consist of:

1. Prelearning: The initiate or novice already possesses some knowledge of what the aspired-to role entails.
2. Separation: The initiate is separated from the wider environment through such methods as sensory deprivation, psychotropic drugs, the imposition of "extreme physical stress, through pain, fatigue, sleeplessness, hunger and thirst, or even actual trauma or illness, in order to restrict attention" (1966: 240), and the "presentation of monotonous and repetitive stimuli, such as drumming, flashing lights, and dancing, which (as in hypnosis) helps to induce trance" (1966: 240). Examples throughout medical school and residency are the frequent clinical slide lectures, often held in large, darkened auditoriums, in which the lecturer presents an onslaught of slides and a wealth of yet more medical "facts" to master and store for recall at a moment's notice.
3. Suggestion: Once the trance state is achieved, the initiate is highly suggestible (including by autosuggestion because the participant deeply *wishes* to succeed in the aspired-to role). The new self restructures beliefs and values and separates from the old self.
4. Execution: When the resynthesis has been achieved, the initiate is expected "to act in accordance with the new cognitive structure" (1966: 241).
5. Maintenance: This often depends on posthypnotic suggestion. But "for 'permanent' change, it is necessary either to renew periodically the ritual itself, or to provide the subject with tangible experience that will serve to maintain the new structure, or both" (1966: 242). In medicine, this maintenance and constant renewal are achieved through limiting association to mostly other clinical colleagues; by regular clinic and hospital staff meetings at which role boundaries are reaffirmed; by a constant "keeping up to date"

with the current, official biomedical literature (journals, books, tapes) that affirm doctrine; by continuing medical education (CME) programs to which one often travels considerable distance to hear medical topics reviewed and updated.

According to Roger Burton and John Whiting, during the liminal period in rites of passage, "the hazing, sleeplessness, tests of manhood . . . together with promise of high status—that of being a man if the tests are successfully passed—are indeed similar to the brainwashing techniques employed by the Communists" (1961: 90). The official American doctrine of individualism notwithstanding, it is in the *group* cauldron of medical school, especially during the internship year, that one is exposed to the constant prospect of public humiliation through the press of sleeplessness, long periods of little or no food, long hours of work, harsh training rituals, and the urgency to perform impeccably and come up with the right answers in the eyes of numerous superiors. In this environment the individualist physician identity is forged, and the drive for self-reliance, the need for absolutes, the renunciation of uncertainty, the fear of failure, and the need to be decisive and virtually self-sufficient are established.

The ritual process of becoming a physician thus involves, among other things, the interplay between the experience of outer assault and inner vulnerability. Masterson writes that "the less intrapsychic structure an individual has, the more he turns to seemingly stable factors in the external world for stability to help him contain and adapt" (1985: 110). From his clinical work he writes that the borderline patient "requires a stable object or an authority to fill his defect in object relations, as well as an external set of rules of guidance to deal with his defects in ego functioning" (1985: 110). People with impaired self-structures are drawn to sects or movements that externally offer functions that the individual lacks internally: a stable, often omnipotent object and a stable auxiliary ego that offers a guide for living and the fantasy of love and affection if the individual adheres to the stringent code of behavior and loyalty.

Masterson describes the dynamic ritual process by which this conversion takes place and allegiance is cemented. In discussing the brainwashing of American prisoners of war in Korea and Vietnam, he writes:

> It could be called psychotherapy in reverse. The individual is not physically tortured, but is deprived of sleep and food, thus weakening his ego resources. He is then isolated with a single interrogator who alternately interrogates and rewards. Over a long period of time the weakening of ego resources and the isolation will impel a borderline individual to unconsciously internalize the wishes of the interrogator in order to relieve his separation anxiety and depression. In this way he is converted. The dynamic for this operation is called identification with the aggressor (1985: 111).

Although I would certainly not apply the label "borderline" to the numerous medical students, interns, and residents in medicine in whom I have seen this transformation from laypersons into physicians, I can attest to the dynamics

Masterson describes. I have long observed—the increasing presence of women in medical school, residency, and medical practice notwithstanding—that medical socialization has been and remains largely a male military experience—for the making of men and women into "medical men." I have likewise long noted the deep cycles of deprivation and indulgence that medical students, interns, and residents go through—be it of sleep, sex, food, alcohol intake, and so forth.

Very early in medical school students learn to learn (Bateson 1972)—that is, they quickly acquire the rules, assumptions, and methods that underlie the acquisition of biomedical knowledge and decisionmaking and technical skills. One of the first lessons is how knowledge is to be categorized. For instance, one category is the "interesting case." The "interesting case" has cognate or related quasimedical terms such as "fascinoma" and "zebranoma" (the suffix "-oma" denoting a tumor, but here used more widely to connote "case," an object of medical "fascination"; "zebra" referring to a rare, exotic disease). It establishes the ground rules, so to speak, for physicians' subsequent interest or lack of interest in "cases." During their training and in practice, nothing can more mobilize many physicians' attention, interest, cognitive skills, willingness to read and conduct literature searches, and collaboration with colleagues than the patient with a biomedically vexing set of "signs" (defined as objective) and "symptoms" (defined as subjective, presented by the patient) that do not suggest a definitive single diagnosis. Occasionally, part of the impetus for the chase comes from physicians' agony over the patient's suffering and their inability to relieve it via a correct diagnosis. More often, the thrill of the etiological fox hunt is cognitively separated from the person of the patient.

At teaching conferences, no stone is left unturned, as faculty question if not "pimp" residents and others for possible leads. Various "war stories" or "horror stories" of possibly similar exemplary cases ("I once had a case something like that") are offered as potentially helpful if not paradigmatic. Participants typically will consult the Washington *Manual of Medical Therapeutics* (Campbell and Frisse 1983), books on problem-oriented medical diagnosis, volumes on particular organ systems, journal articles, and other resources as the teaching conference proceeds. Ardent engagement with the group alternates with silent withdrawal for hurried reading.

Medical faculty ask residents and others to give a differential diagnosis. The group detective work proceeds to rule out diagnostic categories that fit less well than others with the constellation of symptoms. If the central ritual of the teaching conference is the differential diagnosis, then the pièce de résistance is the moment when a definitive diagnosis has been established and confirmed. Discussion of therapy is often an anticlimax or a footnote. There is great exhilaration at having transformed a mass of unexplainable symptoms into a disease-entity with boundaries and a name. Invariably, all leave the conference room exhausted but refreshed, proclaiming what an "interesting case" it had been and eagerly anticipating the next challenge. Conversely, the greatest fear is that of "finding nothing," that is, finding no "real disease" that accounts for the signs and symptoms.

Paradoxes in Medical Training

Two of the most poignant paradoxes that pervade medical education and practice are the self-image and myth of the practitioner proud of his or her independent clinical judgment. The image and myth are paradoxical because they are founded upon unremitting humiliation and the threat of fear to medical student, intern, and resident. Many instructors begin the first day of medical school warning the auditorium filled with one hundred fifty or two hundred already anxious, if also idealistic, students that there will be a prodigious amount to know, that they must know it all, that they cannot possibly know it all, that exams will be tough, and that medical school will be a test of their commitment to medicine. The inculcation and exploitation of vulnerability persist (in a typical curriculum) throughout the two years of "basic," preclinical sciences, the succeeding two years of clinical rotations, the year of internship, and the three to five years of residency. Physicians are expected by their patients and society, and expect themselves, to be autonomous, decisive, creative, and alert. Yet they must spend most of their training practicing for docility.

Creating a practitioner role is not a simple, straightforward process. In medical culture, as in wider American culture, there is chronic conflict between inculcating individual autonomy and ensuring conformism to group norms. As long ago as early 1830s, Alexis de Tocqueville foresaw a society "where the authority of the majority is so absolute and so irresistible that a man must give up his rights as a citizen, and almost abjure his quality as a human being, if he intends to stray from the track which it lays down" (1945: 167). The more the corporate team player becomes a reality in medicine, the more tenaciously many physicians (and other health practitioners) adhere to the image of the practitioner as Lone Ranger—either as an ideal or as an object of nostalgia. Medical school, internship, and residency cannot help but replay earlier developmental and familial dramas. In these contexts one is offered and expected to make free choice *after* clinical teachers and training institutions are satisfied that the trainee is thoroughly regulated.

In his still revolutionary essay, "Reflections on the American Identity," Erikson contends:

> A movement in child training began which tended to adjust the human organism from the very start to clock-like punctuality in order to make it a standardized appendix of the industrial world. This movement is by no means at an end either in this country or in countries which for the sake of industrial production want to become like us. In the pursuit of the adjustment to and mastery over the machine, American mothers (especially of the middle class) found themselves standardizing and overadjusting children who later were expected to personify that very virile individuality which in the past had been one of the outstanding characteristics of the American. The resulting danger was that of creating, instead of individualism, a mass-produced mask of individuality (1963b: 293).

Patricia Harvey, a student of Jules Henry (who wrote about American educational training for submissiveness and conformity, 1963, 1973), remarks that

> Henry's notion of docility used to describe the American classroom becomes the description of response to the stimulus of fear. The immediate consequence is temporary reduction of fear, which can be reactivated at any time. Henry rightly saw the longer term consequences of learning through docility—learning to be stupid. The longer term consequences for the individual and society include loss of creativity and the sense of self, being duped by advertising, business and government, madness, and willingness to support a chronic climate of potential war. . . .
>
> [Jules Henry believed that in education,] the inquiring mind must question questionable truths and that the pursuit of better questions and answers should not be extinguished by the pains of humiliation and fear nor the deadening process of establishing form (conformity) over content and process (1987: 15, 16).

Ironically—and dangerous clinically—biomedical education sows the very self-restriction, standardization, subordination of thinking to authority, and "tyranny of the majority" (de Tocqueville 1946: 167) that are the antitheses of careful scientific discipline, curiosity, and sound clinical judgment in contextually complex medical cases.

Generations of medical students, interns, and residents pass on to one another the common "survival" rule: "Don't ask questions. If you ask questions, you'll either look stupid because you're already supposed to know what you're asking about, or you'll embarrass the teacher into thinking you know more than him (or her)." The physician is able to be independent, creative, and inquisitive only after these very traits have first been suppressed by an intolerance for uncertainty and indecisiveness. The Lone Ranger image of the doctor is a conformist behind the mask. Possession of autonomy of clinical judgment often has a "protest" quality to it. Equally often, when it is the genuine article, it poses a great threat to medical consensus and to one's status on hospital staff.

Richard Shweder and Edmund Bourne (1984) make the important, and somewhat paradoxical, point that individuality must itself be fostered, that is, it does not developmentally occur automatically. I would only add to their observations that when individuality manifests itself as an exaggerated protest, such bravado suggests a failure to achieve separateness and genuine autonomy. Shweder and Bourne write, "It is sobering to acknowledge that our sense of personal inviolability is a violatable social gift, the product of what *others* are willing to respect and protect us from, the product of the way we are handled and reacted to, the product of the rights and privileges we are granted by others in numerous territories of the self (Goffman 1971)" (1984: 194).

From the viewpoint of scientific advance and humanitarian clinical relationships, it is fortunate that many student and resident physicians resist the security and tyranny inherent in group consensus-seeking. To the extent that they are successful, they have preserved some degree of individuality and with it independence of clinical judgment, nurtured by inner confidence from the family past, by marital and family support in the present, by some peers throughout medical training, and by a sprinkling of wide-ranging clinical teachers whom medical training institutions ambivalently attract and employ, if only for a brief time.

Time: A Metacurriculum Within Medicine

One of the overarching "subjects" taught in the medical, internship, and residency curriculum is time. Indeed, a large part of the metacurriculum is *the experience of time.* In the typical seven-year (or more) process of medical training, students, interns, and residents are preoccupied with time. There is never enough time to do all that one wants, is asked, and feels responsible to do. Throughout medical education, students, interns, and residents reckon time via a "countdown" of how long they have to go before some end is reached. Time is marked in short-term intervals, from one hurdle to the next.

The sequence of learning in medical school embeds cultural values through the organization of time. Generally, during the first two years of medical school, one first learns the basic sciences. Even when some lectures or seminars on "clinical interviewing" are offered in the first year, students widely meet a formaldehyded corpse (their cadaver for dissection) before they speak with any patient. The body is a lifeless machine before "it" is a person. In biomedical training, death and deconstruction precede, and set the tone for, life with all of its "conditions."

Early in the basic science years, time is measured in terms of the next exam, the end of the semester, and the major landmark—the successful completion of the first year. The second year repeats the cycle, but with the added anticipation of starting one's clinical years. During the third and fourth years, time is measured in terms of the length of clinical rotations, required or elective. Each rotation typically lasts four to six weeks and exposes the student to the functioning and rigors of varied subspecialties within medicine (pediatrics, emergency room medicine, and so on). Time is reckoned in days and, near the end, in hours. Fourth year medical students interview early for residencies, so that much of the latter half of the year is spent in anticipation of being out of medical school and starting one's internship and residency years.

The duration of internship and residency varies according to the requirements of differing medical specialties (a typical family medicine residency is three years; an orthopedics residency is five years). These years are built around the ebb and flow of the call schedule—that is, those continuous hours during which one must be accessible, "on call," at a moment's notice. During hospital call, one stays onsite in the hospital seeing patients or utilizing a small "call" room with a bed. During home or outside call, one can be paged or telephoned at home or elsewhere (during any and all human activities).

Internship and residency years begin on July 1. The year, while itself a "horizon" or goal, is made more bearable by dividing it into numerous temporal landmarks. Interns and residents not only work long weekday hours on hospital services and in outpatient clinics; they have grueling "call schedules" for nighttime, weekends, holidays, and blocks of time during which they are often expected to be performing other clinical duties as well.

Typically, intern call is every fourth day for a thirty-six-hour period, and resident call is sixteen to eighteen weeks a year. Time during internship and residency is thus reckoned in terms of on call and time off, the number of days until the end of the current rotation, and the weeks or days until the end of the year. Not only is time consciousness one of the predominant ways of organizing one's life; so widespread is the notion of medical training as "doing time," that one is tempted to link medical education with a prison sentence. This punishing schedule, however, presumably assures one a glorious exit into a promising career if one is willing to endure the temporary privations and put in the time.

Although so much of medical training occurs in cycles, students, interns, and residents adhere to a relentlessly segmented, yet lineal view of time. Anticipation of what they will complete in the next brief interim, and what they will start anew, orders their universe. They are constantly looking forward to the next short-term horizon—in large measure for relief from their previous one.

Insight into the experience of time and time management by physicians was provided by my often futile attempts to schedule residents and physician faculty for Balint groups. Not only were the twice-monthly times clearly enunciated during organizational meetings by administrators who were also participants in Balint, but times and places for these meetings were publicized in weekly printed conference schedules distributed in all department members' mail boxes on Monday morning so that all concerned could (if they wished) plan for their entire week. As this did not lead to larger numbers of Balint participants (resident or faculty), I began sending out reminder memoranda, which failed to improve the results. One resident finally urged me to page or "beep" residents and faculty several hours prior to the Balint meeting. At first I balked, protesting that physicians were already inundated with "beeps," that I did not want Balint to be a nuisance. She insisted that this was probably the only way that interested participants would remember to come, that they appreciated rather than resented the reminders, and that they probably had not even waded through their mountains of mail to notice the schedules and memoranda.

As was later confirmed in a Balint group discussion, my desire to be considerate had in fact been counterproductive in terms of the organization of time in medical culture (not limited to the culture of medical education). Residents and faculty constantly apologized to me and to the "group" for tardiness, for forgetting that Balint was occurring that day, and so on. Their world was constructed on a lineal principle of patient load rather than on the basis of clock hours, days, or weeks. The pace, accelerated by medical faculty, nursing staff, and receptionists' scheduling, was a harried, relentless one. Patient care was the timetable and hub of the wheel around which even teaching conferences were tacitly organized and to which needs conference attendance took second place. Numerous residents and medical faculty expressed gratitude for the schedule reminders, explaining almost unanimously that they lived and functioned by their beepers, telephones, and by patient examination schedule. After I had (at first begrudgingly) learned to work within biomedicine's time conception and modus operandi, Balint seminar attendance improved considerably and mutual frustration about scheduling diminished markedly.

An intern in January said optimistically, "Five months to go." A new resident referred to himself as "twenty-four [months] and counting." A second year resident in January, after a difficult weekend of "moonlighting" and feeling guilty that she could not cure everyone, said, "Only eighteen months to go" (until completing her residency). A third year resident in January looked ahead to having only "six months to go" (until she would be out of the program). As the third year of residency progresses, residents have a steady countdown of weeks, days, and final hours.

Medical training is replete with numerous "finishing lines" to cross and obstacles to ever getting there. Many medical students, interns, and residents try to manage their anxiety, to keep from getting lost in the details and in the endless change, by keeping each finish line ever in their line of sight. There is the expectation and wish that once an obstacle or challenge has been successfully surmounted, "there will be open range ahead." At the end of the long arrow of time lies the promise (or hope) of freedom, dignity, control over one's own life and others' as well, and respect as a "real doctor."

Medical students, interns, residents, and practitioners alike fervently wish for a *lineal* experience, and command, of time. Instead, what they find is an experience of time as endless repetition, the cycles of which are resistant to closure. For example, family medicine interns' mood periodicity rests upon the cycle of rotations on such clinical services as internal medicine (three months), obstetrics (three months), pediatrics (three months), surgery (two months), emergency room (one month), and family medicine (one month). Now, admittedly, the range of variation is limited or widened depending upon the choice of specialty and its associated organ systems and methods. Family physicians, general internists, and pediatricians, for example, tend to have a wide range or breadth of knowledge about biomedical and psychosocial matters but lack the depth of some of their subspecialist colleagues (such as pediatric surgeons, cardiologists, gastroenterologists). The converse is likewise true. What is not treated will be consulted or referred to another specialist. Nonetheless, physicians, nurses, PAs, medical assistants, and others are expected to be able to draw upon, in a moment's notice, a prodigious amount of information, skills, and emotional responses in order to be able to deal with each patient in limited time sequences (every seven to ten minutes in some outpatient clinic practices, fifteen to twenty minutes in others).

Alertness, flexibility, and readiness to respond to any medical situation at any moment are premium values that relate to physicians' experience of time. Not only must a physician be able to respond to "anything" with a given patient; he or she must be able to "wipe the slate clean" or "shift gears" and start the decisionmaking process anew as soon as he or she goes to the next examining room or walks to the bedside of the next patient on the hospital ward. Moreover, partly in response to the sheer volume of patients that need to be seen, and partly in response to the internalized clock that marks the expected pace of medicine, clinical thinking and clinical action are expected to be fast and efficient. Clinical work is expected to be accomplished in a brief block of time so that one can in seemingly linear fashion move on to the next small block of linear time.

Like new recruits to military training, interns are often called grunts by residents and faculty physicians. They often regard the type of tasks they are required to perform—menial, procedurally unglamorous, dirty—as grunt work. An intern begins each new rotation with total disorientation (The first question is, "Where is the bathroom?"). One must quickly become oriented and be ready to respond to anything because the intern is "treated as one of the lowest forms of human life" (as interns often say) on hospital services. As the weeks pass, if one is tactful and competent, one starts to feel accepted, allowed·to do more procedures (not just to watch or do "scutwork"), and recognized for what one does. No sooner, however, does one start to feel at home and good about oneself, one's acceptability, and one's skill, than one must prepare to leave, say farewell, grieve (or postpone grieving) and start all over somewhere else.

One family medicine intern said that "family medicine interns get a lot of experience in other people's services. We're always saying good-bye. We start getting good at something, getting recognition. You're starting all over just when you get comfortable. The first five days of a new rotation are hell. We're the new kid on the block every month." Another intern asked, "What do you do to get ready to start another service, another month? Dread, that's how I feel. I woke up the first day of surgery. I said to myself: 'Today is day one, sixty-one to go [on the two-month rotation]. I need to have a good attitude, or I'd be depressed all the time.'" In discussing her treatment of an elderly woman who had a recent history of substernal chest pain and several prior myocardial infarctions, a family medicine intern said, "I fulfilled everyone's expectations but mine. . . . Medical procedure is easy. The main problems were being told what to do by upper level residents, cardiac catheterization fellows, attendings, etc. Knowing our role as the low person on the totem pole was a real eye-opener."

Medical students, interns, and residents alike humorously mark time by labeling various milestones as "syndromes." For instance, interns experience (in North America at least) the "winter depression syndrome," which occurs around January and February of the internship that began the previous July. For interns, February is the cruelest month. They are starting to know the ropes, to have enough clinical skills and experience under their belts to begin feeling that they really are doctors, not just playing at the role. But their frustration and sense of disparity between what they feel they are capable of and how they are treated—by the training institution and patients alike—are at an apex. The "magical" six months, and its association with the Christmas/New Year season of renewal, has failed to put them "over the hump." In the northern latitudes, too, the weather is dismal and discouraging. It is cold. Snow, sleet, and ice make it difficult to get to the hospital and clinics; now travel takes even more time, and time is such a scarce commodity.

Interns are typically angry and depressed. One intern complained, "I bust my ass trying to be a good doctor, and it doesn't make a difference. Here I'm being manipulated by the patients and by the whole damn staff. This is not medicine. But I'm just a scut-monkey, worse (less) than a medical student." Another intern spoke of his, and his colleagues', anger and impatience about how interns are treated. He wondered apprehensively, "Does it get better July 1st [when interns become bona fide residents]?"

One family medicine intern was outraged at his recent six-week experience on a surgery rotation and feared that he had come close to losing his identity as a family doctor:

> I was on call at night, and got yelled at for starting an antibiotic on a septic patient. I couldn't figure out why I couldn't satisfy them. They were so upset, but everything

> I did was medically right. . . . I won't tolerate not being taught, just doing histories and physicals for them. They're rushed in surgery, I know that. No time to teach. I got tired of being dumped on. . . . I was physically beat down. I was feeling disgusted with nurses' calls in the middle of the night. I started *acting* like a surgeon. I became less tolerant. I started feeling the pressure of time. . . . I counted the days and hours and minutes. I got done and got out. That's how I cope—that's how we've learned to cope with the system. Getting through: That's the goal. I was losing my identity, becoming nothing more than a piece of meat. For a while I was in the doldroms. My expectations of surgery were different. I wanted to learn about breast masses and cancer, outpatient surgery. Instead, they took away my dignity. At the end of the surgery rotation, I felt stronger for having survived. Nothing scathes me now!

This intern's temporary protection against the experience of abuse was to identify with those whom he perceived as his exploiters, only later to despise himself for having done so. He obtained closure on this painful episode by branding surgery bad and family medicine good. To him, having survived a grueling rotation was as high a goal as mastery of clinical content. (Survival is also an overarching value in medical socialization.) Finally, he triumphed over vulnerability by immunizing (or anaesthetizing) himself against feeling.

In February, interns' prejudices flare; they are most savage and sarcastic in their remarks about patients (and categories of patients) whom they despise. They become painfully aware of the disparity between their ideals (their ideal self-image as physician) and what (and who) they are horrified they are becoming. "What's happening to me?" is a common, chagrined exclamation. At this time, vituperation against patients whom they brand as scumbags and dirtballs is at its most vicious and unforgiving. Latent racial, religious, age, gender, and IQ prejudices rise and are hurled with full force in discussions about patients, whether in private counseling, consultation, or Balint groups: "I delivered a baby at 4 A.M. and the mother resented having to feed her baby. I felt like saying to her, 'Well, hell, I have to be here, too, and I don't like it either.'"

A second intern complained of having little continuity with patients: "We see most patients for just a moment in time and have no sense of their history. Maybe if we knew them better, we'd have some idea of why they're acting that way." Still another said, "In private practice, you can say 'No' to patients, but not here at the Mecca [high status tertiary care center; note also the allusion to religious pilgrimage: urban medical center as secular Mecca]. There's this long list of people we've got to say 'Yes' to."

Interns find their rotation on obstetrics among the most grueling: "OB is labor intensive. In labor and delivery, we see women at their worst. You see the worst of eight to ten women per day. From 4:30 A.M. to 5:30 P.M. or later you've got to take all this shit. And you're lucky if you get out by 5:30. It's a factory line." They dislike what they are feeling: "Are we bad people to say these things?" "It gets to be too much trouble to care. We're overworked. We never get a chance to know patients well. We're too tired for empathy."

Typically, in individual and group discussions such as these, "patient bashing" through a series of interns' war stories or horror stories escalates into a virtual us-versus-them position. At some point, however, an intern or faculty member inquires, "Why now?" One intern or faculty member points out that this training environment is an artificial one: "In real life practice, you will have a lot more control over your practice and over who your patients are." Interns ask medical faculty, "Did you feel like this [hatred toward indigent patients, for example] when you were an intern?" Invariably the answer is, "Yes." The interns begin to feel somewhat less isolated or irredeemably evil. They begin to examine the larger picture to which their railing is a response.

Feeling treated like worthless scuzzballs themselves by the medical hierarchy, they displace and project their sense of hurt and worthlessness onto those available minority groups with whom it is culturally safe to do so. One asked tentatively, "What's it like to live as a black person in a white society?" Another protested, "It takes energy to try to get to know patients." I briefly interjected that one consequence, if not intention, of our "pressure cooker" educational style is to induce conditions that distance students, interns, and residents from patients and that make trainees take refuge in the "medical guild."

One especially competitive intern commented that "for a senior resident to pick up something [such as a diagnosis] that I didn't get is unacceptable." A second intern insisted haltingly, "*They're* the bad people; I'm not." A third added, "You start feeling guilty toward patients for disliking them. I ask myself, 'Am I judging them too harshly, or are they just trash?'" A fourth intern interjected, "A scary thought for me is, 'Maybe *they're* [the patients] the normal ones!'"

During the course of many such individual and group discussions, the initially rigid boundaries between us (physicians, the good people) and them (patients, especially indigent and racially different ones, the bad people) soften. The interns begin to genuinely grapple with prejudice rather than only give vent to it to expel bad feelings. At least for a time, many participants recognize what current circumstances fuel the rage against patients and minorities and why it erupts when it does. However briefly, faculty and interns are able to situate their volatile emotions and actions within the larger training culture.

Sometimes the end of a new rotation or clinical experience is, or seems, clearly in sight. Then the young clinician begins to think, "It's all downhill from here," only to despair that the end is after all, at least temporarily, an illusion. During the second half of the internship and the first two-thirds of residency, residents will increase their competence and sense of confidence in themselves as physicians. An intern, seven months into internship, reflected on the fact that he and his fellow interns, privately and in Balint groups, had done their emotional "venting" earlier in the year about bad, manipulative, demanding patients, but that the target of the dissatisfaction and invective had in recent weeks been turned against upper level residents, attending physicians, and nurses:

> We now know enough to call ourselves doctors. At first, we were just moles, lower than medical students half the time. Now, we feel more competent and confident. We know our role more. We've handled some difficult situations; we've got a few skills we can use. But that doesn't make a difference to a lot of attendings and residents. Nurses treat us as hired help. "Teach me; don't bark at me." That's what I'd like to say to them. Before, we only had the patients to get mad at.

Upon completing internship rotations and taking the medical licensure exam, one becomes a second year resident. Finally, one feels entitled to call oneself a real doctor. The cycle of what they call "forgetting" (repression, denial, projection) almost invariably begins anew with the start of the second year, with residency proper. New second year residents go to great pains to "forget," to avoid thinking and talking about, what it was like for them to be interns. When medical socialization is at its most "successful" (by official standards, at least), identification with the aggressor eliminates many of the earlier qualms and identity panic. Residents, feeling themselves to be real doctors, can exact from interns what was not so long ago exacted from them. These issues become grist for additional individual and group discussions.

One third year resident in primary care, aware that I am an anthropologist, explained the emotional transition from intern to resident in terms of an appeal to human nature:

> It's an inherent part of human nature for people to affirm their own group at the expense of another group, like family medicine in relation to the other specialties. When you've finished internship, you know that you've made it as a member of the tribe. It's a stressful rite of passage. You say to the new interns: "We passed through [the fire], now you pass through it. I've paid; now you pay." I want things better for the people who come after me. But there's also some malicious enjoyment. "What right do you have to want it better? You gotta pay your dues." It's an ugly, dark side of human nature, the desire to make other people suffer.

In a similar vein, at the conclusion of a long workshop on stress during internship, with the first glimmerings that the future might be dignified and brighter than the dismal present, several members of the group broke into catty, tauntingly humorous remarks about how new interns, four months from now, should be treated. "Only four months left in internship," one intern triumphantly realized. "You can make it for four months," she exclaimed. Another added, "Seeing the twos (second year residents) I realize that you guys made it, so can we." He shortly thereafter added sarcastically, "In a few months we'll be able to say, 'Those *poor* interns!'" A third intern said mockingly, "You'll have to be *nice* to them!"—at which point the group burst into laughter.

Residents refer to the "eighteen-month syndrome" that hits them at the halfway point in their (three-year) training. As one family medicine resident put it, with terror in her voice:

> Oh shit, I have eighteen months to go and I'll be totally responsible for somebody's life. Just when I start feeling confident about my clinical skills, especially in moonlighting [serving as emergency room physician, during which time one is truly in charge of medical care], I begin to realize that in another eighteen months I'll be all on my own, nobody to look over my shoulder. I panic. Where are my blind spots? What diagnoses will I miss? Suddenly, time feels so short when I have to know so much.

Many years ago, one astute resident, upon assuming the third and final year of his training, whimsically referred to his own cohort as "old dogs" and to the second year subgroup as "young pups." This image crystallized my longstanding impression of family-style sibling rivalry in residency training. Numerous residents who, throughout their second year, had in all aspects of decisionmaking and patient care been cautious, deferential, quiet, unobtrusive, even meek, upon becoming third year residents seemed to undergo a dramatic character change, becoming assertive, more self-assured, outspoken, decisive, bossy, even obnoxious. What I had initially mistaken to be a sign of internal "personality" change I came to recognize as a developmental sequence of role transition in the medical training hierarchy. These role attributes pervaded diagnosis, interpersonal style, and administrative behavior alike. Just as on July 1, former grunts began to feel more like real doctors, so with equal cultural logic, on the same day erstwhile young pups mutated into old dogs.

Yet another milestone is the "six month syndrome" (only six months to go before completing residency and going out into "the real world" of medical practice). It is similar to the eighteen month syndrome, except that the height of the self-confidence (often bordering on manic denial of the need for help from anyone) and the depth of self-doubt (verging on a wholesale questioning of one's clinical abilities) are dramatically greater. During a discussion about a patient who had recently died, a resident suffering this syndrome said:

> It's not just this patient. It happens to all of us. It's not just a medical issue. [I asked, "What bothers you the most?"] Something you do or do not do that contributed to her death. . . . I knew her two and a half years. I had continuity of care. She was my favorite patient. . . . There's a feeling that I killed her. The terrible retrospectoscope, it's our worst torturer.
>
> I didn't know well how to deal with this disease [the patient's problems included a history of diabetes, hypertension, schizophrenia, and longstanding asymptomatic resting tachycardia]. I did a lot of reading. Our relationship with our consultants is not good. How much can you depend on your consult when you differ with the consult's opinion?
>
> Should you know everything? How do you forgive yourself when your patient dies? The courts don't always forgive you. When should you "go" with your own feelings versus when to take the consultant's advice?
>
> If I had pinned down the consultant, I'd ask why she thinks the way she thinks. I feel bad that I didn't stand up to the consultant. Getting a consult is going to the oracle.
>
> I wish I could do something more, to fix her. I was not confident in the assessment. I could have gotten a CAT scan. . . . I am grieving over the loss of a *real* person. I didn't expect her to die. Some physicians avoid this involvement. It's protection. How do you not be overconcerned about omissions and commissions?
>
> I don't want to get complacent. As long as I get close to people, their dying is going to hurt. And we're also going to kill people. That's how it feels. It can't be avoided somewhere along the road.

During the final half-year of residency, residents waver from panicky self-doubt ("I thought I was a real doctor, but I'm beginning to realize how much I still don't know") to contemptuous dismissal of all faculty ("I've still got four months to go, I know more than the ones who trained me, but I've still got to put in my time and make it look like I'm interested in learning"). One third year family medicine resident said, "I'm afraid of going in a practice where the other docs know more than I do. All my colleagues know more than I do. It would be nice to have magic—rattles and chains, some magic dust. My biggest fear is that I don't know enough."

This resident, like countless "threes" (third year residents) in their final months, wildly vacillated between quiet confidence, boisterous cockiness, and the pang of terror that asks, "Where's the magic?" The last half of the final year of residency exhibits the mood and behavioral extremes of turbulent adolescence: from desperate clinging to utter repudiation of parentified faculty, who are either viewed as rescuers from ignorance and error or useless impediments to autonomy of clinical judgment. Thus, just as residents are about to cross the "finish line" of their formal training—the whole object of the "countdown"—many experience a stark uncertainty about whether they are ready to go through with it. The ambivalence of regressive pulls and progressive pushes lasts to the very end, if not beyond.

The rhythm, tempo, and pattern of priorities indoctrinated in medical school persist into residency and on into the first years of practice. There is never enough time to get all the work done: seeing patients and families in the clinic often far after official closing time, making rounds on hospitalized patients, meeting with a growing number of hospital committees, attending medical society meetings, interrupting sleep or mealtime or leisure to answer the telephone or to rush to the hospital, keeping up with mounds of medical journals. For many, the long cycles of time continue to be structured largely according to the extremes of self-privation and indulgence, professional asceticism and private saturnalia.

Six months from completing her residency, one family physician talked with me about coming from a family with high expectations. Self-depreciatory, she brooded about whether she knew enough, whether she would know when she knew enough! Then:

> Screw it! That's what another part of me says. When I finish, I'm going to take my time before I settle into a practice. I'll do some dress-making and some travel. In medicine we've no normal sense of time. We have to pack in so much in the few minutes after we get out of bed in the morning. There's so little time for female physicians to spend on feminine rituals [bathing, makeup, and sartorial concerns]. When I finish residency, I want to ski the Himalayas, go to New Zealand, do things I've been putting off eleven years. The residency program sets you up to go into practice. But this delayed gratification has to get satisfied somewhere. So I'll really do it up before I settle into a practice.

Clinicians in training, together with their families, live through a progression of anticipated turning points after which "it's got to get better." At each turn, the expected miracle fails to manifest itself. With the third year of medical school, then internship, later residency, finally group, private, or corporate practice, they console and reassure one another that the future will differ radically from the present. Disappointment leads only to a recalibration of the timetable, not to disillusionment with the timetable itself. "Once we're settled," third year medical students and interns promise themselves or their spouses, "we'll be able to do everything we wanted to do." Each successive "bend in the river" and "top of the next hill" alter little in the overall momentum of the cycles of time. Straight lines invariably turn out to be circles.

Forgetting and Splitting as Tools of Professional Socialization

Thus far in the discussion of time experience among medical students, interns, and residents, I have limited myself primarily to conscious perceptions of time and how it is categorized. There is, however, an additional dimension of the time experience that is at once more long-term, subtle, and largely unconscious—the personal transformation from being a member of lay, popular culture to being and feeling oneself to be a real physician, a member of professional culture. During this process, one not only learns the content of the new culture but in large measure also learns to "forget," repress, and disparage much of the cultural content and meanings of one's erstwhile "lay" identity—and in turn do likewise through one's patients in medical care.

In this sense, the new, professional culture supplants or supersedes the foundation of one's culture(s) of origin. To a large degree, one seeks to leave one's "popular" culture behind in learning and assuming the identity of biomedical practitioner. I hasten to add that this is not everywhere a total, complete process. Nevertheless, medical education and years of apprenticeship largely function to reorient medical students and practitioners to time; the old time dominated by subjectivity is left behind, and the new time regulated by objectivity is entered. There is often a complementarity between the action of the training environment and the young physician's motivation: If medical socialization seeks to remove the apprentice largely from his or her past, the trainee also uses professionalization to escape the personal past.

My first example of this phenomenon comes from teaching in the Department of Psychiatry (housed in the community mental health center) at Meharry Medical College in Nashville, Tennessee, from 1972 to 1978. A wide spectrum of black practitioners and students ideologically championed the cause of historically deprived, if not impoverished, blacks. For many, however, this identification and advocacy occurred more in the abstract and in curriculum/policy meetings than in day-to-day concrete interactions with actual patients or clients. Social distancing manifested itself in such ways as difficulty accepting individual patients and their families, residential choice in affluent black or white neighborhoods far from one's ideological "brothers and sisters," the use at clinical conferences of disparaging language about noncompliant black (or white poor) patients, and the like (see Stein and Hill 1977). Certainly, this did not characterize all my black colleagues (or, for that matter, white colleagues and students who also had a range of commitments to the black movement). But at the time I was surprised and bewildered by the disparity between public espousal and private behavior among many.

Only as I was able, at first very tentatively and diffidently, to voice my perceptions with colleagues, and to deal with them in depth in counseling situations with students and residents, was I able to uncover a developmental compartmentalization.

The often impoverished, conflict-ridden, racially ambivalent life they strove to leave behind was separated from the professional, acculturated, and mainstream American (white) life they unconsciously embraced and hoped to achieve through professionalization and its benefits. As I helped many students and colleagues discover and work through this split between past and present, many were able to integrate these parts of their lives and become more compassionate and responsive toward their black—and white—patients.

During my first years teaching in community-based, largely rural family medicine settings in Oklahoma (Enid and Shawnee, during the late 1970s), I discovered a similar disparity among white family medicine residents, many of whom came from wheat farming families. I noticed at first that the residents became irate about the failure of patients to make or keep return appointments, about patients' poor compliance behavior (with respect to taking medication or scheduling surgeries), and about an occasional death they felt could have been averted. As I took an interest in these "communication" problems, I discovered that the cultural nexus of Oklahoma wheat farming families was a useful framework for describing, interpreting, and predicting health-related behavior and, by extension, for treating many of these patients in this milieu (Stein 1982b, 1987c). The *timing* of health action (or inaction), for many within the white Great Plains ethos, was rooted in the annual agricultural cycle of planting and harvesting as a reticulated system of meaning. Perceived sickness did not invariably lead to illness behavior (such as assumption of the sick role or utilization of medical facilities) because other values predominated (Mechanic 1968; Rosenstock 1960; Kleinman 1980).

Among white Great Plains farming families, health is an instrumental, subordinate value. In their cultural ideal, health is prized as a means of being able to keep active and physically productive and thereby safeguard and demonstrate one's independence. But health, per se, as a medical value is not pursued because health belongs to the moral rather than the medical domain. The ability to do is itself taken to be a sign of healthiness, a condition synonymous with resiliency, toughness, robustness. Too great a concern for health per se is ridiculed and censured. It is seen as doting upon oneself instead of making oneself useful.

From this ethnographic data, I concluded that the beginning of culture-appropriate health planning lay in the awareness by biomedical practitioners that many wheat farming families lived by different rules and priorities from those that governed medicine—and that these decisively influenced health-related behavior. Practitioners' health planning usually did not take into account the competing demands within wheat farming families *and* when it did tended to assume that medicine's priorities should take precedence. Much of physicians' exasperation derived from unsuccessful struggles for control between theirs and patients' world-views.

When I formally presented my observations about the Euro-American regional cultural pattern to residents and faculty physicians, they expressed surprise, delight, bewilderment. They commented that although many of them had lived and grown up in this part of the country, they had so taken it for granted that they had never given any thought to it. They were pleased yet astonished that an outsider could even discover the patterns. Why, they wondered, had *they* not realized these cultural factors? They felt my presentation helped them understand not only their patients but themselves as well. They realized that they had selectively forgotten (repressed) aspects of their own culture of origin discrepant with their new professional identity. Patients had come to represent a past that physicians did not want to be reminded of, or tethered to, even as some of them still relished wheat farming and harvest activities. My presentation struck them as "uncanny," in the sense of familiar yet somehow forbidden (see Freud 1919). With both a sense of grace and some effort, they reassembled, if only temporarily, the "not me" with the "me" of themselves (here, the preprofessional with the professional self).

From my experience in both urban and rural health care training, I have also noted that in the urban medical center training ambience, resident and faculty physicians often rely upon consultations with and referrals to specialists in other roles to perform functions that they include only with reluctance in their own role perception or self-image. That is to say, the division of labor among various biomedical and psychosocial specialists serves emotional as well as practical purposes. In two family medicine residency training settings in which I have taught, residents spend their second and third years of postgraduate training in a community-based rural setting following an internship in an urban tertiary care center. On several occasions shortly after moving to the rural practice-training site, residents demanded, "Where is my medical social worker (or clinical psychologist, or family therapist, or home health nurse), so that she/he can take over when I'm through with the patient?" When I replied that they would of necessity be their own medical social worker and overall community networker, they were horrified at the prospect of being asked to be so intimately involved with their patients' lives. (I hasten to add that many other residents eagerly looked forward to incorporating these facets into patient care.)

In addition to obvious real economic and time considerations, such a question also reflects the difficulty many physicians have (a difficulty that is institutionally supported by a rigid division of labor in urban training centers) integrating the more personal and social aspects of patient care (personality, family situation, economic-employment condition) into the largely doctor-patient relationship (see Eisenberg and Kleinman 1981; Katz 1984a; Stein 1985g; Stein and Apprey 1985). The local, small, and institutional group dynamics formalize and sanction a splitting of mental functions into official clinical roles. Many young physicians who establish practices in rural environments relinquish this splitting of roles with great difficulty. Others avoid the sense of threat altogether by attempting to conduct a strictly biomedical practice (such as relying heavily on prescribing medication rather than counseling with patients).

As Katz (1984a) and Fox (1957, 1959) document, biomedical decisionmaking is rife with choice, ambiguity, and uncertainty. Biomedical trainees and practitioners alike often strive heroically to wrest definitive knowledge and direction from the pharmacopeia of choices. Consider the following event at which I was a participant. At a family medicine grand rounds, the presiding physician quizzed the residents, "What's the best antibiotic for use above the diaphragm? For below the diaphragm? For this exercise, don't think in terms of dollars, just medical efficacy."

The purpose of the exercise was to train the residents to simplify and hone their thinking. The veteran practitioner went around the table asking each resident to commit himself or herself to a choice, then offer a rationale. Following the round robin, we viewed a thirty-minute videotape on first, second, and third generation cephalosporin antibiotics (when to prescribe, efficacy with what infectious diseases, limitations, and so on). Following the videotape session, I went to breakfast with several of the family medicine residents.

I wondered how they would compare their own antibiotic-related decisionmaking with the decision tree offered on the video. Speaking from the perspective of a resident in a community (rather than urban, tertiary care) training program, one resident said, "When we were in the city [at the tertiary care center for internship and medical school], and when we are rotating with community physicians here, you do what they did, and don't ask any questions. You see the kinds of infections the attendings [M.D. faculty] see, and you prescribe the way they do." A second resident added, "I'd like sometimes to ask my attendings why they prescribe the way they do, but it's too late now. I should have asked those 'why' questions when I was still in the city. If I ask questions like that now, I'd just look foolish, and you try to avoid that at all costs."

Although this interchange might be situation specific and unique in terms of medical content, it represents a type of clinical reasoning that I have heard articulated countless times and in a broad range of clinical situations. Two recurrent themes stand out: (1) identification with authority figures (doing as they do) and (2) suppressing (perhaps later, unconsciously repressing) questions, doubts, and self-doubts out of fear of looking foolish, wrong, or recalcitrant (to oneself and to one's medical superiors). Both maneuvers successfully keep any oedipal conflict from flaring and assure the perpetuation of the clinical decisionmaking style represented by their teachers. In stabilizing "personality," these largely out-of-awareness attempts at self-protection likewise stabilize medicine's associated "culture" and "social structure." G. Gayle Stephens, M.D., writes:

> We catch our philosophies from other people in our medical hierarchies, teachers we admire (or hate), residents just ahead of us in the pecking order (those who have either befriended or abused us), and from our fellow students. This process has been studied well by social scientists (Becker et al. 1961). We learn what to do, how to do it, and how to feel about it in the crucible of crisis medicine at 3 A.M. We learn how to behave as a physician informally; the process is called professionalization, and it determines our most deeply held but usually unexamined assumptions (1988a: 5).

One of the major ritual tasks inherent in medical education is to establish various distinctions between us and them: lay public/medical science practitioner, patient/physician, and "my" specialty/"their" specialty (for instance, family medicine/internal medicine, obstetrics, or surgery; psychiatry/family therapy or clinical psychology; and so forth). The ritualization of differences into consolidated boundaries of the self is one of the key processes and structures that unify medical education. To think as a we makes one less lonely, less personally responsible, and less insecure than to think as an "I." Erik Erikson describes boundary-making as "a sense of irreversible difference between one's own and other 'kinds,' which can attach itself to evolved major differences among human populations or, indeed, to smaller and smallest differences which have come to loom large" (1977: 76).

Although this type of analysis has traditionally been restricted to ethnic, religious, and national cultures, it applies to issues of self and group identity among medical professionals as well. For with these as with other categories of human beings, the valued "positive identity" is inextricably tied to the devalued "negative identity" (Erikson 1968). The me is simply not felt to exist without its counterplayer, the not me. In contexts of invidious comparison, mutual envy and jealousy are rarely acknowledged. Through the rigors, deprivations, and triumphs of medical education, physicians learn to incorporate biomedical orthodoxy into the core of their selves. Throughout their lives as practitioners, physicians devote a considerable amount of time and energy to "keeping up with the exponential increase in medical knowledge." But practitioners quickly learn to discriminate between types of knowledge that count and types of knowledge that do not. This, in turn, is a distinction born less of disinterested science than of cultural commitments to being a member of us rather than of them.

Excremental Symbolism in Biomedical Training

In earlier chapters, we encountered biomedicine's obsession with purity, certainty, control, and beneficence, and we investigated the fecal underside of this obsession. What Volkan writes about the dehumanization of the "enemy" in interethnic and international relations holds, I believe, for the building and maintaining of the boundaries of the medical professional identity, although not to the extremes of destroying the enemy (competing subspecialties, bad patients) as in warfare.

> A threatened group's preliminary and primary aim is to set up psychological borders in order not to feel the anxiety arising from unconscious expectation that what is externalized and projected will boomerang. Our externalizations and projections are contaminated with symbolizations, and we act as though the enemy has been safely packaged and labeled with the symbols we have created to represent him; in this process he is crystallized and dehumanized. Symbols of the enemy are usually derived from our bodily parts and functions, and reflect the degree to which we valued or shrank from those parts and functions during our childhood psychosexual development. The most denigrating symbols usually refer to anality (1987: 918).

Medical students, interns, and residents frequently describe themselves, their work, their status, their clinical experiences, and last but not least their patients in excremental terms. They feel treated "like shit." They are often asked to do scut work (shit work). Medical invective and obscene humor are forms by which potentially dangerous aggression can be verbally abreacted (if only temporarily) and gotten out so as not to interfere with compassion and objectivity in patient care. Yet it still does.

Near the end of his intern year, one physician in a discussion group said optimistically, "I'll be the new guy on the block [for example, in the medicine or surgery rotation] one more month; then it'll be another intern's turn to be the new guy on the block." A burst of laughter from the group of interns and residents signaled the anticipated triumph over time and pleasure over the fact that someone else would have to bear the brunt of indignities. They would soon be able to mete out humiliation rather than be its victim. One intern continued sarcastically, "Internship is to learn to take all the abuse in the world. You learn to take forty tons of shit on you, so that later twenty tons of shit feels moderate." Another introduced the issue of how responsibility is learned: "You can do everything right and something bad—shit—will happen." "TSH, that shit happens," said a third year resident in an effort to normalize bad medical outcomes.

A second year resident worried about whether he would become like those residents and faculty physicians whose sadism he despised: "Should we forget about being interns? Shit on someone else like you were shit on? I try to remember what it was like. I don't want to be one of those people who dump on others the way I was dumped on." One frequently hears that "we're [students, interns, residents] up to our ass in ______" [upper level residents, medical faculty, problem patients, paperwork, staff problems]. Anything unpleasurable, bad, can represent the excremental. A seventy-five-year-old patient who had lost fifteen pounds in several months refused to permit his physician to perform a rectal exam. Frustrated because he suspected that his patient had a cancer, the resident snarled during a case discussion, "He's got big turd potential" ("He who impedes me could be shit").

An implicit agenda acquired early in medical school, clutched tenaciously throughout medical training, and taken into practice as well consists of learning who is entitled to "shit on" whom. One learns how much shit one must take and for how long. Scatological sarcasm and humor may well be safety valves for medical trainees and practitioners. Nevertheless the all-consuming issue of control and of who will and may control whom likewise goes to the heart of the official clinical enterprise as well. The compliance issue often plays out the drama of intrusion and control—and quite literally for the substance of another's insides.

Through a sometimes subtle and sometimes blatant process of victimization during medical school and clinical apprenticeship, students and physicians experience the process of control and self-control in often angrily fecal terms. One learns a fundamental emotional dichotomy: between exercising total control (over oneself, another) and total loss of control (as in the phrase "I really lost it"). To be controlled by another is to feel massively "shit upon." To control another is to have the indulgence to "shit upon" him or her. The failure to be able to control another (the patient, the disease) legitimately (through medical means) often unleashes vengeful wrath that includes the wish to empty oneself on the noncompliant object—that is, to let go completely of control in an account-settling evacuation.

Throughout medical school and into practice, yet another dimension to the polarity between doctor and patient is internalized: that of those entitled to "shit upon" others and of those who are expected to be the recipient of "shit." To physicians' chagrin, patients continue to "shit upon" them even after they have avowedly earned the right not to have to "take any more shit from anybody," after they have been certified and licensed for admittance to the elite guild of biomedicine. Perhaps the simultaneous presence of the powerful wish to "shit on" another and the powerful prohibition against it acts to make the specter of physicians' anger toward patients especially terrifying. This leads in turn to a denial of anger, to a search for a self-righteous way of expressing it, or to an unconscious acting out toward the patient.

At some level of awareness, and lasting only transiently, medical students, interns, residents, and practicing physicians recognize in themselves what they so disdainfully brand in their patients. This is clearest, and rawest, among interns. Feeling mistreated, abused, misunderstood, lacking power or authority, harassed by everyone above them in the medical hierarchy, interns refer to themselves as "scuzz monkeys," "worms," or "moles." It does not require that one be of Freudian persuasion to detect in such images the qualities of being far beneath human, of being animal, particularly animals that live in the dirt, animals that are small and disgusting. In medical training, one learns how to be a physician and how to occupy one of the highest of American social statuses by beginning as one of the lowest of the low.

The words and feeling tones associated with being an intern are remarkably similar to those colorful invectives used by interns and higher status physicians alike to portray despised patients. For most, this excruciating sense of kinship with the patient is eagerly forgotten (repressed) as they are able to feel and function more as real doctors during their residency. For later moments of vulnerability and fright, they must be able to protect their dignity by having others embody what they have resolved never again to feel about or in themselves. Its bona fide scientific contribution to physicians' thinking notwithstanding, biomedical education also induces deep regression and humiliation that often make the (unconscious) lure of self-protection via identification with the aggressor hard to withstand. It is difficult for someone who has been treated like shit and who feels like shit to be compassionate toward others rather than to search for "suitable targets" (Volkan 1976) for externalization, displacement, and projection so as to avert being shit forever.

Pimping

During the clinical years of a physician's medical education—usually the third and fourth of medical school, the year of internship, and the years of residency—pimping places the demonstration of knowledge in the service of defending oneself from public humiliation. In this pedagogical rite, one is put "under the gun" of a barrage of questions about one's knowledge of medical facts, differential diagnosis, treatment plans, medication levels, outcomes, contingency plans. The ostensible official protocol and purpose of the exercise are for a more seasoned, higher ranking practitioner to drill a younger, less experienced apprentice in order to keep the latter constantly alert to all that needs to be known in order to be a competent doctor.

Medical group teaching and learning activities thus interweave scientific, reality-oriented information with ideological, ritual information. The former comprises the official, explicit group agenda; the latter contains the unofficial, implicit, often difficult to verbalize group agendas.

These interwoven domains of clinical reality are distinct group operations. Bion (1959) calls them "work" (reality orientation, rationality) and "basic assumptions" (fantasy), respectively; La Barre (1972) identifies them as "secular" (ego orientation) and "sacred" (id/superego domination), respectively. In an ethnographic study of psychiatric residency training, Light (1980: 212) astutely notes that the socialization or inculcation of the rules and ways of thinking of the culture of psychiatry is the main concern of training. The diagnostic labeling of patients is secondarily "good for" the patients. It is primarily an affirmation of the cultural worldview and the power of those learning the art of labeling and of those imparting such knowledge. Similarly, in his study of occupational rituals in patient management, Charles Bosk (1980) analyzes clinical decisionmaking rituals in which patient information is transformed into biomedical categories that function to reduce uncertainty and validate the medical status hierarchy.

Pimping falls into the category of implicit, basic assumption activity. It functions as verbal dueling, one-upmanship; it enables the seasoned practitioner to find a student's or resident's soft spot of ignorance or uncertainty and publicly expose it, to display expertise and trip another up (see Freeman 1987). The group uses the scientific, medical content and jargon as a means to and in the service of display and triumph over others. When I attend medical case conferences, grand rounds, and ad hoc clinical teaching sessions, I always ask myself, What kind of information is being conveyed and imparted and at what level? What is the nature of the discourse being conducted and observed? How do the actors account (to themselves) for the discourse?

Resident or faculty physicians often warrant pimping as a method for sharpening a young physician's or medical student's skills in diagnosis, ordering and interpreting tests, and patient management. Concurrent with these, however, pimping also teaches the student, intern, or resident the dire necessity of being right, the conviction that there is a single correct answer to a medical problem, and the belief that one must always appear certain in order to avoid being "one down" to another. To be right is to save face in the faculty's eyes and in those of the group and oneself. To "miss something" or to be wrong is to be utterly humiliated, to lose face, and to be perceived and come to perceive oneself as unprofessional (see Stein 1985b, 1985g, 1986a).

The underlying purpose of the ritual is for the clinical teacher to "break" the younger clinician and for the latter to do everything possible to keep from being "broken." The technique is a ritual attempt to expose, ridicule, and subjugate one's underlings—to do to them what others once tried to do to oneself. Many advanced medical residents and faculty physicians who might otherwise have empathized with the plight of third and fourth year medical students on their clinical clerkships instead do their best to catch them off guard and pillory them before their peers. As one physician described:

> "Pimping" is teaching by intimidation. I had my first personal introduction to it my very first day of my very first rotation during my third year as a medical student. I was on medicine [internal medicine]. We all solemnly entered the conference room and sat down around the table. In came the chief of the medicine service. He put a CAT scan of the head up on the viewing box and turned on the light. The only

CAT scan I'd ever seen before was on "Ben Casey" on TV! It was so quiet you could have heard a pin drop. His first words were, "Give me a differential diagnosis for what you see."

He looked around the table, then his eyes zeroed in on me: "You, give me a differential diagnosis." My mouth went dry. What was I supposed to be able to say? I'd never before even seen one of these things up close. I said, "Brain tumor." He snapped back, "No shit!" Then he persisted: "That's not a differential. Give me a list of all the possible diagnoses you should think of when you see a CAT scan of the head that looks like this." I sat there dazed. How was I supposed to be able to do this on the first day? I didn't even know where the bathroom was on the medicine service, let alone know what pathologies of the head could present like that picture.

I finally said, "I don't know." I knew he thought he won a victory because the goal of pimping is to keep somebody under the gun long enough that they break under the strain, to find a vulnerable spot where they're deficient, and to make a show of it to everyone at the conference. I had a little advantage over most of the others that day because I'd seen that attitude and style in sports for years. I'd spent enough time in football, basketball, baseball, to know that what the chief of medicine was doing was the same as my coaches had done. So I kept my cool, and let his arrogance go in one ear and out the other. But it wasn't easy.

In this manner, tolerance for ambiguity and uncertainty, which is the essence of science and the mark of the scientific spirit (Bronowski 1956), is renounced and banished from the young physician's mental world as an intolerable affront to self-esteem. How can one be scientific if one must always be "right" or at least know where to find "the" answers or to find an even greater authority than oneself who surely has them? Yet biomedical culture appeals to science as the ultimate repository of the knowledge and method that enable one to be right. Ironically, this invocation violates the essence of scientific inquiry as it appropriates science to serve medical orthodoxy.

A passage from psychiatrist Alice Miller helps us to comprehend medical pimping through the eyes and experience of clinical teachers and upper level personnel. In discussing the failure of empathy and the scornfulness parents often show toward children, Miller asks that we

> see the parents, too, as insecure children—children who have at last found a weaker creature, and in comparison with him they now can feel strong. . . . [Miller points to] the sense of strength that it gives the adult to face the weak and helpless child's fear and to have the possibility of controlling fear in another person, while he cannot control his own. . . .
>
> Contempt for those who are smaller and weaker thus is the best defense against a breakthrough of one's own feeling of helplessness: it is an expression of this split-off weakness (1981: 66–67).

In the insecure medical student, intern, or resident, the more senior practitioner sees his or her intolerable image of helplessness, vulnerability, envy, and uncertainty. In treating the person lower in the hierarchy with disdain, in precipitating situations of helplessness, the upper level clinician protects himself or herself from the breakthrough of feelings of weakness by first provoking and then "treating" them in the lower level apprentice and student—who, through identification, do likewise with categories of "contemptible" patients.

In case presentations or discussions in which the physician or medical team has been unable to arrive at a quick diagnosis, the physician may humorously or angrily say, "The patient has gooned me." To "goon" is to make a fool, a sap, out of another person; intentionality is usually assumed by the victim to be behind the act. "Gooning," however, is a term mostly associated with the experience of medical students, interns, residents, and junior physicians at the hands of their superiors. It is the extreme outcome of pimping, when the apprentice has been unable to come up with the right answer (from diagnosis to laboratory values to cost of a given drug) for the interrogator, at the moment, he or she feels "gooned." Phrases such as "set up to be shot down," "shit on," and "screwed" are often associated with being gooned.

Whether one feels gooned by a patient or by a medical superior, one feels a fool, a victim of humiliation, out of control—in short, the reverse of feelings a physician expects to have. Feelings of having been gooned commonly lead to greater effort to find the definitive diagnosis or to prove the superior wrong, that is, to redoubled efforts at mastery. Such feelings likewise commonly lead the victim of gooning to find another person—a medical student, a nurse, a patient, an administrator—to goon in order to be relieved of the sense of inadequacy. Ultimately, a goon has been momentarily deprived of a sense of competence, a sense that male physicians associate with losing their manhood. Efforts rapidly ensue to restore it, often through the verbal "castration" of another, vulnerable male or female.

During the years, senior residents, faculty physicians, and veteran practitioners who supervise medical student electives have said to me (if I might be permitted to crystallize into a single statement countless variants on the theme), "We've got to keep these medical students, interns, and residents on their toes, to make sure that they never get complacent. . . . I don't like the word "pimping"—it makes it sound cruel. I like to think of it as keeping them awake at all times. It's for their own good. You might think it's sadistic, but it's not. They'll come back and thank us someday." That "thanks" eventually assumes the form of identification with the aggressor, through which the outer danger is internalized into an inner one that is lessened by becoming like the original source of threat. Second year residents often adamantly say, "I don't want to think about my intern year ever again," deeply resenting the pimping on the wards and in the clinics. Yet they begin to pimp their juniors in the hierarchy in order to escape remembering their own vulnerability.

In ways cogent to my exploration of the process of becoming a physician, psychiatrist John E. Mack, in a review of Harold H. Saunders's *The Other Walls: The Politics of the Arab-Israeli Peace Process* (1985), writes of the experience of intergroup victimization: "Saunders acknowledges empathically the genuine experiences of victimization of the Israeli and Palestinian peoples, but he also goes on to examine the ways in which those experiences may skew perception and the capacity to adjust to new realities. Both groups even misuse their histories of victimization to justify new cycles of violence that perpetuate the patterns of victimization" (1986a: 744). This juxtaposition of Arab-Israeli conflict, wherein the roles of terrorist and terrorized frequently shift between them, with the inner world of the American medical student, intern, and resident, is not farfetched. For, with medical trainees as with victimized ethno-national-sectarian groups, each appeals to its history of victimization to justify new cycles of brutality that perpetuate the patterns of victimization.

The clinical authoritarian style is further reaffirmed and evoked by many patients who—even as in recent decades they demand greater autonomy and equality in the clinical relationship—expect "magical" cures for all of life's afflictions. Some threaten malpractice litigation if a less than perfect medical solution occurs. Medical training is unconsciously designed to force physicians to shore up their defenses against these old and recurrent threats by first overwhelming trainees and then offering protection against these induced threats. This has the characteristic of a "protection racket" (see Stein 1984) in which protectors first endanger those to whom they subsequently offer protection.

One purpose of pimping is to see how much pressure the student or intern can stand. Then, through the ultimate gesture of one-upmanship and generosity, the teacher offers "the right answer" to the broken intern or resident. Although pimping occurs widely in one-on-one encounters between superior and subordinate, it is most effective (and devastating) when it is a public rather than private display. The one being tested is scrutinized by many eyes and heard by many ears, which heightens the respondent's wariness. At the same time, if one can summon all the right answers and retain one's composure during the interrogation, pimping can heighten one's grandiosity because one has at least momentarily beaten the sly authority at his or her own game.

In its extreme, this widely used medical teaching style keeps the teaching physician in total control and the subordinate physician or group out of control as a way of teaching the subordinate(s) the need to be in total control of himself/herself and others at all times. Pimping asserts one's status superiority over others by putting the medical student or resident constantly on the defensive in order to teach the subordinate how to be "on top of everything" at all times. This ostensibly inculcates self-assurance through unremitting vulnerability and verbal violation. Pimping often combines a sadistic volley of questions with the tactic of withholding crucial information unless the subordinate asks specifically about it, which induces a sense of vulnerability, rage, and compensatory identification.

Such complex dynamics were illustrated at a medical case conference. The topic of the conference was the differential diagnosis of a disease in which the patient presented to the hospital with hemoptysis (coughing up of blood, including the coughing up of gross blood, that is, bloody or blood-tinged sputum).

In a departure from routine procedures, the presenting resident and moderator assigned each participant entering the conference room to a specific locale: residents (numbering about fifteen) at one table; faculty physicians (numbering about five) at a parallel table; non-M.D. faculty (numbering six) at another table; and medical students (numbering about six) to chairs at the rear of the now-crowded conference room. The atmosphere quickly became tense and filled with jabs of humor.

A pall of uncertainty—perhaps the chief bane of American biomedicine (Katz 1984a; Stein 1985g; Stein and Apprey 1985)—haunted the group as the presenting resident formally convened the conference. He announced that he was going to administer a test to the group, one like the much feared National Boards Examinations (comprehensive multiple choice exams given during medical school that are often used to determine class promotion if not graduation). He then described the format the conference would follow: He would offer the group bits of information about different aspects of hemoptysis and a case of hemoptysis, after which he would ask each group to offer in rank order differential diagnoses. Groups were to publicly compete with one another for the correct and quickest diagnosis.

Early in his presentation, he notified the group that when he had worked up this case of unexplained hemoptysis on a pulmonology (lung) hospital service recently, he had understood that "the bomb drops in one and a half hours." He explained this to mean that at the end of one and a half hours, when the attending (faculty) physician came on the service, he was expected to have working diagnoses on this patient and on two new patients as well. He impressed upon us, albeit humorously, that we had until 1:30 P.M. to arrive at *our* diagnosis (if we wished to save face as he had done). On at least one later occasion during the conference the presenter conjured up the specter of "the bomb dropping" imminently.

There was intense group involvement throughout this conference. Participants asked the presenter questions (the replies served as additional information to be used in making the diagnosis). The presenter called upon M.D. faculty members, residents, and medical students to come forward from their seats and perform such tasks as reading (interpreting) X-rays and reading physicians' medical reports to the group. Not only did he arouse "performance anxiety" in the group, but he attempted to channel it into medical learning and decisionmaking activities. He provided the group with far more than his faculty physician had provided for him. For instance, at the beginning of the conference, he gave everyone a handout on which was listed (1) the differential features of hemoptysis (coughing up blood) and hematemesis (vomiting blood); (2) five categories of causes of hemoptysis and further discussion of how characteristics of sputum vary with differing biomedical diagnoses; and (3) brief epidemiological associations of hemoptysis and diagnostic categories. The effect, if not intent, of this onslaught of information and complexity, coupled with the intense anxiety to arrive quickly at the right answer, was to make the group feel increasingly dependent upon the presenter for additional information. If all went well, the group would have the dual outcome of arriving at the right medical answer and publicly saving face.

The presenting physician took delight in parceling out piecemeal only the kind of information that corresponded to the clinical category on which he was preparing to "test" the group. Moreover, he did not offer potentially crucial kinds of data unless participants first raised the appropriate questions. The presenting resident at this conference pimped the participants gently rather than heavy-handedly. He presided over the conference in a relaxed, playful (rather than arrogant or aloof) fashion. Indeed, at the close of the conference, he was pleased not only that *he* had arrived at the right diagnosis (lung cancer) before his faculty physician had arrived on the service, but that at this conference the medical students had been the ones first to reach the correct answer (lung cancer) and keep it at the top of their rank-ordered three diagnoses. By the end of the conference, the bomb that participants had feared would drop on them had been averted, at least this time.

From the outset, the structure and unfolding of the conference evoked in me feelings of anxiety about the adequacy of my knowledge, the pressure of time to provide the "right" answers quickly and confidently, insecurity about how a wrong answer might be ridiculed by the group, the wish to be seen as competent in medical colleagues' eyes, and a sense of virtual timelessness, as in dreaming. I quickly realized that there was little that I could contribute intellectually to the biomedical side of the diagnosis. Once I was able to withdraw myself from that expectation and relax more in the group as observer, I used those feelings and fantasies evoked by the group and its presenter as guides to the process within the group itself. I have never before so vividly and powerfully experienced the "group ego" and "group superego" take form (see Parin 1988). I experienced quite viscerally Bion's point that "emotionally the group acts as if it had certain basic assumptions about its aims" (1955: 476).

From this vantage point, the emotional significance of the hemoptysis conference for presenter and participants alike appeared to be the need or compulsion to repeat and master anew (albeit projectively embodied through the group) previous or recurrent anxieties or traumas. This would seem to serve as the impetus for the specific choice of style and format of the presentation (preparation for the "National Boards" examination by the group, preparation for a bomb to be imminently dropped). In his article "Remembering, Repeating, and Working-through," Freud writes that "the patient does not *remember* anything of what he has forgotten and repressed, but *acts* it out" (1914: 150). He reproduces the past "not as a memory but as an action; he *repeats* it, without, of course, knowing that he is repeating it. For instance, the patient does not say that he remembers that he used to be defiant and critical towards his parents' authority; instead, he behaves in that way to the doctor" (1914: 150).

The presenting physician at the conference, of course, remembered full well the weight of his attending's expectation that he complete a workup on two patients plus the patient who was coughing up blood. But the only hint he gave us as to its emotional significance for him was the repeated ominous fantasy that "a bomb would drop" at the end of that one and a half hours. Indeed, there was little emotion expressed or *discussed* during the entire conference. Instead, the conference had been orchestrated—and was eagerly, enthusiastically participated in—as action. I would interpret this to signify that the presenter, together with the group, reproduced the past not as an affect-laden memory but as an action designed to reenact and gain mastery over that intolerable memory. The conference became a living memory that the speaker, with the cooperation of the clinical group (who had similar experiences and thus "resonated" with those of the speaker), reenacted and used to turn widely shared uncomfortable feelings of being the passive victim of a situation into reassuring feelings that came from the active taking of control in the present (Freud 1920).

The presenting physician served as the shaman or medium for the group to repeat his earlier personal trauma. For any therapy to work, those who participate in it must have some conviction as to its efficacy. The presenting resident's therapy—his pedagogical ritual—worked because it was able to inspire the uncertainty (if not terror) for which he was able to offer the ritual solution as a cure (compare Devereux 1980b). The presenter's identification with the aggressor, his subsequent projective identification into the clinical group, and the group's reciprocal "identification with the aggressor" can go a long way in accounting for the specific dynamics and style of this presentation and group interaction.

I have no question that the case conference performed genuine work group activity (learning differential diagnosis in medical practice). But such rational, biomedical learning was fueled by group needs and served the deeper purposes of fulfilling the group's basic assumption activity: "fight/flight" under circumstances in which it was impossible to take flight. To a degree, a second basic assumption of the group came into play: emotional dependency. The presenting resident became a mother/father nurturer and "provider" of firmer defenses for the group to use in saving face and achieving mastery in the face of dread. At the level of work, the conference occurred within lineal time. At the level of basic assumption activity, the conference seemed to float in a trance or dream in which past, present, and future condensed into one.

Following the conference many participants remarked and wrote in their formal evaluations that they had been highly engaged by it. To my knowledge, no one had dozed (a plight endemic to medical conferences). Nor did participants surreptitiously busy themselves with other projects (opening mail, reading journal articles) while paying perfunctory attention. But the question remains: What happens when groups act out and ritually resymbolize their shared unconscious conflicts rather than rendering them accessible to conscious control through interpretation and the integration of feeling? In the conclusion of his study of a southern snake-handling cult, La Barre asks, "Can a society never modify the cultural superego, the Sacred Past? Not so long as it insists that salvation comes only through allegiance to the sacred past! Cultural compulsions constrain societies as firmly as compulsive systems bind the individual neurotic" (1969: 170). What Parin writes of the ego psychology of role identification seems especially apt for the process of medical professionalization.

> The narcissistic gratification derived from role identification is most striking when the assumption of the role results in other massive frustrations. Recruits who have suffered deprivation of their rights and harassing treatment during military training, remember during their analysis how identification with their role brought them immediate relief. When part of the individual superego can be delegated to the authorities, passive, masochistic homosexual and other regressive satisfactions suddenly become possible. Here, and especially in less disagreeable role assignments, the narcissistic gain is achieved through being a recruit, a doctor, or a father, for example; if we are dealing with more or less permanent identification, the feeling of an identity of one's own is strengthened, no matter how much this identity is founded on unavoidable or even forced adaptation (1988: 121).

Having participated in the conference described previously, I found myself asking, To what environment is this ritual adaptive? To the degree that reality (the coughing up of blood, its explanation, and its treatment) was summoned to bear so heavily the burden of fantasy, of basic assumption, I concluded that hemoptysis was pretext rather than essence, symbol (or vehicle) rather than symbolized. The conference was not primarily about hemoptysis, although it was officially, ostensibly about hemoptysis. The pedagogical ritual was founded (inter alia) upon three defenses: (1) identification with the aggressor, (2) projective identification, and (3) the turning of being acted upon into initiative and taking control oneself. Although these are adaptive to the environment of medical school and residency training, they are maladaptive in patient care. Moreover, they assure cultural continuity of the institution of biomedicine and the intergenerational transmission of its "culturally constituted defense mechanisms" (Spiro 1965) at the price of inner maturity and outer realism. For ultimately, such a culture can only repeat itself by (1) shoring up its members' defenses and (2) claiming that the topic is "medicine" rather than "group."

Shared traumas and conflicts are endlessly repeated. Institutional/professional defenses against them are offered to each generation of professional initiates. Among such defenses are the need for certainty and the belief that it can be found; the need to be right and the belief that through adherence to clinical orthodoxies one is assured of being right. Through this ritual process, succeeding generations are taught what to remember and what to forget and in turn reaffirm in the generations of clinical elders their own remembrance and forgetting.

Through medical education, internship, and residency training, clinical categories of knowledge and skill are acquired and incorporated into the self, becoming part of the practitioner's identity. While one learns much "biomedical science," one also learns that some cultural values and pursuits are even more important than science, even as they may be implemented in the name of science.

Although one learns to learn biomedicine in medical school, the groundwork for the future practitioner's choice of medicine for a career and profession is laid much earlier. In the next chapter, I try to show that the emotional and cognitive plausibility—the sense of rightness or fit of self with imagined career—for role training and identification as a medical professional derives from the interplay between formative childhood relationships and the developing structure of the future physician's unconscious.

SEVEN

THE SELF OF THE PHYSICIAN: LINKS BETWEEN CULTURE AND PERSONALITY

THIS CHAPTER IDENTIFIES developmental precursors and current unconscious conflicts in biomedical practitioners' life experience that set the stage for the choice of medicine and of a particular practice style as in part a solution to these deeply personal issues. In exploring unconscious and family-of-origin issues in the motivation to become a physician (or other type of practitioner), I argue that the "source of the Nile," the *fons et origo* of biomedicine, if not of all culturally constituted symbols and metaphors and practices, lies in those experiences and motivational forces that lead a person to invest in and identify with or to develop a particular set of cultural meanings. This chapter establishes the dynamic link between the personality of the practitioner and the culture of medicine and the society it serves and embodies.

PHYSICIAN, FAMILY, AND CULTURE: OVERLAPPING CONTEXTS IN PATIENT CARE

In recent years, a considerable literature has developed on the influence of physician (or, more generically, clinician/health care practitioner) family-of-origin issues on the clinician-patient relationship and clinical work itself (Christie-Seely et al. 1984; Crouch 1986; Mengel 1985, 1987; Schwartzman 1986). Mark Mengel, for instance, notes that the out-of-awareness repetition of one's early familial relationships and rules in clinical roles often results in physician ineffectiveness (1987). A parallel literature on the influence of unconscious factors in all aspects of clinical decision-making, research, and treatment has developed within the fields of psychoanalysis, psychiatry, and psychoanalytic anthropology (Davidson 1986; Devereux 1967; Freud 1905, 1923; Katz 1984a; Kernberg 1965; Reich 1951; Smith and Stein 1987; Stamm 1987; Stein 1985e, 1985g, 1986c; Stein and Apprey 1985, 1987). Veikko Tähkä (1984), Howard Stein (1985g), Howard Stein and Maurice Apprey (1985), and Karl Menninger (1957) all draw attention to unconscious factors from formative childhood years that are expressed in medicine and that affect professional choice. For instance, conflicts about acknowledgment and expression of aggressive drives might come out in clinical relationships with patients who do not accept or follow medical advice, who do not accept the physician's wish for control, and so forth.

Unexamined responses to patients can range from rejection, indifference, seductiveness, and callousness to oversolicitousness and indulgence of patients' wishes (seeking patient satisfaction and approval). What such responses have in common is that the physician is responding to a past situation or recurrent pattern in the present, not to the distinctiveness of the patient. Actions that stem from unexamined physician subjectivity often feel stressful. The physician feels unwittingly compelled to reenact an old scene or relationship in the present, to right an old wrong, to alleviate a deep hurt, through the patient. To do so, the physician transfers his or her problem onto the patient and treats it in and through the patient. To protect brittle self-esteem (Rochlin 1973), a physician threatened with the sense of failure might be contemptuously rude toward a patient or relentlessly aggressive in pursuing a cure.

The choice of medical profession is both conscious and unconscious. Tähkä identifies "the need to help people, alleviate suffering or influence the community in ways designed to promote the health of its members" (1984: 23) as being some common conscious reasons. When referring to the role of "paragon figures" in such choice, Tähkä writes that the choice might be consciously motivated by the need "to follow in father's footsteps, but it may also be based on an unconscious identification with, for instance, the caring and nurturing mother who alleviated the sufferings of childhood. Conscious and unconscious models and objects of identification may of course be other than one's own parents" (1984: 23).

The strong pull of early, unresolved family influences is exemplified by the dilemma of one resident who was nearing completion of his training. One morning Dr. B. said quietly but urgently to me after medical rounds were over, "Let's go to the coffee shop for breakfast." He was in a crisis about the choice of a practice site (even if only for a time-limited contract) and the choice to stay in primary care (or leave it for a medical specialty with less patient contact). In fact, he wondered why he was in medicine at all.

Dr. B. felt torn between his Christian (and mother-related) sense of responsibility to care selflessly for the sick and his wish to make lots of easy money without having to work much for it (a message from his father since he was small). Dr. B.'s parents had divorced when he was a child. Dr. B. described his mother as sickly, depressive, and manipulative throughout his childhood and early adolescence. Her illness symptoms cleared considerably when she settled into a rigorous, well-paying job she liked. His father was a successful, affluent, and remarried real estate agent who had urged Dr. B. from the beginning to go to medical school and be a doctor and return to live and settle in his hometown.

Dr. B. said that throughout his premedical undergraduate years he had consistently earned a high grade point average. He had done all this to please his father, to show he could do it. When he started medical school, his grades fell. Now, just a few steps from achieving "his" goal, he was not sure he really wanted to be a physician. He felt like running away, unsure of who "he" really was. He had difficulty tolerating prolonged contact with recalcitrant patients. "You want to try to cure people, and some of them just don't let you cure them." He was not sure that he really wanted to be a family doctor, always available to patients. He said, "Now that I'm done, I find that I'm just playing my father's game. I don't know what I want to do with my life. Dad says sign the contract. But it ain't that simple any more for me."

We talked about his having a few years to think about what he wanted to do the rest of his life. He considered it. He also said he was thinking about taking a radiology residency, in which he could have regular hours, no call schedule, time for his family and home. He was also giving some thought to emergency room medicine.

> I need some time to think, and I'm running out of time. I remember an old movie [something from the 1940s] in which X and Y [actors' names] were flying a plane and were downed and stranded in the desert. One of the guys had a knack for tinkering, so he repaired it as best he could. They only had a few chances to fire up the plane. After the first failed attempt, X said that the next ones have to work or it's curtains. But Y used the next firing not to get the plane going but to blow all the soot and dirt out of the exhaust, so that if the plane would have a chance at all, the engine would be cleaned out. The gamble paid off: The last shot they had fired up and the plane took off, the other guys were strapped to the wings, and they all got off. That's my plan: I've got to use my next shot to clean out the cobwebs.

Dr. B's use of the movie scene dramatically illustrates the all-or-nothing way in which he viewed his future: death by reengulfment in his family, life by autonomy (symbolized by successful flight, achieved in perhaps an anally explosive manner). Simultaneously the meaning, practice, and choice of biomedicine were heavily intertwined with unconscious and family significance, which erupted precisely at the moment when he was about to leave the residency training "nest." In his residency training, Dr. B had consistently found most vexing and evoking of his contempt those middle-aged, vaguely somaticizing, seductive, dependent, demanding, unhappily married women whom he could not quickly cure and be rid of—women, in short, as we discussed in numerous counseling sessions, who conjured up the overwhelming presence of his mother, to whose care he had been virtually abandoned while his father was on business trips and during long work evenings of dubious activity. Medicine which had begun for him as a sort of secular way of saving people (earlier in his life he had been an avid evangelical Christian proselytizer) and a culturally acceptable symbolic solution to his identity problems, suddenly itself became a monstrous problem.

In a recent study of the doctor-patient relationship, Ellen Lazarus writes that

> although a wide range of personalities is attracted to the field, as in any profession, the people drawn to medicine have generally been characterized as science-oriented, high achievers—very bright, highly disciplined, goal-oriented people with narrow interests and minimal education in the humanities or social sciences beyond high school. A strong undergraduate background in the sciences predisposes them toward the biomedical perspective (cf. Carver 1981). Physicians on the faculty generally agree with this characterization of doctors. One physician I interview in this study commented, "The personalities and socialization of physicians should include people

> who are willing to have delayed gratification, who value control of the environment, who are compulsive and like to pay attention to detail. They are often sicker than the average, I mean physically ill, and therefore have more contact with the system and put a higher value on the system. Often they are children of physicians and so see the realities pro and con. Like nurses, they self-select. Conditioning reinforces. It's not off target to say it helps to be rich" (1988: 38).

Whereas Lazarus enumerates largely conscious factors that influence the choice of medicine as a career, Tähkä identifies largely unconscious aspects of the regulation of self-esteem that are applicable for all physicians, male or female. These features are at once a part of selecting a medical career and of practice reality itself.

> Doctors usually are people for whom success is important. Virtually without exception future doctors are selected from students who topped their class at school which, besides ensuring a high level of talent, usually also implies above average personal ambition. The socially highly respected position of doctors often seems to correspond to these ambitions. . . . The temporary helplessness and dependence of patients, the respectful attitude of other health care personnel and the special powers conferred by society may foster unrealistic images in the doctor about himself as the omnipotent master of life and death. . . .
>
> Excessive use of childish means of regulating self-esteem is only rarely possible for doctors nowadays. Nevertheless, the doctor is endangered because he rarely receives realistic feedback about his own function and behavior in professional terms. If a barber or a motor mechanic does shoddy work or behaves badly with his customers, he receives immediate critical feedback which forces him to reevaluate and improve either his work or his behavior if he desires to prosper in his trade. Doctors very rarely receive this kind of feedback from their patients because patients feel it may be dangerous or unwise to criticize a person in whose hands they have placed their health. There is a similar relative lack of feedback in hospital communities where the doctor usually is at the top of the hierarchy (cf. Cullberg, 1970). It is difficult to see one's own limitations and deficiencies when others do not point them out. Hence, a special alertness is demanded of doctors that they maintain a realistic image of their own capabilities and limitations. . . . If the doctor's self-esteem is too dependent upon his ability to cure, the center of gravity of his professional practice will be skewed from helping patients to using them as exhibits in evidence of his professional skill. This may easily lead the doctor to vent his irritation on those patients who do not improve as expected and to the avoidance of those groups of patients for whom complete recovery is no longer possible (1984: 25–26).

A primary care intern who had previously earned a number of academic degrees presented to me and to a group of his physician peers a case of a six-year-old girl dying of a congenital enzymatic disorder.

> Her six foot, four inch father, wearing coveralls, and who states that he has three or four Ph.D.s, insists that he "knows" what's going on medically. He wants a "roundup" to kill all the bugs: "I want an X-ray," he tries to order. He constantly beeps the doctor, certain that there's something that can still be done to save his daughter. "I want her on everything, and now," he demands.
>
> The supervising physician is extremely irritated with the father, who threatens to call the hospital patient representative unless he gets his way. As intern, I'm only

an observer in this case, but cases like this make me feel backed in the corner. At this point in our training we don't want to admit, "I don't know." The parent's intimidation and frustration play on the doctor's frustration to gain control. What do you do, tell the patient to find another doctor?

[Another intern added, "I'd rather have Dad be pushy than fall apart. I dread patients going boo-hoo. Sure we're taught to let them cry and grieve, but it makes you feel helpless. . . . What are we going to fill that void with when that boil bursts?"] So each intern puts in his time and puts off talking with Dad about his grief. Let the next intern take it. As soon as you start to get to know a patient or a family, your time's up. So you don't get involved and just pass it on. It's easier on you that way.

[Another intern interjected, "What do you do if he CRIES? . . . Crying takes *time*. We're worried about residents and attendings seeing us just holding hands and comforting instead of acting like real doctors who are supposed to do something"] The parent wants control; the doctor wants control. The parent wants to take control from you. Interns have more problems with this because they have absolutely no control in the hospital services. We don't even know if we can control *ourselves*.

Later on, privately, as clinic consultant, I speculated to this same intern about yet another issue that might have upset him in this case—that he had multiple higher education degrees and a notable professional work experience and was now "just an intern," reduced to feeling like "a mole." His eyes brightened: "Maybe I'm really identifying with the father's sense of vulnerability and powerlessness. Maybe I see myself in his situation." He then reflected that his wife was pregnant with their first child, which might have added to the identification.

The intern's outrage over this parent's repugnance at the care his daughter was receiving almost literally melted from his face as he came to realize and feel his own overlapping issues. He recognized more fully how helpless, humiliated, and enraged *he* felt as a "mere" intern—just as the patient's multiply-degreed father felt himself to be a "mere" father, powerless to save his daughter. Physician interns and residents, seasoned medical practitioners, indeed clinicians of all types, are emotionally vulnerable to overidentification with and revulsion toward patients whose life situations and stages resemble their own. These awaken in them what they are struggling to repress.

In discussing "the myth of altruism" in social work (Lawton 1982), psychoanalyst Rochelle Shatzman makes some cogent observations that also apply, in my experience, with equal force to men and women within medicine:

All psychological processes are transactional events, a recent discovery. . . . The social worker's desire to help is recognized as a manifestation of the social worker's need to control irresponsibility and disorderliness in himself, thereby gaining self-approval, and possibly the approval of society (parents). We see the undesirable impulses in his intense efforts, in his extreme efficiency, in his "selfless" devotion to duty, in his moral rectitude. The need to strenuously control his own impulses is revealed by the sternness of the demands he places on himself. . . . The social worker is not speaking only for himself, he is not revealing only his own impulses and defenses: he is speaking for the individuals who make up the society itself. . . . Since we cannot successfully control our own narcissism, it must be controlled in others.

> Thus we see that the definition of "true" helping, altruism, denies the helper any right to *want* to have his efforts praised; by some logic, if he wants to be praised, his desire to help is despicable and his help worthless (1983: 382).

The control of the patient through compliance becomes many a physician's principal and relentless preoccupation. Just as "the parent uses the child to 'cure' himself, demanding that the child control himself because the parent cannot control himself" (Shatzman 1983: 384), many physicians unwittingly use the patient to "cure" themselves of the problem of control.

The problem of self-control in the physician and the problem of control in the wider society are inextricably linked. The physician, struggling for self-control, is delegated by society to control the patient in behalf of a society that can scarcely control itself. Such widespread diagnoses as hypertension, diabetes, obesity, bulimia, anorexia nervosa, alcoholism, drug abuse—all problems of control—signify how pervasive is the culturewide problem that medicine is singled out to solve.

From within the sacred microcosm of the clinical relationship—officially regulated by confidentiality and patient advocacy—the physician often attempts unconsciously to achieve (tenuous) self-control and to serve as an agent of social control. The patient, who is the official focus of patient care, is in fact often a medium through which the physician and society struggle with the problem of self-control. What Meyer Gunther (1976: 205–206) describes as a professional hazard for the psychoanalyst—"***the inevitable threat of narcissistic disappointment or humiliation***"—is likewise true of any practitioner who works with refractory patients such as chemical abuse addicts. Gunther, following Heinz Kohut, refers to the analyst's demanding self-expectations in therapy, which are evoked by patients' demands, but further recapitulate the analyst's own prior experience of anxiety and humiliation as a child upon being unable "to meet his own (depressed) mother's demands for understanding and comforting" (1976: 216). I find this pattern to be common among biomedical physicians as well (Stein 1985e, 1985g).

To the threat of narcissistic injury is added the fact that the instinctual indulgence the addict engages in—or seemingly so to the physician or counselor—challenges the clinician's imperfect personal and professional renunciations, reaction formations, and attempts to control others' saturnalias. Problems of addiction among physicians themselves attest to the difficulty of their social role. Since the early 1980s, the new cultural diagnostic and syndrome category "impaired physicians" has even emerged and with it an array of detoxification and rehabilitation institutions. Patient types whom physicians condemn the most roundly and forgive the least are often shadows of what many physicians are tempted to become. Psychopathic tricksters everywhere test and strain the mettle of society's moral police.

A compulsive need to treat patients who resist (or whom the counselor perceives to resist) cure may lead to escalating aggressive zeal by clinical staff (see Lerner 1979). Such redoubled zeal in the face of failure—and to virtually all American clinicians, failure spells intolerable defeat—may mask unconscious guilt and rage toward patients who fail to respond (Lerner 1979). These overdetermined emotional responses and accompanying therapeutic activism in turn often rest upon unconscious projective identification with the patient as a representation of a parent or of a repudiated aspect of oneself. In work with patients who are experienced as thwarting or defying the therapist's effort (including substance abusers, hypochondriacs, noncompliant hypertensives and diabetics, and chronically ill and disabled patients who fail to respond to rehabilitation efforts), "treatment efforts easily become irrational, excessive, overly intrusive, and punitive" (Lerner 1979: 467). Families, therapists and society alike vacillate between identifying momentarily with the addict-violator and identifying with the vindictive superego representative of the imperfectly internalized parent.

No amount of "rectification of names" (from compliance to adherence, contract, and self-regulation) can efface the psychological issues underlying compliance. To this must be added the widespread sense among Americans that the social order itself is out of control! The cultural burden of medicine has indeed become great; patients, families, insurance, government institutions, and the wider culture together call upon medicine to bring order and structure to people's lives. No single institution, no matter how dedicated or zealous its practitioners, can single-handedly eradicate the problems that lie with the ethos of the culture.

The Unwelcome Incursion of the Past into the Present

Often in medical education and practice, as in other areas of life, people experience and act upon inner emotions and thought processes as if these were wholly located in the outer world. Freud writes that "before [a language of abstract thought had been developed] owing to the projection outwards of internal perceptions primitive men arrived at a picture of the external world which we, with our intensified conscious perceptions, have now to translate back into psychology" (1913: 64). He also writes that "the ego is first and foremost a bodily ego; it is not merely a surface entity, but it is itself the projection of a surface. . . . [Freud adds a footnote stating that] the ego is ultimately derived from bodily sensations, chiefly from those springing from the surface of the body. It may thus be regarded as a mental projection of the surface of the body, besides, as we have seen above, representing the superficies of the mental apparatus" (1923: 26). Finally, Norman O. Brown contends that "human culture is a set of projections of repressed unconscious. . . . Like the transference, human culture exists in order to project the infantile complexes into concrete reality, where they can be seen and mastered" (1959: 154).

The human body, interpersonal relationships (such as physician-patient), and society all can be consciously experienced as screens upon which inner unconscious thoughts, affects, fantasies, and conflicts can be projected and played (acted) out. Throughout my career as a behavioral scientist, first in psychiatry, later in family medicine and occupational medicine, I have counseled and provided quasitherapeutic consultations with interns and residents about difficult, vexing, and bad patients. Interns and residents have likewise sought me out for occasionally long-term counseling with respect to strong emotional reactions they have had toward patients. They sought to better understand and control these reactions so that they could be more effective and more compassionate physicians. In the course of such consultations, during which pertinent life history materials were elicited, I have noted recurrent family patterns among interns and residents. Such patterns were also expressed through an extremely aggressive, macho medical style that eagerly embraced the sports, military, and mechanical metaphors and their associated values discussed earlier in this book.

Many of these individuals remembered their mothers of childhood as controlling, dominating, predatory, manipulative, and sometimes seductive women who were sometimes emotionally very close and at other times punitive if not brutal. Many of the mothers were described as sickly and/or depressed and turned to their offspring, usually sons (the future doctors), for comfort and treatment. The fathers tended to be away for long hours at work (including farm work, in which the fields and the company of other men were an often sought refuge from wife and family; see Stein 1987a, 1987c). In turn, they tended to be aloof and passive when at home, occasionally bursting out with explosive anger and recrimination, if not meting out beatings.

Prior to his case conference presentation about a child whom he had diagnosed as having failure to thrive, one resident, Dr. M., agitatedly requested that I talk with him. We entered the conference room and did a "dance" of where to sit; he was very uneasy. He had already put a thorough three-generation genogram on the magic marker board, having just talked with a patient, Beth (whose baby, Julie, he had just delivered the previous day). He also had several pages of notes.

Dr. M. said that Beth's extended family characterized itself as close-knit yet did not seem to be available to Beth when she needed them. Her first baby, Doug, had failed to thrive in a period during which Beth had been using narcotics. Dr. M. had involved himself with removal of Doug from Beth's care. But the child had continued to have lethargy-vomiting spells every eight to ten days under foster care, the same as under natal care. Now Beth appeared to have ceased using hard drugs and was negotiating for Doug's return with the help of her attorney.

Dr. M. talked about his fear of "being put on the stand" and seeing Beth and the judge "pronouncing judgment over me." As he went over the genogram, I gently asked him where he "fit" into it all because he had written "me" with arrows beneath the mother and two children. He started talking about himself and his family, then switched back to Beth's family, using the genogram to create distance.

> When I was little and I wanted to say anything, I had better be right. My mom and dad would ask me something, and when I answered the question, I'd better come up with the right answer or they'd hit me upside the face. [I pursued him on the phrase "upside the face."] I'd get beaten and sometimes it was on the face. You learned never to speak just glibly 'cause the consequences were great. You learned to watch yourself and keep your mouth shut unless you were sure of yourself.
>
> With Doug, I started out thinking that his failure to thrive was psychosocial in origin, but then I became less sure. It's true that the mega workup on him produced nothing. Just before his hospitalization for tests, he went through one of his episodes, and sure enough when he was in the hospital he was just normal—and as soon as he returned home ten days later he started getting lethargic and nauseous! I started to think that I should have given more credence to the medical side of things. Maybe I could have come up with the right answer that way. I could just see Beth,

> the judge, and jury looking at me and saying, "Why didn't you get more aggressive with the medical stuff?"
>
> I think that's why I have this medical/psychosocial split. I started thinking initially that I could come up with the right answers with psychosocial stuff, but then I got scared—thinking about being up there on the stand. It was either/or, and the psychosocial had let me down. It was frightening because I was expected to come up with the right answers—or else, "Whop upside the head."

I interpreted: "Just like when you were small." He gave a loud "Yeah" of recognition. Several times in this discussion, I brought him back to his feelings (anxiety, dread, fear of judgment, rage about helplessness) and to his original family situation. He began to realize that one of the major (mental) functions of the medical model and of medical decisionmaking was to provide him the authority and certainty so that he would not be wrong and would thereby avoid being helpless at the hands of successors to his parents. Through medicine, he would have the chance of not being wrong and therefore of preserving himself from beatings and humiliation. One of the culturally elaborated ideal roles within medicine, in fact, is for the physician (and other health care personnel as well) to "have the right answers" to give to authority figures (successors and representatives of parents) and in turn to function as authority figures. At a deeper level, this averts punishment, humiliation, and threat of abandonment (see Katz 1984a; Stein 1985g; Stein and Apprey 1985).

The present case resembled and evoked the past. For a while, Dr. M. was back in the past all over again. I mused that perhaps he felt like an endangered Doug. He stood up and went over to the genogram, saying:

> There's more here than meets the eye. When I was two or three, my parents divorced. My dad, whom I can't remember, just up and left. He left for another woman, leaving my mom high and dry to take care of everything. I had two sisters. Mom had to take all the responsibility. A year or so later, she married. My stepfather says he loves me, that he's glad we're now his family, and all that. But I've often wondered whether that's just what he thinks we'd like to hear. I don't know what he really thinks and feels about me, whether he ever really wanted me.

I pointed out the parallel between this and Beth's family's myth of closeness and actual abandonment or vacillation. He recognized the parallel. He really seemed to be mastering this old trauma, seeing what in the case had terrorized him. During the subsequent case conference, although he was well organized and vigilant, he did not seem to be repeating the family situation in which he was the helpless child and the other participants were dangerous, critical parents. This was one of the most emotionally demanding and stretching experiences with a resident I had had in a long time.

For male physicians, I frequently discern a dynamic of what Ralph Greenson (1968) and Robert Stoller (1985) call a difficulty in disidentifying with a mother to whom they were closely tied. Medicine for them was a way to gain distance from the controlling mother, to prove that they were real men. Mothers had supervised and regulated everything and had exercised dominion over their bodily functions as they grew up. Identifying with this, these young clinicians eagerly became executives of compliance in later work with their patients. But also, especially when the mother had been sickly and dependent on them for "parentified" care, they identified themselves in their medical role as the one responsible for "repairing" their patients' bodies and lives in ways better than they had been able to do for their mothers.

In American society, long described as rife with "momism" (Wylie 1979; Erikson 1963b), one available mechanism for males to disidentify with "mom" and her inner presence is through the rigors of medical training and practice. This serves the function of rites of passage and intensification of the American cult of masculinity. In medical training and practice, clinical valor is performed and praised in the language or idiom of military and sports valor. In the past decade, with the success of the women's liberation movement in America, women have become an increasing presence in medical school and practice. In my experience, this imminent threat to the "men's club" and virtual "secret society" of medicine has been met by men's attempt to incorporate women (insofar as they are willing) as "one of the boys." This involves a masculinization that reaffirms the male-female antagonism and polarization. By "really" becoming a malelike physician (with the virtues of aggressiveness, the love of procedure, the avoidance of intimacy with patients, disdain for "wimpy" patients and homosexuals), female physicians become less of a source of pollution and paradoxically affirm male role security.

The issue of cross-sex identity and its resolution has been much discussed in the cross-cultural literature developed and inspired by J.W.M. Whiting (1960; see also Whiting, Kluckhohn, and Anthony 1958; Munroe, Munroe, and Whiting 1981; Snarey and Son 1986, 1987). John Snarey and Linda Son summarize this approach as follows:

> Whiting's theory indicates that in cultural groups where father participation in childrearing is absent and where a close mother-son relationship is present, boys will develop an unconscious primary feminine identity. This cross-sex identity becomes a source of conflict during adolescence when emulation of their mother is culturally forbidden and conscious identification with the father is expected. Whiting goes on to say that in these cultural groups boys are typically provided with an initiation ceremony at puberty that functions to resolve this conflict. These ceremonies of initiation into manhood may include painful hazing by men of the society, tests of endurance, seclusion from women, or genital operations. In the absence of such male initiation rites, boys may act out their feminine identity when social sanctions are not oppressive. If a male dominant image is highly valued, however, the boy's primary feminine identity may be acted out through hypermasculinity—overdetermined attempts to prove one's masculinity through physical violence, aggressiveness, or military valor (1987: 72–73).

Snarey and Son argue that in societies in which cross-sex (feminine) identification is strong among males as a result of early childhood socialization, its outcome in adulthood "depends on the cultural mechanisms available for resolving or acting out the conflict. The absence of effective male initiation rites and the presence of strong social prohibitions against homosexuality, for instance, predict the presence of hypermasculinity" (1987: 73–74).

For these men—and for those women in medicine who aspire, through medicine, to become "one of the boys"—the medical profession itself functions as a masculinity cult (see Brandes 1979; M. Gilmore and D. Gilmore 1979; D. Gilmore and Uhl 1987; Ingham 1964) in which the demonstration of bravery and aggression is accomplished through clinical prowess in diagnosis and treatment. Likewise, for them, medical school, internship, and residency are not only a rite of passage from lay to professional status but a ritual of manhood (compare Herdt 1982) that heightens the boundary between female and male. David Gilmore and Sarah Uhl (1987) point out that it is invalid to extrapolate the classic Latin-Mexican type of machismo (Ingham 1964) to the rest of the ethnographic world in which some sort of masculinity complex occurs. Nonetheless, cross-cultural evidence (as in D. Gilmore and Uhl 1987; Gregor 1985) strongly suggests that a difficulty in establishing a male gender identity, resulting from the establishment of a strong "protofeminine" identification through closeness with the mother, will lead the male to seek (if group ritualization is not provided) forms to bolster his disidentification and counteridentification.

One would suspect that male sports, businesses, and military organizations perform similar functions because medicine borrows some of its most potent metaphors from them. Where gender identity conflict is not dramatically, even brutally, ritualized and a masculine identity affirmed, individuals are left to improvise on their own or to find groups or organizations that will offer them a rigid boundary definition. In more compassionate settings, gender identity conflict (expressed as feared, repressed femininity and passivity versus aspired-to hypermasculinity) can be understood and worked through (as in psychoanalysis; see Apprey 1981; Snarey and Son 1987).

Forbidden Tools of the Self

In medical training, linkages between current clinical interactions and past influences are complex. Often the linkages emerge in layers. Consider the following example. An irate third year and chief primary care resident fumed during a counseling session:

> Dr. X. [a second year resident in her specialty] is arrogant, an SOB, an asshole. He's so manipulative. He asks, "When is checkout?" [from the hospital service]. I answer that if patients need admitting [to the hospital], you need to take care of them. If things get busy, you have to stay around. He didn't care and left. It is an occupation-of-origin issue for me [an allusion to some prior work experience, to which subject she returned much later in the meeting]. He's refused to tell me a patient's blood gases. He treats me like I'm the enemy. My obligation is to the medical service; that's where his is too. . . . I'm so fucking pissed at him. . . . He's angry. He makes me so angry. It's not a difficult service [the primary care inservice]. What's the issue, then? How do I handle him when what he's doing makes me go nutsy?

This resident wrestled with questions of her own authority over a junior resident, her position in the administrative order of the primary care clinical division and the department.

> Either I'm in charge or I'm not. Dr. X. is in a rage, out of control. I'm expected to ignore his hostility. He's in danger, crying wolf, stabbing me in the back. I'm afraid for him. He's a time bomb. My days are good or bad on the service depending on how he acts.

She then spontaneously introduced the mysterious subject of "occupation of origin." I asked her to explain.

> It's an employment-of-origin issue. When I was a social worker, I worked with a woman who was nuts, who made my life miserable. I finally filed for unemployment on grounds of mental cruelty and I won a unanimous decision. It was like living with terror, working for her. He—Dr. X—could twist things to get me in trouble with the attendings. We're in the middle of some procedure and he takes off to have a donut. Just give me a clue. I'm going crazy.

Thus far, she had made the association, even blurring, between her frightening former job situation and her present work with Dr. X. I tried to focus on why this resident had emotionally "gotten to" her now. I asked her, "What was different? Is it because you are now chief resident? Is your image of how things ought to happen part of it, since you're a very responsible physician?"

> I'm being reasonable for the most part, lenient, flexible, and *then I get walked over!* I'm getting ballsy [having balls, like a male physician, also becoming assertive or aggressive]. I'm taking charge on the service. That's quite an accomplishment for a woman. Then he says to all this, "Fuck this."
>
> He reminds me of my brother. He's either totally good or totally bad. He's out of control, hostile, so much of the time. In my family, everybody loves to hate my brother. Just like Dr. X. You feel so sorry for him, my brother. With Dr. X., I want to stand up for myself; then I got shit upon. How am I supposed to handle my hostility, and I don't have a penis? Maybe I'll bring in my three-foot wooden phallus that I have at home; it's an African wood carving. [She soon began to wonder aloud:] Why does this set me off? I didn't have to deal with him, to take all that crap from him. Yet I do.

I started to focus on the practical issue of whether she could permit herself to set limits on Dr. X and what the consequences of this would be in the medical service. I asked her how direct she had been with him when he was being inappropriate. Suddenly her loud anger, accompanied by agonized bending forward and putting her head in her hands, abruptly changed. She became quiet and stared out into space. She protested, "To say 'No' is cruel to someone who is sick. I've survived twenty years with my brother. I can survive as many years as he needs."

I pointed out the poignant equation in her mind between saying "No" and "cruelty," and I wondered why she felt the need just to survive. Was that all she was good for or worthy of? As the discussion continued, I explored with her the issue of setting limits, that it might even be good for the resident rather than a sign of cruelty. She persisted, however, fighting the confrontation: "I feel trapped. I'd be willing to be skewered for my brother."

I encouraged her to explore further the meaning of her role as the one who expects herself, and is maybe expected by others, to be skewered for her brother's sake. By the conclusion of an emotionally vacillating counseling session, she began to permit herself to see options other than submitting to the terrorism of the resident. She came to recognize that terrible as her current predicament was, it was burdened both by what she had called her employment-of-origin situation and her family-of-origin situation. In the latter, to set limits for her emotionally "sick" brother would violate the family rule that he was too disturbed to have limits set for him. Yet by being so lenient and permitting him to walk all over her, she had built up a self-fulfilling prophecy of hatred and ultimately wanted to be cruel to the very person who needed protection from cruelty.

She came to realize that the current practice and training situation was to her an intolerable repetition of an earlier, now internalized, family situation that had made her feel powerless and enraged. By better understanding and emotionally reexperiencing the original traumatizing situations, she was able to consider alternatives to it in her relationships with medical colleagues. In this, the resident began by reliving in the present her original home situation—it was a reign of terror to which she was expected to respond with leniency rather than any hostility. That her supposedly disavowed anger was breaking through was her initial symptom, which she at first displaced by asking me how to handle the recalcitrant resident. Although much of this case is idiosyncratic, it links personal, familial, and former and current occupational situations. Further, it illustrates the frequent linkage between the taboo on expression of hostility in family of origin; its repression, denial, and projection in a physician's character structure; and its vicissitudes in difficult relationships with fellow clinicians, patients, supervisors, and subordinates.

That the choice of biomedicine as a career, and one's practice style, can largely function as an unconscious counterdependent strategy and in turn help one cope with unsettling family-of-origin issues is illustrated by the following excerpt from counseling I did with a physician in her forties. She had recently resigned from the HMO that had employed her for several years. Defining her current feeling as burnout, she explained that "I don't like dealing with patients any more." Shortly thereafter she added, "A lot of physicians in HMOs go through this." She continued:

> Part of it is a midlife crisis, I'm sure. My image of myself got very blurred. I was doing everything badly. There were so many demanding patients. They asked me for things I wasn't giving to my family. I got angry. . . .
>
> [I asked her how much she thought her difficulties stemmed from the demanding HMO environment and how much from herself.] I was expecting perfection from myself. I didn't want to make mistakes. I got arrogant telling patients and staff what I had said seven times. I expected them to get things after fewer times than that! I was demanding and critical. Then I stayed away [from meetings and conflicts], not wanting to face rejection. . . . I don't work well with other people telling me what to do. . . . I'm afraid of becoming like my father. [I asked her to explain.] He's there, part of me. He got his prejudices from his mother. I don't want to be paranoid. She was a bigot. German farm woman in the Great Plains. She hated herself because she was a woman. She was full of "shoulds." I'm not proud of any of the family. All they do is criticize. . . . Dad had problems with Mom; now [that]

I'm living with her, I see she's part of the problem. . . . I want to work a way out of all this. I need to see new solutions. . . . Physicians live by moment-to-moment decisions, but doctors can't plan long range. I don't make plans that last. I need to have more choices. I've not made good choices. If I'd focus and concentrate, maybe I could come up with better choices [career, love]. My choice of medicine was not good for me. [I asked her to explain further.] Mom was always critical of Dad and of marriage. She complained of being helpless. For me, medicine was a way of being in charge, not dependent on anyone else.

What Obeyesekere (1981) terms "personal symbols," that is, symbols whose meanings have deep, unconscious motivational significance, and cultural symbols, which is to say symbols which have widespread currency in a society, are often aspects of the same mental process and structure. What is private is often displaced and projected onto, and becomes embodied in, what is public; and what is public is frequently incorporated and identified with, because it serves inner needs (see review of Obeyesekere by Lock 1983). The question "What sustains the cultural system?" can in part be answered by the discovery of a fit among personal, institutional, and macrocultural issues. Even if imperfectly, this fit often builds on the repetition of early, traumatic developmental situations, inner conflicts, and subsequent defenses against them. But the fit between individual psychodynamics and cultural representational or ritual systems is never perfect (Spiro 1982b). Nevertheless, cultural continuity is in large measure contingent upon the ability of a cultural symbol and ritual system to represent, express, and to a degree bind the anxiety, shame, guilt, and core fantasies derived from growing up in that society. Despite the United States' much touted cultural pluralism and diversity, a fit between early childhood experiences and medical socialization and practice can be identified.

Early in the second year of his residency training, Dr. H had "accumulated" (his term) several middle-aged patients whom he characterized as demanding, dependent, and manipulative and as taking great amounts of his time. A young, married physician, he and his wife were expecting their first child. He aspired to be a devout Christian, emphasizing the formula JOY (Jesus first, Others second, Yourself third) as the organizing principle in his life. He had a strong wish to "fix" and "cure" all patients and expressed difficulty in setting limits and saying, "No." He became depressed and angry with himself and resentful toward patients who did not improve or try to help themselves.

His Christian self-for-others attitude combined with an explicit mixture of biomedicine and homespun politics: "Where I come from, everybody is expected to pull their own weight and not live off the fat of the land." He made himself selflessly available to patients (taking lengthy telephone calls at home; permitting patients to talk for one-half to one hour in his office even when he had vowed to limit the visit to fifteen minutes) and then bitterly complained that *they* had not stopped talking. He wondered:

What do you do when you try to set limits—say, on the number of office visits per week a patient can have or on the amount of time you spend with them—and they keep calling or coming in or talking? How do you make plans for them or

> with them, like for them to take the medicine you prescribe, and they don't carry out the plans? There's a lot of patients on welfare and I'd like to say to them, "Go out and get a job, become economically self-reliant, and that will increase your self-esteem." With a lot of patients, I'm the parent. When they don't listen, punishment might bring them around to my way of thinking. What kind of punishment? Not writing prescriptions for them, firing them from the clinic.

I asked Dr. H to describe a little about how he grew up, the atmosphere in his home. He was the youngest of three siblings. His father was a rancher. Both his father and mother were active outside the home in their local community, rarely sitting down, for instance, just to watch TV. His family, past and present, was actively involved in a rural evangelical Protestant church, attending worship services several times per week. He said:

> People in my family rarely get sick. We keep too busy. You don't have time to think about yourself. [I asked him if he could recollect punishment when he was small.] Whenever I did anything wrong, I got whipped. I've always been big. My mother use to give me beatings until I was around twelve or fourteen. One day I had her pinned to the refrigerator. That was the last time she tried to beat me. After that my father did all the whipping when he got back from work.
>
> I sometimes wish that I could take the stick to patients the way they did it to me. Maybe it could make them listen better. But you can't do that. I don't mind seeing patients back every week or for months so long as we're making progress. But what are we accomplishing and what am I accomplishing if all the patient does is come here [to the clinic] week after week and have a social visit?

I mentioned some of the work of Otto von Mering and William Earley (Earley and von Mering 1969) in which they state that many patients go to the doctor as their only or rare social visit. I wondered aloud whether he might rethink his expectations of such patients. He continued, however:

> I've gotta feel that we're achieving something. I can take even small steps, but I don't see the point to continuing seeing patients if there's no progress. That's what I mean about the doctor being the parent for many patients: When you're the parent, you have certain expectations of the child. If they do something right, they get a reward; if they do it wrong, they get punished. I guess I just haven't yet found an adequate way to punish patients who just keep coming back to see me and aren't working on getting better.

Dr. H consciously accepted a parental, caretaking role. In unconsciously identifying the parent with the aggressor, he sought a role with his patients as his parents had with him. But it was imperfectly internalized. He did not just punish; he struggled with the idea of punishing. If anything, rather than punishing, he was overly indulgent with patients (reaction formation) who took advantage of him, which made him wish to punish more.

Society and health professionals alike have an ideal image of physicians that conflicts with the reality of the full spectrum of human feelings and fantasies. Much of the power of this image can be traced to childhood expectations and family experiences. Professional training in medicine builds on this earlier core.

During professional training, health professionals learn to become superb observers of patients and of diseased organs and tissue but have little training in how to observe themselves; they therefore have poor access to their own feelings and fantasies, in part because they are not supposed to have them (in the official view these all interfere with one's professionalism). Even classroom use of such tools as the genogram (McGoldrick and Gerson 1985) may be taught as an exercise that utilizes pervasive defenses within medicine that distance clinicians from time-consuming interaction with patients.

As medical trainees become professionals, they are taught objectivity and detachment; these become internalized as paramount values. There develops a shared wish that emotional responses do not exist or that they exist only in the sick and infirm, that is, in patients and families. The desire to act professionally often leads to the disowning of powerful feelings. But feelings, wishes, and fantasies that are split off, repressed, denied, and counteracted do not disappear; they reappear through the acceptable disguise of patient care. Clinicians can often use patients and patient care as a means of gaining distance from their own feelings and conflicts. Issues that cannot be acknowledged and examined as existing inside are displaced and projected onto the screen of diagnosis and treatment. In the rush to action, the clinician "treats" his or her unresolved conflicts outside, in the person and body of another.

In an insightful vignette, psychoanalyst Jay Katz illustrates how unconscious father-son conflicts in surgeon George Crile, Jr. affected his eager embracing of radical mastectomy as a means of totally denying uncertainty.

> Crile [Jr.] wrote that his father, George Crile, Sr., a renowned surgeon of the early twentieth century under whom he trained, "*never* did a radical mastectomy" [Crile 1973]. Instead, his father always employed a less mutilating surgical procedure. George Crile, Jr., continued, "During my residency at the Cleveland Clinic, I was also exposed to the influence of Dr. Tom Jones, who *always* did a radical mastectomy. Being a rebellious child, I discounted my father's ideas, adopted the Jones technique, and for seventeen years I performed only radical mastectomies." Now, however, Crile concluded, "conventional radical mastectomies are not done" at the Cleveland Clinic.
>
> Having been trained by his father and Jones, Crile was aware of the uncertainties that surrounded the proper treatment of breast cancer, but he was compelled to deny uncertainty and substitute an uncompromising certainty in its place for powerful personal reasons. . . . I . . . encourage a more self-conscious and reflective recognition of the constant presence of uncertainty in medical practice. Such heightened awareness may alert physicians to the fact that something may be amiss whenever single-mindedness dominates their therapeutic interventions (Katz 1984b: 38).

Sociologist Renee Fox (1959) and psychoanalyst Jay Katz (1984a, 1984b) separately show that peremptory clinical activism may serve as a defense against uncertainty. It sustains and in a sense creates "dogmatic certainty" (Katz 1984b) through the exercise of power and control. The resulting flight into action may create a medical cascade that renders any caution, prudence, or delay intolerable. Katz concludes that

> if greater [physician] awareness and acknowledgement of uncertainty are too much to ask, at least it must be recognized that, in physician-patient interactions, professionals' defenses against ignorance and uncertainty are a greater problem than patients' ignorance. . . . Patients' supposed intolerance of medical uncertainties may thus turn out to be a reflection less of an inherent incapacity to live with this tragic fact and more of an identification with the perceived incapacity of physicians to live with it. Patients' supposed intolerance may turn out to be significantly affected by a projection of physicians' intolerance onto patients (1984b: 44).

The aggressive drives are part of medical practice, medical education, and inherent to the very dynamics of medical groups. Tähkä writes that

> being effective as a doctor usually involves the ability to take initiative, courage to make decisions and to perform tasks with often far reaching intrusion on the body of the patient. . . . The practice of medicine in general does require an adequate amount of neutralized aggressive energy as a power source for activity. If instead the aggressive drives are tied up in various conflicts and thus inhibited from supplying power for determined activity, the result may be various inhibitions of function, difficulty in making decisions or excessive and guilt-ridden worry about the well-being of patients.
>
> On the other hand, the aggressive drives of the doctor may be incompletely sublimated, in which case they do not provide the driving power for exclusively appropriate activity in the practice of his [or her] profession. The non-sublimated aggressive drives in the doctor may then seek a target in the patient and emerge as a form of direct or indirect physical or psychological ill-treatment of the patient. It may for instance be expressed by humiliating or annoying the patient, in causing unnecessary pain or discomfort or simply in direct bursts of anger at the patient with no consideration for the framework of professional behavior (1984: 26).

A markedly aggressive approach to medical treatment resembles, if not derives, from what deMause refers to as an "intrusive" mode of childrearing (1974b). The goal and process of this approach to socialization are to conquer the child's mind, "control its insides, its anger, its needs, its masturbation, its very will" (1974b: 52). The intrusively raised child is often hit but not regularly whipped (in contrast to earlier, more primitive modes). Further, the child is made to obey his or her care-givers promptly with threats of guilt. The parents are also more capable of genuine empathy than those who project their own unconscious issues onto their children. A yet more advanced childrearing mode, which deMause terms the "socializing" (1974b), teaches the child by training, guiding, and urging conformity.

Although it is all too easy to try to force data gained through observation and participation into a favorite procrustean theoretical bed, my familiarity with the family background of many of the psychiatry and family medicine residents with whom I have worked the past sixteen years persuades me that much of the ideological struggle in medical practice and medical education—and within individual physicians—about what approach to use with patients, and therefore the controversy over compliance, rests upon formative experiences these physicians have had in their families of origin. How a physician will respond to and feel about a patient will often be a replay of her or his own family experiences, evoked by and projected upon the patient. Through the doctor's countertransference responses, the patient embodies the refractory child in the doctor and alternately summons up the self-righteous parent with whom the doctor has identified. In my experience, although many physicians would like to see themselves as truly guiding, training, socializing—if not helping—their patients, they find themselves drawn into the role of taskmaster in trying to regulate in the patient what the patient cannot—and the physician experiences as "will" not—control for himself or herself. The cultural language of biomedicine—and the preferred metaphors of war, technology, sports, and economics—strongly persuades me that much of the practice of American medicine is a playing out of residues from intrusive/socializing childrearing in the physicians' own lives. Consider the following physicians' stories.

VIGNETTE 1

The following tragic case is taken from a volume on the psychology of ethnonationalism that I co-authored with a distinguished group of psychiatrists (GAP Committee on International Relations and Stein 1987). It shows how personality conflicts, family-of-origin experiences (especially those in relation to the physician's mother), ethnicity, and the occupation of physician were interwoven in the physician's diseases and, ultimately, in his death.

> A sixty-year-old physician sought psychiatric treatment for increasing anxiety and depression that made him drink to excess. His symptoms were recent and quite disconcerting as he had hitherto been successful and well disciplined. After completing his medical education in his native city, he had begun practice in a city several hundred miles away and quickly established himself. A good public image was important to him; he made the most of his blond good looks, Anglo-Saxon name, athletic ability, and membership in the Episcopal Church.
>
> Though his manner was poised and persuasive, he had some undesirable personality traits, being rather deliberate and a bit too controlling with his patients, who considered this as evidence of his interest in them. Few saw that behind his facade he was actually quite dependent on them. To his wife and son he appeared to be domineering and demanding, but the former finally recognized the dependency he could not himself acknowledge. She herself was very dependent and reared their children with some difficulty; when they left home, she stopped trying and lapsed into using alcohol and tranquilizers, which her husband supplied. In an effort to save herself, she finally left him and got along better without him. His clinical problems began when he was left alone.
>
> His public personality was designed to disguise what he thought of as his problem—he was Jewish. His father was a successful but striving professional, and his mother also was never content, always demanding more from her family—"typically Jewish—pushy and possessive"—he said. "She was a teacher and very controlling. I couldn't wait to get away from home." As a boy he had been "fat and ugly, so ashamed I'd never get into a swimsuit."
>
> Feeling overfed, feminized by his mother, and too fat, he reacted in high school by becoming athletic, remaining so all his life. After medical school he distanced himself from his family psychologically and socially as well as literally, but was clearly unable to escape his dependency on his mother, his denial of it, and his controlling nature. He made no attempt to analyze the reason for these troublesome traits, but

> stereotyped them as being Jewish and ascribed them to his mother. He used Jewish ethnicity to deny and externalize parts of himself he hated, and adopted WASP ethnicity to achieve and support his ego ideal.
>
> His personality conflicts were his ultimate undoing. The main artery of one leg became so constricted that he had to abandon his vigorous games of handball, so he had surgery to correct it. He foolishly began playing handball again too soon after the operation, and the artery ruptured and his leg had to be amputated. "I should have known better," he mourned. His image was shattered; he saw himself as flawed, ugly, weak, childish, and feminine. Becoming dependent on drugs and alcohol, he died in circumstances that suggested suicide (1987: 68–69).

Although the case highlights ethnic symbolism in the expression of personality conflicts, it likewise clearly shows how the identical issues of controlling/being controlled, masculine/feminine, WASP/Jewish were played out in this physician's own body image and in his professional work. It would be tempting to distance ourselves from this case, if not dismiss it as an exception or as an instance of the increasingly popular category "impaired physician," were it not for the fact that in all our lives, facets of our early development in our families, what we make of our cultural legacies, and our occupational choices and experiences are all tightly interwoven. The type of physician, or other practitioner, one is cannot be separated from the type of man or woman one is.

VIGNETTE 2

Dr. Z is a fifty-three-year-old, second generation Polish American family physician. He spent his formative years in the Chicago Polish community, became a general practitioner, and during the 1970s received board certification in family medicine. He is now a practicing family physician and academician. During his twenty-five years in medicine, he has become increasingly concerned with issues of legitimacy for family doctors and family medicine departments within mainstream biomedicine. His model of "real medicine" is that of the internist and surgeon. An avid supporter of research in family medicine, one of his principal goals is to demonstrate to those in medical subspecialties that family physicians can perform complicated obstetrics, read electrocardiograms and X-rays, and perform other difficult diagnoses and procedures as well as their colleagues. He labors indefatigably to prove the worth and elevate the status of family medicine as a bona fide discipline.

In his family of origin, he was always very close to his mother and remote from his father. Although she was a devout Polish Catholic, she made it her mission in life to Americanize him. One of her ambitions was for the family to move to a respectable, middle-class American neighborhood away from inner-city Chicago. It was important for her that she and her family look and act as American as possible. Manners, demeanor, grooming, cleanliness, and style of dress and speech were all of utmost importance to her so that she and her family could demonstrate they were loyal Americans, as good as anyone, even if they were "Johnny come latelys." Many of her ambitions toward legitimacy and respectability were carried forward by her son, who in his efforts on behalf of family medicine relentlessly championed her cause.

In his professional realm, one of Dr. Z's favorite mottos is the need "to clean up family medicine" and make it into a "real" specialty that family practitioners can stand up and be proud of. He only halfheartedly supports including psychology, social work, family studies, family counseling, and the like as part of family medicine's core. "We're not going to be able to stand up and be counted unless we have the hard data to prove we're not second-class doctors." "Just keep your noses clean," he admonishes. His clinic office and home are monuments to the display of status and respectability. Yet, in his view, despite all his tireless efforts, his family medicine seems never to have arrived with sufficient triumph as a legitimate, full-fledged member of the biomedical family of specialties.

From this brief description, I have interpreted Dr. Z's occupational choices and meanings as partial reenactments of early family and ethnic issues. The split between ethnic and American parallels that between dirty and clean, behavioral science and real medicine, and soft data and hard data. Just as his mother was zealously ambitious for him, so he is now ambitious in behalf of family medicine so that, like him, it will become respectably, unquestionably mainstream and American. His worst fear is that no matter how hard he scrubs his beloved family medicine, it will remain the alien outcast he still fears himself to be.

Vignette 3

One resident physician in her mid thirties spoke repeatedly during her counseling of the supreme value she placed upon "unbroken unity" in all of her relationships. Whether in intimate relationships with men, in occupational groups of medical peers, or in her religious community, she sought the "feeling of family" that she never had in her family of origin. She conducted an anguished search for idealized relationships in which she could merge and through which she could acquire a self. Bypassed in a recent promotion to chief of medical service, she felt jolted out of her quest, deprived of what she felt to be rightfully hers, and "discounted" (a word she frequently used to describe how she felt treated in relation to others who were given preferential treatment despite her hard work, superiority, and merit).

During the ensuing weeks in counseling, only slowly and with difficulty did she recognize and acknowledge the anger behind the hurt and the family origins of her futile quest. She had long insisted that her parents "had done the best they could; they just didn't know better" in order to avoid looking at the early family source of her intense separation anxiety, her dread of rejection, her fear of being overlooked, and her vacillation between clinging to relationships at any cost and renouncing everything for professionalism. Gradually, in discovering her rage, she discovered her self, that is, her personal distinctiveness. She voiced anger and terror at her father's "emotional abandonment" of her and her mother's "consuming" of her. Gradually she began to need less and to look less for the security of perfect relationships in which she would find unity in her orientation to her work environment and other social contexts.

In light of these vignettes, let me briefly summarize an impression I have had from working as teacher, supervisor, and counselor with many residents in psychiatry and family medicine and from discussions with a number of psychoanalysts. (1)

Repair of the patient may serve to repair the self of the physician. For example, just as the child feels called upon to nurture, sustain, if not altogether "parent" the depressed or chronically sick mother so that the mother will be able to better minister to the child's needs, so later the doctor often unwittingly repeats the earlier child-parent relation in clinical practice, hoping to repair the patient in order that (unconsciously) the patient may be able to repair the doctor's own fragile cohesiveness. This can, of course, occur in clinical relationships irrespective of the age or sex of the patient. (2) Emotions and fantasies associated earlier with the (usually mothering) parent are reawakened and projectively identified with the (often refractory) patient. (3) Through the patient and the disease(s), the physician contends with the ambivalence toward the parent whom he or she felt to be emotionally inadequate. (Does this, at least in part, account for the longevity of the appellation "inadequate personality" that physicians continue to use in relation to patients with whom they feel inadequate?) (4) The symmetrical struggle with the patient for compliance and control often unleashes inwardly turned rage that originally could not be directed against the mothering parent, who could not be repaired by the child's earlier efforts.

VIGNETTE 4

There are further issues to consider in understanding the pervasiveness and tenacity with which clinicians' personal, familial issues influence the doctor-patient relationship. The externalized control of such disavowed personal characteristics or impulses as rage, greed, dependency, and weakness is only part of the story in the struggle for control. Yet another level is the reparative meaning medical practice holds for many physicians. While doctors refer to many procedures as repair in the more mechanistic sense, they often act as if far more is at stake in terms of their own sense of wholeness than whether the patient's machinery is back in order.

In the late 1970s, I had been supervising a family physician with a young couple whose stormy, brief marriage had been characterized by a fear of intimacy, extramarital affairs and provocations, mutual recrimination, and so forth. Following one particularly difficult session, the physician and I left the consultation feeling glum and (as is my practice) discussed various aspects of the session. He said, dejectedly, "Something's wrong today. Before today we've always ended on an upbeat note. It's as though today we weren't able to do anything for them." I commented, "I'm feeling it's as though today they weren't able to do anything for us—that's my problem." He exclaimed, "That's it!" with a recognition of our unconscious investment in the direction and outcome of the marriage therapy.

We then devoted the remainder of the "debriefing" to a discussion of our reaction to the couple, the implicit values of marriage and of counseling that we were inadvertently imposing upon the couple, and so forth. We spoke of the Hollywood and Walt Disney sentimentality on the movie screen and on television that "confirms" our childhood wishes and expectations for couples somehow to "live happily ever after." We discovered the extent to which, even momentarily, we were dependent upon the couple's ability to resolve their profound problems—that is, the extent to which we had projected our wishes and agendas onto them and into the therapy in which we had to "do something" to rescue them. Therapeutic intervention had become projective intrusion. If ever so briefly, we became part of their problem, implemented by our value orientation. Our discussion felt as if we were awakening from a dream or trance.

VIGNETTES 5 AND 6

A physician and his wife had been trying to get pregnant for two years. When she finally did become pregnant, they were happy; but the happiness lasted only two weeks. The pregnancy turned out to be ectopic (the fertilized egg was implanted outside of the uterus). The physician later said that during his wife's bleeding and surgery, he did not have much feeling, but "then it hit me, and I've been grieving over it." He finds work in the newborn nursery most taxing emotionally. "I was a father for two weeks. . . . I'm appalled when I see mothers who are deserting their infants, mothers who don't want their kids, where we wanted a kid so bad." He voiced how difficult it was not to turn against these mothers for neglecting or rejecting a child when he and his wife were deprived of the child they wanted. Here, he was intellectually aware of his feelings, although unsure whether he could control them in the doctor-patient relationship, interviews, and patient care.

Similarly, a behavioral scientist was consulting with a married, female family medicine resident who was irate about a pregnant Chinese American woman who refused to take the prescribed iron-enriched vitamins and who seemed otherwise noncompliant and uninterested in her own pregnancy. The patient had evidently not wanted to become pregnant and now wanted to have her baby and be over with it (abortion was out of the question). A consultant was brought in to mediate the conflict. The consultant spoke with the patient in Chinese and learned that in her culture, pregnant women do not take vitamins. The consultant discovered, however, that within the patient's framework, seaweed figured prominently in her diet, and the consultant and the resident successfully got the patient to increase her intake of seaweed to give her the necessary iron supplement.

Although the resident was glad that her patient was getting the iron [in a culturally acceptable form], she still found herself disliking the patient and not looking forward to OB visits with her. Following the delivery, the resident and behavioral scientist visited the neonatal unit, and as the resident looked longingly at the baby she said to her colleague (something like), "I wish *I* could have a baby like that. Why do people who don't want babies get them and others can't have them?" The resident had thus far been unsuccessfully treated for infertility. Although at a relatively surface level the case was a conflict in explanatory models, at a deeper level it represented her envy of her patient for having the child she could not have, her projective identification of the patient with bad aspects of herself (and perhaps her own mother).

VIGNETTE 7

Storytelling and listening between clinician and patient (or client, family, fellow clinician, and staff member) can ***facilitate or prohibit the emergence of the deeper intrapsychic story***. Ironically, often one of the latent functions of clinical practice is to protect the clinician via the patient from the painful reemergence of his or her own intrapsychic story. Patient care often serves as an interpersonally regulated defense mechanism. Thus, what the patient needs to be healed (if not cured in the biomedical sense) is precisely what the clinician defends against in himself or herself most. In *Countertransference and Psychotherapeutic Technique*, for example, James Masterson admonishes therapists that "to the degree to which you have not resolved your own depression (not necessarily an abandonment depression), you will have great difficulty tolerating your patient's depression, because it stimulates your own. It resonates with a lot of the things which you experienced as a child which you have repressed, and it stimulates them and starts tugging on them; they start pushing up, trying to get release" (1983: 188). For clinician (therapist, physician, nurse) and patient alike, the implicit and explicit stories together constitute the "whole" story. Moreover, the mental organization of clinician and patient will determine the "choice" of story (similar to symptom choice) that can be articulated, elicited, or heard.

Dr. J. is a physician practicing in a small rural Oklahoma town. In a dinner conversation with physician colleagues and myself, he discussed the case of an eighty-year-old female patient of whose diagnosis he was uncertain. Dr. J. sometimes thought it was Alzheimer's disease; other times he thought it was cognitive/affective change based on anxiety. The patient had an older brother who was severely demented and who had to be constantly cared for by the family, at great expense to them. He said, "I took the attitude that we're going to lick this. So I made my plan to try every anxiolitic if I had to. It's like I lined up the medicines from the PDR [*Physician's Desk Reference*] in my mind and said, first we'll try this. If it doesn't work, we'll try the next one. And so on."

Following some open-ended questioning on my part, Dr. J. associated that in his family of origin he had a grandmother who in her old age had become psychotic and a burden on the family. He said that he was becoming "obsessed with this patient, trying to find something that would work, and still unable to make a definitive diagnosis of Alzheimer's." He became a little tearful as he talked about his grandmother. He also remembered that in obtaining a history from the patient's family, the patient had been rather anxious, worried, agitated, not exactly the Oklahoma pioneer woman type. He then spoke admiringly of another elderly patient who had recently died. This patient had exemplified the endurance and dignity into old age that he attributed to a healthy rural life. He admired that the patient's family had allowed the death to occur at home.

I recalled aloud that only a few months earlier his father had undergone some abdominal surgery and that the surgery had gone well. I wondered whether his father's aging was part of this "obsession" with the patient and the need to find something that would make her less "off the wall." Something resonated in him. He started talking about his father's surgery, that the growth in the abdomen was not a malignancy, that his family had been reassured by the biopsy. But "it's real hard for me to see my parents age. It's starting to show in their pace, an occasional lapse in memory. I find myself wanting to shake my father and say 'Come on, you could remember that if you tried harder.'"

In an earlier part of the discussion while we were eating, much of our conversation was occupied with cholesterol/triglycerides, discussing how high or low our levels were (I did not know mine). We wondered what food to order from the restaurant. Three of us ordered a half-order per person of corn chips heaped with cheese, chili, hamburger meat, and spices, not exactly a vegetarian dish! Thus, part of the context of the discussion was this physician's realization of his own aging and fragility. Perhaps (I did not explore this) he also feared the prospect of becoming psychotic ("like" his grandmother) as he aged further.

Our discussion did not provide Dr. J. with a new diagnosis or treatment plan. It helped him, however, to realize that much of what haunted and drove him about this case—and his need to make something work for this family—was its resemblance to earlier and current issues in his personal/family life. He left better able to look at the patient and family for who and what they were, less contaminated with what they represented to him.

Vignette 8

Despite defenses erected from childhood against identifying too closely with and experiencing patients' suffering, and despite the officially taught "professional distance" of the clinical role, physicians and other biomedical practitioners do in fact often manage to bridge the experiential chasm between themselves and their patients. A common pathway is one whereby a physician undergoes an experience that he or she had hitherto minimized or discounted in patients and for which he or she had berated if not condemned patients for seeking medical help. Many interns and residents, male and female alike, have said as follows:

> I used to resent these moms and dads who would call you at home, or have you paged in the middle of the night, to come in to the emergency room because they were worried about their kid. Maybe it was a sore throat, or the ear was too pink, or they weren't eating right, or fever. The mom and dad could never find time during the day, when the clinic was open, to bring in the kid. There was always some excuse: had to work, couldn't find a sitter for the other kids, or it looked worse. Most of the time, the kid didn't really need to be brought to the ER, and there wasn't anything more we could have done there than we'd have done at the clinic. Sure you could give them reassurance. But it sure was expensive, either to them, or to the insurer, or to us taxpayers if the patient was on welfare or Medicaid. I always wondered about what kind of people would be so inconsiderate of *my* time.
>
> Then my wife and I [or my husband and I] had our first child. And everything changed. I used to be to the [political] right of Atilla the Hun when it came to wanting to really put these parents in their place. Now, *we're* the ones who get bent out of shape when our daughter [son] is crying at night and we don't know why, when we try to take care of things as long as we can, but sometimes run out of tricks in the middle of the night. When it's your own kid, and you're the parent who's worried, a lot of the objectivity goes out the window. You don't think according to the Washington *Manual of Medical Therapeutics*. You wonder, "Is my kid going to get worse? What might happen if we do wait?" Then we're the parents who call the doctor at the wrong time! I've been more accepting and tolerant of new parents who get me out of bed in the middle of the night, because now I've been there myself.

This example illustrates how a life-cycle transition experience often leads to greater compassion toward patients in similar developmental stages. For cases of how a physician can use his or her own illness experiences in the service of empathy, see Hahn (1985a).

Self and Clinical Role

In biomedical practice, the clinical relationship is an inseparable part of any technique or procedure. The true "self" of the provider is part of what the clinician provides to the patient—or, alternately, withholds or conceals (see Candib 1987). Attentive listening is itself also an act of intimacy and reciprocity. One "tells" or discloses much about oneself by what one can and cannot afford to allow the patient to say or to permit oneself to hear and respond to.

The self-insight of the physician—of any clinician—is a powerful diagnostic and therapeutic tool. In permitting intimacy and reciprocity through the use of one's own depths in medicine, the clinician acknowledges a shared, common humanity with the patient despite the necessity of divided function and unequal roles. In permitting and fostering intimacy with the patient (and, for that matter, with other medical colleagues and staff or between medical educator and resident), the clinician avows that "my experience could help illumine theirs and help them to perceive and feel for themselves." The reverse is likewise true, as Searles (1975) writes in "The Patient as Therapist to His Analyst." To heal is not only to ply a trade or a technique. It is to be moved by the one whom one would heal. Healing, in this sense, validates and transforms both healer and patient (and family).

As I have shown, such an approach to healing and physician-patient communication is far from the dominant cultural model. Powerful cultural currents, sown in childhood and reaped in adulthood, militate against greater access to and use of these aspects of the self. This, I believe, is one conclusion that can be drawn from the linkage I have identified among the majority of the life history vignettes presented in the chapter, the factors in medical socialization, and the values and metaphors discussed earlier in the book. In a sense, one's early years and their legacy, the intense professional training ritual, the institutional and ideological structure of biomedicine, and the American ethos together "conspire" to split off, project, and repress much of those very instruments of the self that could be mobilized in the healing relationship. Childhood, family, unconscious, medical education, and the cultural organization of American medicine and its society intertwine to make as certain as possible that the unconscious is kept securely at bay—only for it to find indirect expression in the very out of control acts and the fear of loss of control that medical professionalism is designed to prevent. Childhood, early family experiences, and their intrapsychic elaborations set the stage for adult culture in which they are again met and reenacted in new guises, in which repetitions are solutions, and in which a tie with the past is preserved through the present. Breaking the cycle in medical practice and training is prodigiously difficult precisely to the degree that the larger culture remains committed to keeping that cycle intact in order not to unearth the deeper meanings and feelings against which culture vigilantly defends.

To complete this cultural study of biomedicine, I now conclude by briefly exploring the utility of a psychoanalytically informed ethnographic approach to future research, teaching, and practice in American biomedical culture.

CONCLUSION

Implications of an Anthropological Approach for the Study, Teaching, and Practice of Biomedicine

THIS BOOK BEGAN WITH A SERIES of questions, which the ensuing chapters attempted to address if not to answer, about American biomedicine in particular; about biomedicine as an ethnomedical system; about the fit between individual and culture, between institution and society; about the process of becoming both a member of society and a member of a clinical profession; and about the process (methodology and theory) by which one comes to learn about these.

This book has thus attempted to accomplish several things. First, it has offered a broad and deep ethnography of the culture of American biomedicine, including a description of the selection and socialization process by which one comes to be a member of the medical guild. Second, it has attempted to locate the professional culture of biomedicine within the larger cultural currents of American society. Third, it has attempted to link the developmental line of individual practitioners, professional socialization, institutional dynamics, the dynamics of the culture of medicine, and those of American culture (including its values and metaphors). Fourth, it has attempted to illustrate how idiographic research can be reconciled with nomothetic research. Fifth, although largely an intensive study of a single culture and an interpretive exploration of biomedicine, it has addressed such cross-cultural issues as the symbolization of distress (cancer, AIDS, alcoholism), the relation between the culturebound and the universal, benevolence and aggression in the practitioner and in the social image of the practitioner, and the ritualization of manliness. Sixth, it is simultaneously an anthropological account of medicine and of how the author worked in medicine as part of the data-gathering itself. In this respect, it aspires to integrate applied medical anthropology, critical medical anthropology, and clinical anthropology. Seventh, it has advocated a psychoanalytically informed ethnographic method by which a researcher and/or clinician might obtain similar data (or the perspective within which additional data would be gathered) to go beyond the findings of this book.

The ethnographic method, which is the foundation of anthropological fieldwork and theory building, is quintessentially contextual and open-ended. In looking, one never knows quite what to look for and can therefore discover what others have overlooked. Likewise in hearing, one cannot know in advance what to listen for. Systematic observation based on participant observation within a group leads to an uncovering of patterns and levels of meanings and relationships that are often not discernible by standard (and standardized) American cultural techniques of data collection. Through immersion in the group, often for long periods of time, one learns how that system and its many subsystems are organized (Geertz 1973; LaBarre 1978; Spiro 1982a: xv; Stein 1982e, 1983a). I have urged that in order for this ethnography to be deep as well as broad, it must include an openness to a psychoanalytic perspective on the culture under study. In studies of medical systems, the ethnographic method permits an investigator or clinician to grasp the breadth, complexity, and depth of symptom formation, persistence, and treatment.

In this concluding section, I urge the adoption of this approach in clinical research, teaching, and practice in American biomedicine. This is not a brief for employing great numbers of anthropologists and other behavioral scientists in medical settings. It is not a plea for more "turf." It is rather a plea that all medical research, patient care, and medical education could benefit from acknowledging and eliciting the contextuality inherent in every aspect of medicine (as in every aspect of life). For the physician, nurse, PA, physical therapist, or administrator to conduct ethnographic inquiry into American medicine, he or she need not abandon other "routine" medical activities and do something separate called "ethnography." It is less a matter of who utilizes this approach (anthropologists, physicians, psychoanalysts) than of what can be incorporated in any day-to-day framework of activity. That is, this approach is a perspective and way of thinking and working that merits inclusion in the tool kit of all health care professionals.

Just as it is imperative for better health care that biomedicine expand systems thinking beyond the biomedical disease and the patient to subsume the patient's world, we must likewise insist on the same inclusiveness—which is to say, rigor—in exploring the health care side of the clinical relationship. Until the 1980s or slightly earlier, most anthropologists in medical settings taught physicians and other biomedical personnel about ethnic, religious, familial, social class, and other features of the *patient* population. The patient, the patient's family, and the disease consist of several subsystems in the always present larger social system that includes the cultural world(s) of the investigator, practitioner, and teacher. A truly clinical ethnographic systems approach is as much interested in the physician's (and any other practitioner's) view of and feelings about himself or herself, the physician role, the culture of medicine, the patient, and the disease, as it is interested in the world of the patient.

G. Gayle Stephens, M.D., writes of the relationship between the medical profession and the wider society:

> I have no need to whitewash the medical profession or to deny the reality of individual failures to live up to its highest ideals, but the magnitude of the problem is too great to be explained by that. Blaming individuals will get us nowhere. The facts are that the medical professions, the lay public and the institutions of society (hospitals, health insurance companies, businesses, the courts and units of government,

> etc.) are inextricably bound together in creating the system in which we all move and have our being, and there is more than enough blame to go around. In one sense it may be said that we have a system, for good or ill, that we all have a vested interest in, one that represents the plusses and minuses of our demands, expectations, beliefs, and self-interests (1985: 11).

To one knowledgeable of the history of medicine, the naturalistic, ethnographic approach proposed here would be congruent with if not simply an extension of the inquisitive naturalism associated in biomedical history with such luminaries as Hippocrates, Leonardo da Vinci, Bernardino Ramazzini, Sir William Harvey, John Snow, Rudolf Virchow, Sir Alexander Fleming, Louis Pasteur, and Robert Koch. It simply expands our interest in human suffering from its manifestation at the cellular and anatomical levels in the body to its expression in the persons of all participants to the clinical relationship, whether they be identified as the afflicted, the family, or the practitioner and his or her medical culture (see Stein 1982i). The use of the ethnographic method to describe and explain the small and large group dynamics of medical practice would be a valuable tool for practitioners, teachers, and researchers who wish to help American medicine to become truly context sensitive in clinical decisionmaking, treatment, and social policy planning.

In *Naturalistic Inquiry*, Yvonna Lincoln and Egon Guba (1985) urge that science as a whole can advance only through the adoption of more naturalistic research methodologies. Psychoanalyst Sylvia Brody calls for a similar approach to the study of infant development (1982: 586–587). In a series of works I describe the utility of psychodynamically attuned, ethnographically contextual teaching approaches to medical/residency education (Stein 1982e, 1983a, 1985g; Stein and Apprey 1985; Snider and Stein 1987). I also encourage study of one's own family as a tool for understanding the complexities of issues in personal, family, and occupational life that affect behavior that physicians label as medical "noncompliance" (Stein 1988; Stein and Pontious 1985). For the medical practitioner or the medical behavioral scientist, there need be no dichotomy between clinical work and fieldwork.

In a paper on primary care theory and research, Kleinman advocates the ethnographic method as a means of eliciting meanings associated with illness and treatment:

> Qualitative description, taken together with various quantitative measures, can be a standardized research method for assessing validity. It is especially valuable in studying social and cultural significance, e.g., illness beliefs, interaction norms, social gain, ethnic help seeking, and treatment responses, and it is the appropriate method to describe the work of doctoring. . . . If the ethnography of meaning is not legitimated in primary care research, even though it is legitimated in anthropology, sociology, and social psychology, then meaning will not receive a scientifically appropriate assessment in primary care (1983a: 543).

I only urge that this approach be considered appropriate and essential for any medical setting, not that of primary care alone (see Hahn and Gaines 1985).

The ethnographic method proposed here for the study of American medicine is introduced as a potential corrective in clinical research, training, and practice.

It supplements rather than supplants biomedical research designs by making self-reflexiveness the foundation of all knowledge and clinical work. Ideally, at least, it helps the acquisition and validation of knowledge to become more rigorous. There is no necessary antipathy among researchers or clinicians who focus on different facets or levels of a patient's sickness or on different clinical abstractions (gene, molecule, cell, organ, person, family, occupation). The antipathy enters only when researchers or clinicians assume or claim that their part is in fact the whole or the part that merits the highest if not exclusive clinical status. Devereux writes that the use of scientific methodology to reduce anxiety is illegitimate only when methodology is "used *primarily* as an ataractic—as an anxiety-numbing device" (1967: 97). Good methodology "does not empty reality of its anxiety arousing content, but 'domesticates' it, by proving that it, too, can be understood and processed by the conscious ego" (1967: 97). "What matters, therefore, is not whether one *uses* methodology *also* as an anxiety-reducing device, but whether one does so *knowingly*, in a sublimatory manner, or unconsciously, in a defensive manner *only*" (Devereux 1967: 97).

A psychoanalytically informed ethnographic approach to clinical teaching, patient care, and medical research is not only intrinsically worthwhile and methodologically sound. It is also practical. It directs us to become better observers and interpreters of American medicine without prescribing precisely what or who to observe and interpret. It helps us to have a better grasp of the whole system. It allows the nature and extent of that system to be an open question. It is true to the lived reality of all participants to the clinical encounter, while accepting nonexperiential factors (culturally labeled as "biology") as part of the clinical picture.

Philosopher Alfred North Whitehead writes that "a one-sided formulation may be true, but may have the effect of a lie by its distortion of emphasis" (1926: 123). Moreover, "progress in truth—truth of science and truth of religion—is mainly a progress in the framing of concepts, in discarding artificial abstractions or partial metaphors, and in evolving notions which strike more deeply into the root of reality" (1926: 127). This criticism applies to biomedicine's penchant for devoting exclusive attention to disease-entities. It applies as much to medical anthropology and medicine's penchant for focusing attention on the patient to the exclusion of the observer or clinician (and *their* cultures and institutions). It also applies de rigueur to much of medical anthropology's paradoxically narrow if not parochial view as to what meaning-centered or interpretive medical anthropology should encompass. There is no prima facie reason the exploration of meanings and constructions (a current buzzword) of clinical reality should be limited only to certain categories of people (patients, shamans, physicians) and certain types of clinical thought (experiential as opposed to reductionistic or natural science—another false dichotomy, in my view). If everything we all do (inside and outside medicine) is cultural, why should not, say, a microbiologist's search for disease etiology be of as great an interest to those trying to understand meanings (and the search for meaning) as a patient's health belief model? The science of the human animal would do well not to commit the same kind of mistakes of which it accuses biomedicine: the exclusion of some kinds of meanings.

An ethnographic approach helps clinician, clinical teacher, and clinical researcher to ask novel questions rather than insist on the sanctity of culturally routine ones.

Thus, a physician treating a hypertensive or diabetic patient who does not take the prescribed medication might ask himself or herself, "Why am I so utterly focused upon this patient's compliance?" rather than "What's wrong with this patient that he/she doesn't comply?" The physician might further inquire, "What are the meanings and relationships according to which the patient lives and within which my call for 'compliance' does not fit?" Such a perspective permits the physician to escape from the control trap and arrive with the patient at possible alternative, creative solutions. A depth psychology–informed ethnographic approach to all clinical work provides a way of reframing, of imagining anew, how we think about our work, which includes ourselves.

In medical education, research, and practice alike, it behooves us to attempt making explicit what is often culturally implicit, not only in the patient, patient's family, personal network, occupation, and community, but in the world in which the clinical teacher, researcher, and practitioner move as well. It is not enough for the medical anthropologist or academic physician, say, to become knowledgeable about the patient population and to exhort medical students and residents to do likewise. To become a tunnel-visioned "expert" on any one part of the system can give an incomplete, unbalanced, and distorted view of the system as a whole, especially when the worldview the doctor or teacher brings is officially taken for granted rather than approached with as much interest, critical acuity, and compassion as is that of the patient. If I may make an analogy: It is like trying to study the specific gravity of materials by only examining the intrinsic property of the material rather than its relationship to water.

How can we humanize the patient or the family if we do not also simultaneously humanize the doctor, the teacher of medicine, the medical researcher, and the groups we call institutions—that is, inquire into their complex "explanatory models" (Kleinman 1980), "semantic illness networks" (Good 1977), and unconscious influences on all aspects of clinical work (Stein 1985g; Stein and Apprey 1985)? This book has shown that physicians' decisionmaking is scientifically, situationally, historically, and emotionally shaped. The ethnographic method is capable of eliciting all of these ingredients, together with the dynamics or process by which they congeal into specific research designs, treatment plans, and clinical relationships.

Any unit of clinical, didactic research interest (chromosome, cell, person, family, culture) can inadvertently be used by its proponents as a blinder in the guise of illumination. How can these blinders be acknowledged, and their meanings or origins understood, if they are not addressed during professional education and if they are not made a part of ongoing continuing education? A comprehensive ethnographic approach to medical education, practice, and research helps us to transcend any one-sidedness. Specifically, it helps us to understand the world of the patient, the world of the disease, and the world of the doctor, teacher, and researcher ***in relation to each other in a single system, and to help them renegotiate that relationship***. In medical education, the interpretation of one's own professional group (or culture) is at least as vital an educational—and clinical—task as the interpretation of the patient's family and culture. Incidentally, the same is true in international diplomacy for the interpretation of other cultures or nations (see Stein 1980a, 1982a, 1985c, 1985h). The United States could benefit from its "Russia watchers" knowing how and why they are "watching" the "Russians"!

Where might one begin? The further exploration of American medical culture can be found virtually anywhere: in a biochemistry lab, on television commercials, in clinic waiting rooms, at hospital conferences. It is more to the point to observe and analyze clearly what we might have taken for granted or overlooked. In cultural studies, one can start anywhere. The point is to begin and permit oneself to be led by the data (the culture's free associations, so to speak) rather than formulate an inquiry beforehand that precludes the discovery of anything new. With this perspective, one can learn a great deal about medical culture with or without conducting formal studies. All it takes is the wit, courage, and discipline to look beyond the official cultural agenda and notice what has been there all along—the multiple levels on which culture always operates.

At this point, the reader—perhaps a busy practicing physician, the already overworked clinical teacher, or a researcher interested in achieving results—may object to this entire line of reasoning, saying, "It is all very interesting, but it is a time-consuming way of gathering data, one that is certainly not cost effective, especially in these spartan times." I wish that there were an easier, quicker, and less anxiety-arousing way to gain access to our subject—human beings suffering their afflictions and seeking respite if not cure and other human beings engaged in patient care, medical research, and preparation of the next generations for patient care. I must insist, however, that ***our methods must be true to our subject matter.***

A psychoanalytically informed ethnographic framework is simply the best one I know that honors its subject. There are no shortcuts in data-gathering and data-reporting that do not falsify the elusive clinical reality we are trying to chronicle and explain. Whether we like it or not, there is no way to read others' minds or lives. To pursue what Tullio Maranhão wryly calls a "snapshot anthropology" (1984: 270)—a concise formula about every group—as if it offered accurate portraits of people's lives is to confuse the pursuit of convenience and the flight from our anxiety (see Devereux 1967) with the nature of the subject we are trying to comprehend.

What Gregory Bateson wrote in 1972 for behavioral scientists applies with equal force to physicians, practitioners of other biomedical specialties and allied health professions, and to clinical teachers of all fields:

> Let me then conclude with a warning that we social scientists would do well to hold back our eagerness to control that world which we so imperfectly understand. The fact of our imperfect understanding should not be allowed to feed our anxiety and so increase the need to control. Rather, our studies could be inspired by a more ancient, but today less honored, motive: a curiosity about the world of which we are part. The rewards of such work are not power but beauty (1972: 269).

We moderns are perhaps existentially more in the same boat as the Nibelung dwarf Alberich, thief of the Rhinegold in Richard Wagner's opera *Das Rheingold*, than we would care to admit. The price of Alberich's wealth and power was the renunciation of love. The evil that ensues during the dramatic tetralogy all ultimately traces to that original fateful choice of greed over intimacy. Paradoxically, in medicine as in other pursuits, when power is less doggedly sought it is often more mightily achieved. This does not argue for the abdication of those medical and widely social metaphors discussed throughout this volume. Rather it argues for a clinical imagination greater than the metaphor. Bateson's curiosity about the world of which we were a part, after all, is responsible for some of the seminal insights and discoveries of the greatest pioneers of biomedicine.

The practice of medicine, medical education, and medical research in the United States are all being subjected to increasing simplification and regimentation of clinical thought, standardization, centralized outside control, mechanization, and minimalist philosophy of responsibility (see Kormos 1984; Stein and Hill 1984; Stephens 1984a, 1984b, 1984c). If these ominous and swift cultural currents are to be reversed, all of us who work within medicine and who seek the personalization of medicine must address, within the house of medicine as well as without, why these currents that are so patently debasing and destructive are felt by increasing numbers within medicine and in the wider society to be a compelling solution to our time of troubles. This book has offered an interpretation of these dangerous currents. If hope is to be more than chimerical, it lies in helping—in part through the ethnographic approach—the institution of medicine and the wider culture to become more conscious of those inner meanings and feelings that have profoundly affected, if not determined, the shape of contemporary American medicine.

Although this has been primarily the intensive ethnographic and interpretive study of a single ethnomedical system, I wish to conclude this book on a theoretical and comparative cross-cultural note. A lively controversy in medical anthropology and transcultural psychiatry abounds regarding the concept (and the meaning) of "culture-bound syndromes" (Devereux 1980a; DiNicola 1988; Hahn 1985c; Kenny 1978, 1983; Kirmayer 1987; Prince 1985, 1987; Prince and Tcheng-Laroche 1987; Simons and Hughes 1985; *Social Science and Medicine* 1985; Yap 1969). Among the indigenous terms grouped (and debated) within this rubric are ***latah***, ***susto***, ***amok***, ***arctic hysteria***, ***taijin kyofusho***, ***ghost sickness***, ***cargo cults***, ***koro***, (in the West) ***anorexia nervosa***, ***bulimia***, ***obesity***, and ***premenstrual syndrome***. The fault lines, so to speak, in this controversy, form around such issues as localism or relativism versus universalism, behavioral criteria versus meaning-centered criteria, culturally unique features versus more widespread features, cultural explanation versus psychological or biological explanation, emic versus etic frameworks. In short, approaches range from one end of the spectrum where the observer or clinician is little interested in local meanings given to the putative syndrome, to the other end of the spectrum where the observer or clinician views a syndrome as exclusively relative to, circumscribed by, and the outcome of the society that is its host and medium. The former aspires to explanation through decontextualization (at least in the sense that the local accounts are viewed as misleading). The latter defines explanation exclusively in terms of cultural contextualization (once the cultural embeddedness of the syndrome is traced, explanation is complete).

Although in this book I have not focused directly on culture-bound syndromes, in exploring American biomedicine I have attempted to demonstrate that biomedicine is relative to American culture and that the very culture is likewise relative to strong underlying protocultural (or culture-formative) currents that can be variously labeled "psychocultural" or "psychohistorical." Although at one level I have viewed culture as context, at another level I have also explored culture in context (see

La Barre 1980). For instance, earlier discussion of running/jogging and the fitness/wellness/health movement were analyzed as American in content and in stylization and as responses to widespread regression, guilt, and anxiety (also see Yates, Leehey, and Shisslak 1983). I demonstrated that the study of how "culture shapes" and how "culture is shaped by" are two facets of the same dynamics of meaning in ethnomedical as in other cultural systems. In my view, the Western medical or clinical term *syndrome* is a subset of the larger conceptual and comparative issue of identifying cultural forms and searching for—and sometimes imposing—common denominators. Thus, for example, whether one regards nationalism to be a syndrome, it is a now-widespread social form. Although the musical content of Wagner, Smetana, Verdi, and Sibelius differed greatly, they all drew their inspiration from the same psychocultural well springs of nationalism.

The approach I have taken views any local cultural configuration ultimately in the context of the human condition, of which recurrent themes the local group is a variation. For instance, in challenging the Whorfian equation of language (cultural symbol) with thought, Devereux (1980a) "sought to define criteria of normality and abnormality in pan-human terms, such that cultural values could then be understood in a larger context of human nature" (Kilborne 1988: xv). He inquires into the unconscious significance of diagnosis, discovering, for instance, that its principal purpose is not so much to name a disease as to differentiate between the person (and his or her reference group) performing the diagnosis and the person (and his or her group) who is diagnosed—that is, to sharply distinguish between who is and who is not labeled sick, deviant, criminal, or polluted (Devereux 1980a). Further, in meditating on the extent of human destructiveness, he notes that not all widespread and massive destructiveness is conducted by those labeled or diagnosed as sick, criminal, crazy, antisocial, or otherwise deviant. It is far too anxiety arousing for most observers and clinicians to recognize the extent of pathology in normative behavior.

In an essay on cultural relativism, Melford Spiro approaches the local/universal issue from the viewpoint of psychocultural functionalism:

> Given [the] limited and limiting perspective [of epistemological relativism] how could it be denied, for example, that the doctrine of karma is unique to the religious tradition of India? Or that, even within that tradition, its meaning in Buddhism may be different from that in Hinduism. Or, for that matter, that even within Buddhism (Spiro 1982a) and within Hinduism (Keyes and Daniel 1983) it again has different meanings.
>
> If, however, the concept of karma is understood in the context of Hindu and Buddhist praxis—that is, functionally—it is then apparent that, at only a slightly more abstract level, it bears a striking family resemblance to concepts found in many other cultural traditions. Consider, for example, such concepts as luck, fate, predestination, God's will, kismet, fortune, destiny, or, for that matter, cultural determinism! Although formally and semiotically different from each other, and they in turn from karma, all of those concepts, just like karma, provide an explanation for the vagaries of an actor's "life chances" (as Weber called it) without recourse to the agency (and therefore the responsibility) of the actor himself (1986: 267-268).

From the viewpoint of a number of writers (La Barre 1954, 1972; Devereux 1967, 1980a; Spiro 1979a, 1979b), saying that a given cultural form (ethnomedical system, religion, politics, music, art) is embedded in a specific local culture is not incompatible with also saying that it is simultaneously relative to the human condition. Members of all groups are wrestling with similar characteristic issues. More than three decades ago, for example, Devereux suggested in an argument similar to that of Spiro that a psychological trait "can appear as a ***custom*** in tribe A, as a ***myth*** in tribe B and as a ***neurotic fantasy*** in members of tribe C" (1955: 111).

It is both ironic and paradoxical that in a book in which I have often described American biology as cultural ideology, I should conclude on a note that asks for more, rather than less, biological groundedness. One of the central contributions to knowledge of both the Freudian and anthropological revolutions is the exploration of the kind of animal, the kind of primate, we are and of the consequences of our place in the animal kingdom for all that we do. If physicians—and their counterparts such as shamans, medicine men and women, witch doctors, "curers" all—are frequently seen by their constituencies as less than humane, that can never imply that they cease to be human. For it is that very humanness that derives from having grown up in a gendered body, from experiencing the world through that body, and from being that very body in a family setting, that produces the very best and very worst in us all.

If biomedicine has erred, it is from not having taken the biological dispensation far enough. Constrained in its visual field and other sensorium by the values, metaphors, and meanings identified throughout this book, biomedical researchers and practitioners have considered only ***the biology of the human body as inanimate "object"*** and have failed to include within their compass ***the human body as "subject."*** To complete its task, American biomedicine needs now to consider the biology of experience as well as the influence of organic entities upon health and sickness and upon experience itself (also see Scheper-Hughes and Lock 1987; Browner, Ortiz de Montellano, and Rubel 1988 [plus commentaries]).

Neither biomedical culture, nor American culture nor any culture, comes from itself or merely from its prior self called "history." The future study of biomedicine, no less than of culture generically, would do well to be founded upon what and who we are as a species, which would with some effort take us to the heart of the matter of what our ethnomedicine, or any culture, is for.

References

Abse, D. Wilfred. 1974. *Clinical Notes on Group-Analytic Psychotherapy.* Charlottesville: University Press of Virginia.

Agar, Michael. 1973. *Ripping and Running: A Formal Ethnography of Urban Heroin Addicts.* New York: Academic Press.

Aleksandrowicz, Dov R. 1962. The meaning of metaphor. *Bulletin of the Menninger Clinic* 26: 92–101.

Alexander, Franz. 1948. *Fundamentals of Psychoanalysis.* New York: Norton.

______. 1950. *Psychosomatic Medicine.* New York: Norton.

______. 1960. *The Western Mind in Transition.* New York: Random House.

Alexander, Linda. 1981. The double-bind between dialysis patients and their health practitioners. In *The Relevance of Social Science for Medicine,* edited by L. Eisenberg and A. Kleinman, pp. 307-329. Boston: D. Reidel.

Anstett, Richard, and Mary Collins. 1982. The psychological significance of somatic complaints. *Journal of Family Practice* 14(2): 253–259.

Anzieu, Didier. 1984. *The Group and the Unconscious,* translated by Benjamin Kilborne. Boston: Routledge & Kegan Paul (orig. 1975).

Apfel, Roberta J., and Susan M. Fisher. 1984. *To Do No Harm: DES and the Dilemmas of Modern Medicine.* New Haven, CT: Yale University Press.

Apprey, Maurice. 1981. Family, religion and separation: The effort to separate in the analysis of a pubertal adolescent boy. *Journal of Psychoanalytic Anthropology* 4(2): 137–155.

Aries, Nancy, and Louanne Kennedy. 1986. The health labor force: The effects of change. In *The Sociology of Health and Illness: Critical Perspectives,* edited by P. Conrad and R. Kern, 2nd ed., pp. 196–207. New York: St. Martin's Press.

Arlow, Jacob. 1979. Metaphor and the psychoanalytic situation. *Psychoanalytic Quarterly* 48: 363–385.

Arnold, Matthew. 1869. *Culture and Anarchy: An Essay in Political and Social Criticism.* London: Smith, Elder.

Bakan, David. 1968. *Disease, Pain, and Sacrifice: Toward a Psychology of Suffering.* Chicago: University of Chicago Press.

Balint, Enid. 1974. A portrait of Michael Balint: The development of his ideas on the use of the drug "doctor." *International Journal of Psychiatry in Medicine* 5: 211–222.

Balint, Michael. 1957. *The Doctor, His Patient and the Illness.* New York: International Universities Press.

Barrabee, Paul, and Otto von Mering. 1953. Ethnic variations in mental stress in families with psychotic children. *Social Problems* 1(2): 48–53.

Bateson, Gregory. 1972. *Steps to an Ecology of Mind: Collected Essays in Anthropology, Psychiatry, Evolution, and Epistemology.* San Francisco: Chandler.

Becker, Ernest. 1973. *The Denial of Death.* New York: Free Press/Macmillan.

______. 1975. *Escape from Evil.* New York: Free Press/Macmillan.

Becker, Howard S. 1963. *Outsiders: Studies in the Sociology of Deviance.* New York: Free Press/Macmillan.

Becker, Howard, et al. 1961. *Boys in White: Student Culture in Medical School*. Chicago: University of Chicago Press.

Becker, Lorne. 1984. Personal communication, September.

Becker, Marshall H. 1986. The tyranny of health promotion. *Public Health Review* 14: 15–25.

———. 1987. The cholesterol saga: Whither health promotion? *Annals of Internal Medicine* 106(4): 623–626.

Benedict, Ruth. 1934a. Anthropology and the abnormal. *Journal of General Psychology* 10: 59–82.

———. 1934b. *Patterns of Culture*. Boston: Houghton Mifflin.

Bennett, John W. 1982. *Of Time and the Enterprise: North American Family Farm Management in a Context of Resource Marginality*. Minneapolis: University of Minnesota Press.

Berger, Peter, and Thomas Luckmann. 1966. *The Social Construction of Reality: A Treatise in the Sociology of Knowledge*. New York: Doubleday.

Binion, Rudolph. 1976. *Hitler Among the Germans*. New York: Elsevier.

———. 1981. *Soundings: Psychohistorical and Psycholiterary*. New York: Psychohistory Press.

Bion, Wilfred R. 1955. Group dynamics: A review. In *New Directions in Psycho-Analysis*, edited by M. Klein, P. Heimann, and R. Money-Kyrle, pp. 440–477. New York: Basic Books.

———. 1959. *Experiences in Groups*. New York: Basic Books.

———. 1961. *Experiences in Groups and Other Papers*. New York: Ballantine Books.

Bliersbach, Gerhard. 1987. My introduction to the psychohistorical outlook. *Journal of Psychohistory* 14(4): 336–339.

Bloch, Donald A. 1984. You can tell a book by its cover. *Family Systems Medicine* 2(2): 123–124.

———. 1987a. Editorial. *Family Systems Medicine* 5(2): 147–149.

———. 1987b. Editorial. *Family Systems Medicine* 5(4): 403–405.

Blumhagen, Dan. 1980. Hyper-tension: A folk illness with a medical name. *Culture, Medicine and Psychiatry* 4: 197–227.

Bock, Philip K. 1988. *Rethinking Psychological Anthropology: Continuity and Change in the Study of Human Action*. New York: W. H. Freeman.

Bornemann, Ernest. 1976. *The Psychoanalysis of Money*. New York: Urizen Books.

Bosk, Charles. 1980. Occupational rituals in patient management. *New England Journal of Medicine* 303(2): 71–76.

Bowen, Murray. 1978. *Family Therapy in Clinical Practice*. New York: Jason Aronson.

Boyer, L. Bryce. 1979. *Childhood and Folklore: A Psychoanalytic Study of Apache Personality*. New York: Library of Psychological Anthropology.

Brain, James L. 1977. Sex, incest, and death: Initiation rites reconsidered. *Current Anthropology* 18(2): 191–208.

Brandes, Stanley H. 1979. Drinking patterns and alcohol control in a Castilian mountain village. *Anthropology* 3: 1–16.

Brocher, Tobias. 1984. Diagnosis of organizations, communities, and political units. In *The Irrational Executive: Psychoanalytic Studies in Management*, edited by M.F.R. Kets deVries, pp. 373–391. New York: International Universities Press.

Brodey, Warren M., Marjorie Hayden, and Othilda Krug. 1957. Intra-team reactions: Their relation to the conflicts of the family in treatment. *American Journal of Orthopsychiatry* 27: 349–355.

Brody, Howard. 1987. *Stories of Sickness*. New Haven, CT: Yale University Press.

Brody, Sylvia. 1982. Psychoanalytic theories of infant development and its disturbances: A critical evaluation. *Psychoanalytic Quarterly* 51: 526–596.

Bronowski, Jacob. 1956. *Science and Human Values*. New York: Harper & Row.

Brown, Norman O. 1959. *Life Against Death: The Psychoanalytic Meaning of History*. New York: Viking Press.

Browner, C. H., Bernard R. Ortiz de Montellano, and Arthur J. Rubel. 1988. A methodology for cross-cultural ethnomedical research. *Current Anthropology* 29(5): 681–702.

Burda, David, and Suzanne Powills. 1986. AIDS: A time bomb at hospital's door. *Hospitals* 60: 54–61.

Burnside, John W. 1983. Medicine and War—A Metaphor. *JAMA* 249: 2091.

Burton, Roger V., and John W.M. Whiting. 1961. The absent father and cross-sex identity. *Merrill Palmer Quarterly of Behavior and Development* 7: 90–98.

Calogeras, Roy D. 1982. Sleepwalking and the traumatic experience. *International Journal of Psycho-Analysis* 63: 483–489.

Campbell, J. William, and Mark Frisse, eds. 1983. *Manual of Medical Therapeutics*, 24th ed. Boston: Little, Brown.

Candib, Lucy M. 1987. What doctors tell about themselves to patients: Implications for intimacy and reciprocity in the relationship. *Family Medicine* 19(1): 23–30.

Carlyon, William H. 1984. Disease prevention/health promotion: Bridging the gap to wellness. *Health Values: Achieving High Level Wellness* 8(3): 27–30.

Carth, Elaine, and Rudolf Ekstein. 1966. Interpretation within the metaphor. *Journal of the American Academy of Child Psychology* 5: 35–45.

Carver, Cynthia. 1981. The deliverers: A woman doctor's reflections on medical socialization. In *Childbirth: Alternatives to Medical Control*, edited by S. Romalis, pp. 122–149. Austin: University of Texas Press.

Cass, Alvah. 1988. Personal communication, May 5.

Caster, John H., and Eugenie Gatens-Robinson. 1983. Metaphor in medicine. *JAMA* 250(14): 1841.

Chernin, Kim. 1981. *The Obsession: Reflections on the Tyranny of Slenderness*. New York: Harper & Row.

Christie-Seely, Janet, R. Fernandez, G. Paradis, Y. Talbot, and R. Turcotte. 1984. The physician's family. In *Working with the Family in Primary Care: A Systems Approach to Health and Illness*, edited by J. Christie-Seely, pp. 524–546. New York: Praeger.

Clark, M. Margaret. 1973. Contributions of cultural anthropology to the study of the aged. In *Cultural Illness and Health*, edited by L. Nader and T. W. Maretzki, pp. 78–88. Washington, DC: Anthropological Society of Washington.

Cohen, Carl I., and Ellen J. Cohen. 1978. Health education: Panacea, pernicious or pointless? *New England Journal of Medicine* 299(13): 718–720.

Cooper, Kenneth H. 1978. *The Aerobics Way*. New York: Bantam Books.

Crawford, Robert. 1980. Healthism and the medicalization of everyday life. *International Journal of Health Services* 10: 365–388.

______. 1985. A cultural account of health: Self-control, release, and the social body. In *Issues in the Political Economy of Health Care*, edited by J. McKinlay. London: Tavistock.

Crile, George, Jr. 1973. How much surgery for breast cancer? *Modern Medicine* (June 11): 32.

Crouch, Michael. 1986. Working with one's own family: Another path for professional development. *Family Medicine* 18: 93–98.

Cullberg, J. 1970. Panel discussion: Patientpsykologin inom invärtesmedicinen. *Läkartidningen* 67: 5929.

Dale, Philip Marshall. 1987. *Medical Biographies: The Ailments of Thirty-Three Famous Persons*. Norman: University of Oklahoma Press.

Davidson, Ronald H. 1986. Transference and countertransference phenomena: The problem of the observer in the behavioral sciences. *Journal of Psychoanalytic Anthropology* 9(3): 269–283.

Deal, Terrence E., and Allan A. Kennedy. 1982. *Corporate Cultures: The Rites and Rituals of Corporate Life*. New York: Addison-Wesley.

Delmar, Diana. 1987. Family physician finds HMO is his kind of practice arrangement. *Family Practice News* 17(19): 1, 46.

deMause, Lloyd. 1974a. The evolution of childhood. In *The History of Childhood*, edited by L. deMause, pp. 1–73. New York: Psychohistory Press.

———., ed. 1974b. *The History of Childhood*. New York: Psychohistory Press.

———. 1977. Jimmy Carter and American fantasy. In *Jimmy Carter and American Fantasy: Psychohistorical Explorations*, edited by L. deMause and H. Ebel, pp. 9–31. New York: Two Continents/Psychohistory Press.

———. 1979. Historical group-fantasies. *Journal of Psychohistory* 7(1): 1–70.

———. 1982. *Foundations of Psychohistory*. New York: Creative Roots

———. 1984. *Reagan's America*. New York: Creative Roots.

———. 1988. "Heads and tails": Money as a poison container. *Journal of Psychohistory* 16(1): 1–18.

Dete, Mary K. 1987. Professional and community resources. In *Primary Care in the Home*, by L. H. Bernstein, A. J. Grieco, and M. K. Dete, pp. 63–70. Philadelphia: J. B. Lippincott.

de Tocqueville, Alexis. 1945. *Democracy in America*, edited by P. Bradley, 2 vols. New York: Knopf.

Devereux, George. 1955. Charismatic leadership and crisis. *Psychoanalysis and the Social Sciences* 4: 145–157.

———. 1956. Normal and abnormal: The key problem of psychiatric anthropology. In *Some Uses of Anthropology: Theoretical and Applied*, edited by J. B. Casagrande and T. Gladwin, pp. 23–48. Washington, DC: Anthropological Society of Washington.

———. 1967. *From Anxiety to Method in the Behavioral Sciences*. The Hague, Netherlands: Mouton.

———. 1980a. *Basic Problems of Ethno-Psychiatry*, translated by B. Miller Gulati and G. Devereux. Chicago: University of Chicago Press.

———. 1980b. Normal and abnormal. In *Basic Problems of Ethno-Psychiatry*, by G. Devereux, pp. 3–71. Chicago: University of Chicago Press (orig. 1962).

De Vos, George. 1966. Toward a cross-cultural psychology of caste behavior. In *Japan's Invisible Race*, edited by G. De Vos and H. Wagatsuma, pp. 353-384. Berkeley: University of California Press.

———. 1975a. Affective dissonance and primary socialization: Implications for a theory of incest avoidance. *Ethos* 3(2): 165–182.

———. 1975b. The dangers of pure theory in social anthropology. *Ethos* 3(1): 77–91.

———. 1980. Ethnic adaptation and minority status. *Journal of Cross-Cultural Psychology* 11(1): 101–124.

Diamond, Michael A. 1984. Bureaucracy as externalized self-system: A view from the psychological interior. *Administration and Society* 16(2): 195–214.

———. 1988. Organizational identity: A psychoanalytic exploration of organizational meaning. *Administration and Society* 20(2): 166–190.

Diamond, Michael A., and Seth Allcorn. 1986. Role formation as defensive activity in bureaucratic organizations. *Political Psychology* 7(4): 709–732.

DiNicola, Vincenzo F. 1988. An essay review on *Hunger Strike: The Anorectic's Struggle as a Metaphor for Our Age*, by Susie Orbach. *Transcultural Psychiatric Research Review* 25(1): 47–54.

Drucker, Peter F. 1954. *The Practice of Management*. New York: Harper.

Dubos, René. 1959. *Mirage of Health: Utopias, Progress, and Biological Change*. Garden City, NY: Doubleday/Anchor.

Dundes, Alan. 1984. *Life Is Like a Chicken Coop Ladder: A Portrait of German Culture Through Folklore*. New York: Columbia University Press.

______. 1985. The American game of "smear the queer" and the homosexual component of male competitive sport and warfare. *Journal of Pyschoanalytic Anthropology* 8(3): 115–129.

Earley, L. William, and Otto von Mering. 1969. Growing old the outpatient way. *American Journal of Psychiatry* 125(7): 963–967.

Ebel, Henry. 1980. Notes toward a psychohistory of some major institutions: The psychohistory of money. *Journal of Psychohistory* 8(2): 227–230.

______. 1984. Yes, but whyever did it happen? *Journal of Psychoanalytic Anthropology* 7(4): 416–420.

______. 1988. Personal communication, August 13.

Edgerton, Robert B. 1967. *The Cloak of Competence: Stigma in the Lives of the Mentally Retarded*. Berkeley: University of California Press.

______. 1976. *Deviance: A Cross-Cultural Perspective*. Menlo Park, CA: Cummings.

Eisenberg, Leon. 1977. Disease and illness: Distinctions between professional and popular ideas of sickness. *Culture, Medicine and Psychiatry* 1: 9–23.

______. 1988. Science in medicine: Too much or too little or too limited in scope? Appendice in *The Task of Medicine: Dialogue at Wickenburg*, by K. L. White, M.D., pp. 190–217. Menlo Park, CA: Henry J. Kaiser Family Foundation.

Eisenberg, Leon, and Arthur Kleinman. 1981. Clinical social science. In *The Relevance of Social Science for Medicine*, edited by L. Eisenberg, and A. Kleinman, pp. 1–23. Boston: D. Reidel.

Ekstein, Rudolf. 1966. *Children of Time and Space, of Action and Impulse: Clinical Studies on the Psychoanalytic Treatment of Severely Disturbed Children*. New York: Appleton-Century-Crofts.

Elkisch, Paula, and Margaret S. Mahler. 1959. On infantile precursors of the "influencing machine." In *The Psychoanalytic Study of the Child* 14: 219–235. New York: International Universities Press.

Ellul, Jacques. 1964. *Technological Society*. New York: Knopf.

Engel, George. 1977. The need for a new medical model: A challenge for biomedicine. *Science* 196(4286): 129–136.

Erikson, Erik H. 1958. *Young Man Luther: A Study in Psychoanalysis and History*. New York: Norton.

______. 1959. *Identity and the Life Cycle: Selected Essays*. New York: International Universities Press.

______. 1963a. *Childhood and Society*, 2nd ed. New York: Norton (orig. 1950).

______. 1963b. Reflections on the American identity. In *Childhood and Society*, by E. H. Erikson, 2nd ed., pp. 285–325. New York: Norton (orig. 1950).

______. 1964. *Insight and Responsibility*. New York: Norton.

______. 1968. *Identity: Youth and Crisis*. New York: Norton.

______. 1974. *Dimensions of a New Identity*. New York: Norton.

______. 1977. *Toys and Reasons: Stages in the Ritualization of Experience*. New York: Norton.

Estroff, Sue E. 1981. *Making It Crazy*. Berkeley: University of California Press.

———. 1984. "Who are you? Why are you here?": Anthropology and human suffering. *Human Organization* 43(4): 368–370.

Etzioni, Amitai. 1961. *A Comparative Analysis of Complex Organizations*. New York: Free Press.

Evans-Pritchard, Edward E. 1962. Anthropology and history. In *Social Anthropology and Other Essays*, by E. E. Evans-Pritchard, pp. 172–191. New York: Free Press.

Fabrega, Horacio, Jr. 1975. The need for an ethnomedical science. *Science* 189: 969–975.

Falk, John L. 1983. Drug dependence: Myth or motive? *Pharmacology, Biochemistry and Behavior* 19: 385–391.

Feder, Stuart. 1978. Gustav Mahler, dying. *International Review of Psycho-Analysis* 5(125): 125–148.

Federn, Paul. 1952. *Ego Psychology and the Psychoses*. New York: Basic Books.

Fenichel, Otto. 1945. *The Psychoanalytic Theory of Neurosis*. New York: Norton.

Fingarette, Herbert. 1985. Alcoholism and self-deception. In *Self-Deception and Self-Understanding: New Essays in Philosophy and Psychology*, edited by M. W. Martin, pp. 52–67. Lawrence: University Press of Kansas.

Ford, Julian D. 1978. Therapeutic relationship in behavior therapy: An empirical analysis. *Journal of Consulting and Clinical Psychology* 46(6): 1302–1314.

Fornari, Franco. 1974. *The Psychoanalysis of War*. New York: Anchor Books.

Foster, George M. 1976. Disease etiologies in non-Western medical systems. *American Anthropologist* 78: 773–782.

Foster, George M., and Barbara Gallatin Anderson. 1978. *Medical Anthropology*. New York: Wiley.

Foulkes, S. H. 1948. *Introduction to Group-Analytic Psychotherapy*. London: Heinemann.

Fox, Renee. 1957. Training for uncertainty. In *The Student-Physician*, edited by R. Merton, G. Reader, and P. Kendall, pp. 207–241. Cambridge, MA: Harvard University Press.

———. 1959. *Experiment Perilous: Physicians and Patients Facing the Unknown*. Glencoe, IL: Free Press.

Freeman, Sarah. 1987. Physicians' explanations: Discourse framing and breakdown of coherence. Presentation at the Eighty-sixth Annual Meeting of the American Anthropological Association, Chicago, Illinois, November 19.

Freidson, Eliot. 1970a. *Professional Dominance: The Social Structure of Medical Care*. New York: Atherton Press.

———. 1970b. *Profession of Medicine*. New York: Harper & Row.

Freud, Anna. 1965. *Normality and Pathology in Childhood*. New York: International Universities Press.

Freud, Sigmund. 1900a. The interpretation of dreams. In *The Standard Edition of the Complete Psychological Works of Sigmund Freud* (SE), translated by J. Strachey, vols. 4 and 5. London: Hogarth Press, 1953.

———. 1900b. The primary and secondary processes—repression. In *SE*, vol. 5, pp. 588–609. London: Hogarth Press, 1953.

———. 1901. The psychopathology of everyday life. In *SE*, vol. 6, pp. 1–279. London: Hogarth Press, 1960.

———. 1905. Jokes and their relation to the unconscious. In *SE*, vol. 8, pp. 3–236. London: Hogarth Press, 1960.

———. 1908. Character and anal erotism. In *SE*, vol. 9, pp. 169–175. London: Hogarth Press, 1959.

———. 1910. The future prospects of psycho-analytic therapy. In *SE*, vol. 11, pp. 139–151. London: Hogarth Press, 1957.

———. 1912. Recommendations to physicians practicing psycho-analysis. In *SE*, vol. 12, pp. 109–120. London: Hogarth Press, 1958.

———. 1913. Totem and taboo. In *SE*, vol. 13, pp. 1–161. London: Hogarth Press, 1955.

———. 1914. Remembering, repeating, and working-through. In *SE*, vol. 12, pp. 147–156. London: Hogarth Press, 1958.

———. 1919. The "uncanny." In *SE*, vol. 17, pp. 218–252. London: Hogarth Press, 1962.

———. 1920. Beyond the pleasure principle. In *SE*, vol. 18, pp. 7–64. London: Hogarth Press, 1955.

———. 1921. Group psychology and the analysis of the ego. In *SE*, vol. 18, pp. 69–143. London: Hogarth Press, 1955.

———. 1923. The ego and the id. In *SE*, vol. 19, pp. 3–66. London: Hogarth Press, 1961.

———. 1927. The future of an illusion. In *SE*, vol. 21, pp. 5–56. London: Hogarth Press, 1961.

———. 1930. Civilization and its discontents. In *SE*, vol. 21, pp. 64–145. London: Hogarth Press, 1961.

Friedman, Meyer, and Ray H. Rosenman. 1974. *Type A Behavior and Your Heart*. New York: Fawcett Columbine Books.

Fuchs, Victor R. 1974. *Who Shall Live? Health, Economics and Social Change*. New York: Basic Books.

Gaines, Atwood D., and Robert A. Hahn. 1985. Among the physicians: Encounter, exchange, and transformation. In *Physicians of Western Medicine*, edited by R. A. Hahn and A. D. Gaines, pp. 3–22. Boston: D. Reidel.

GAP Committee on International Relations, and Howard F. Stein. 1987. *Us and Them: The Psychology of Ethnonationalism*. Group for the Advancement of Psychiatry (GAP) Report no. 123. New York: Brunner/Mazel.

Gardner, Leonard. 1977. Humanistic education and behavioral objectives: Opposing theories of educational science. *University of Chicago School Review* 85(3): 376–394.

Gazda, Thomas D., Rollin M. Gallagher, III, David N. Little, and Marga S. Sproul. 1984. The group practice seminar: A Balint-type group in the setting of a family medicine training program. *Family Medicine* 16: 54–58.

Geertz, Clifford. 1972. Deep play: Notes on the Balinese cockfight. *Daedalus: Journal of the American Academy of Arts and Sciences* 101(1): 1–37.

———. 1973. *The Interpretation of Cultures: Selected Essays*. New York: Basic Books.

Gerber, William G., and Carlos E. Sluzki. 1978. The physician-family relationship. In *Family Medicine Principles and Practice*, edited by R. Tayler, pp. 216–220. New York: Springer-Verlag.

Gilmore, David D., and Sarah C. Uhl. 1987. Further notes on Andalusian machismo. *Journal of Psychoanalytic Anthropology* 10(4): 341–360.

Gilmore, Margaret, and David D. Gilmore. 1979. Machismo: A psychodynamic approach (Spain). *Journal of Psychological Anthropology* 2: 281–300.

Ginsberg, Eli. 1983. Allied health resources. In *The Handbook of Health, Health Care, and the Health Professions*, edited by D. Mechanic, pp. 479–494. New York: Basic Books.

Glenn, Michael L. 1988. The resurgence of the biomedical model. *Family Medicine* 20(5): 324–325.

Goffman, Erving. 1963. *Stigma: Notes on the Management of Spoiled Identity*. Englewood Cliffs, NJ: Prentice-Hall.

———. 1971. *Relations in Public*. New York: Basic Books.

Golub, Ellen. 1981. Cancer and death in the Promethean age. *Journal of Popular Culture* 14(4): 725–731.

Gonen, Jay Y. 1975. A *Psychohistory of Zionism*. New York: Mason Charter.

Good, Byron J. 1977. The heart of the matter: The semantics of illness in Iran. *Culture, Medicine and Psychiatry* 1: 25–58.

Gosling, R., D. Miller, D. Woodhouse, and P. Turquet. 1967. *The Use of Small Groups in Training*. London: Tavistock.

Green, Donald R. 1976. Personal communication, May. Quoted with permission.

Greenson, Ralph R. 1967. *The Technique and Practice of Psychoanalysis*. New York: International Universities Press.

______. 1968. Dis-identifying from mother: Its special importance for the boy. *International Journal of Psycho-Analysis* 49: 370–374.

Gregor, Thomas. 1985. *Anxious Pleasures: The Sexual Lives of an Amazonian People*. Chicago: University of Chicago Press.

Grinker, Roy, Sr. 1973. *Psychosomatic Concepts*. New York: Jason Aronson.

Gunther, Meyer S. 1976. The endangered self: A contribution to the understanding of narcissistic determinants of countertransference. *Annual of Psychoanalysis IV*. New York: International Universities Press.

Gussow, Zachary, and George S. Tracy. 1968. Status, ideology and adaptation to stigmatized illness: A study of leprosy. *Human Organization* 27: 316–325.

______. 1976. The role of self-help clubs in adaptation to chronic illness and disability. *Social Science and Medicine* 10: 407–414.

Hahn, Robert A. 1984. Rethinking "illness" and "disease." In *South Asian Systems of Healing*, edited by E. V. Daniel and J. F. Pugh, pp. 1–23. Leiden, Holland: E. J. Brill.

______. 1985a. Between two worlds: Physicians as patients. *Medical Anthropology Quarterly* 16(4): 87–98.

______. 1985b. A world of internal medicine: Portrait of an internist. In *Physicians of Western Medicine: Anthropological Approaches to Theory and Practice*, edited by R. A. Hahn and A. D. Gaines, pp. 51–111. Boston: D. Reidel.

______. 1985c. Culture-bound syndromes unbound. *Social Science and Medicine* 21(2): 165–171.

Hahn, Robert A., and Atwood D. Gaines. 1982. Physicians of Western medicine: An introduction. *Culture, Medicine, and Psychiatry* 6: 215–218.

______, eds. 1985. *Physicians of Western Medicine: Anthropological Approaches to Theory and Practice*. Boston: D. Reidel.

Halenar, John F. 1979. Big business turns up the heat on doctors. *Medical Economics* (July 9): 109–121.

Hall, Edward T. 1977. *Beyond Culture*. Garden City, NY: Anchor Press/Doubleday.

Harvey, Patricia. 1987. Jules Henry's warnings on docility, stupidity, and risk in education and life. *High Plains Applied Anthropologist* 7(1): 15–18.

Havighurst, Clark C., and Glenn M. Hackbarth. 1979. Private cost containments. *New England Journal of Medicine* 300: 1298–1305.

Hay, Thomas H. 1971. The Windigo psychosis: Psychodynamic, cultural, and social factors in aberrant behavior. *American Anthropologist* 73: 1–22.

Hayden, Gregory F. 1984. What's in a name? "Mechanical" diagnosis in clinical medicine. *Postgraduate Medicine* 75(1): 227–232.

Heath, Dwight B. 1985. In a dither about drinking. *Wall Street Journal*, February 25, p. 28.

Heilbroner, Robert. 1988. Economics without power. *New York Review of Books* 35(3): 23–25.

Helman, Cecil G. 1987. Heart disease and the cultural construction of time: The Type A behaviour pattern as a Western culture-bound syndrome. *Social Science and Medicine* 25: 969–979.

Henry, Jules. 1963. *Culture Against Man*. New York: Random House.

______. 1971. *Pathways to Madness*. New York: Random House.

______. 1973. *On Sham, Vulnerability and Other Forms of Self-Destruction*. New York: Random House.

Herdt, Gilbert H., ed. 1982. *Rituals of Manhood: Male Initiation in Papua New Guinea*. Berkeley: University of California Press.

Heschel, Abraham Joshua. 1965. *Who is Man?* Stanford, CA: Stanford University Press.

Hilfiker, David. 1984. Facing our mistakes. *New England Journal of Medicine* 310: 118–122.

Hill, Robert F. 1978. On the meaning of "disability" in the American culture. Manuscript prepared for the Oklahoma Coalition of Citizens with Disabilities project. "Breaking Through" (#76–094), sponsored by the Oklahoma Humanities Committee, Oklahoma City, Oklahoma.

______. 1983. Personal communication, March.

Himmelstein, David U., Steffie Woolhandler, and the Writing Committee of the Working Group on Program Design. 1989. A national health program for the United States: A physicians' proposal. *The New England Journal of Medicine* 320(2): 102–108.

Hocking, B. 1987. Anthropologic aspects of occupational illness epidemics. *Journal of Occupational Medicine* 29(6): 526–530.

Hofstede, Geert. 1980. Motivation, leadership, and organization: Do American theories apply abroad? *Organizational Dynamics* (Summer): 42–63.

Holmes, Thomas H., and Richard H. Rahe. 1967. The social readjustment rating scale. *Journal of Psychosomatic Research* 11: 213–218.

Hook, R. H. 1979. Phantasy and symbol. A psychoanalytic point of view. In *Fantasy and Symbol: Studies in Anthropological Interpretation*, edited by R. H. Hook, pp. 267–291. New York: Academic Press.

Hopper, Kim. 1982. Discussant comments following the organized session, "The Lure and Haven of Illness." Eighty-first Annual Meeting of the American Anthropological Association, Washington, D.C., December 4-7.

Hulka, Barbara S., Lawrence L. Kupper, and John C. Cassel. 1972. Determinants of physician utilization. *Medical Care* 10: 300–309.

Illich, Ivan. 1974. Medical nemesis. *The Lancet* 1: 918–921.

______. 1975. The medicalization of life. *Journal of Medical Ethics* 1: 73–77.

______. 1976. *Medical Nemesis: The Expropriation of Health*. New York: Pantheon.

______. 1982. Medicalization and primary care. *Journal of the Royal College of General Practitioners* 32(241): 463–470.

Ingham, John. 1964. The bullfighters. *American Imago* 21: 95–102.

Janis, Irving L. 1982. *Groupthink*. Boston: Houghton Mifflin.

Jaques, Elliott. 1955. Social systems as a defense against persecutory and depressive anxiety. In *New Directions in Psycho-Analysis*, edited by M. Klein, P. Heimann, and R. Money-Kyrle, pp. 478–498. New York: Basic Books.

______. 1976. *A General Theory of Bureaucracy*. New York: Halstead Press.

Jette, Alan M., K. Michael Cummings, Bruce M. Brock, Maz Crispin Phelps, and James Naessens. 1981. The structure and reliability of health belief indices. *Health Services Research* 16(1): 81–98.

Johnson, Thomas M. 1989. Contradictions in the cultural construction of pain in America. In *Advances in Pain Research and Therapy*, edited by C. S. Hill, Jr. and W. S. Fields, vol. 2, pp. 37–47. New York: Raven Press.

Jonas, Steven. 1986. Health manpower. In *Health Care Delivery in the United States*, by Steven Jonas, with contributors, 3rd ed., pp. 54–89. New York: Springer.

Jones, Ernest. 1948. *Papers on Psycho-Analysis*, 5th ed. Baltimore, MD: Williams and Wilkins.

Kafka, John S., and Joyce W. McDonald. 1965. The latent family in the intensive treatment of the hospitalized schizophrenic patient. In *Current Psychiatric Therapies*, edited by J. H. Masserman, vol. 5, pp. 172–177. New York: Grune and Stratton.

Katon, Wayne, and Arthur Kleinman. 1981. Doctor-patient negotiation and other social science strategies in patient care. In *The Relevance of Social Science for Medicine*, edited by L. Eisenberg and A. Kleinman, pp. 253–279. Boston: D. Reidel.

Katz, Jay. 1984a. *The Silent World of Doctor and Patient*. New York: Free Press/Macmillan.

———. 1984b. Why doctors don't disclose uncertainty. *Hastings Center Report* 14: 35–44.

Kaufman, Sharon. 1988. Toward a phenomenology of boundaries in medicine: Chronic illness experience in the case of stroke. *Medical Anthropology Quarterly* 2(4): 338–354.

Kaufman, Sharon R., and Gay Becker. 1986. Stroke: Health care on the periphery. *Social Science and Medicine* 22: 983–989.

Kelly, Jeffrey A., Janet S. St. Lawrence, Steve Smith, Jr., Harold V. Hood, and Donna J. Cook. 1987. Medical students' attitudes toward AIDS and homosexual patients. *Journal of Medical Education* 62(7): 549–556.

Kenny, Michael G. 1978. Latah: The symbolism of a putative mental disorder. *Culture, Medicine, and Psychiatry* 2(3): 209–231.

———. 1983. Paradox lost: The Latah problem revisited. *Journal of Nervous and Mental Disease* 171: 159–167.

Kernberg, Otto F. 1965. Notes on countertransference. *Journal of the American Psychoanalytic Association* 13: 38–56.

———. 1975. *Borderline Conditions and Pathological Narcissism*. New York: Jason Aronson.

———. 1984. Regression in organizational leadership. In *The Irrational Executive: Psychoanalytic Studies in Management*, edited by M.F.R. Kets deVries, pp. 38–66. New York: International Universities Press.

Kets deVries, Manfred F.R., ed. 1984. *The Irrational Executive: Psychoanalytic Studies in Management*. New York: International Universities Press.

Keyes, Charles F., and E. Valentine Daniel, eds. 1983. *Karma: An Anthropological Inquiry*. Berkeley: University of California Press.

Kiefer, Christie W. 1976. Review of *Morita Psychotherapy*, by D. Reynolds. *Medical Anthropology Newsletter* 7(4): 11–12.

Kilborne, Benjamin. 1988. George Devereux: In memoriam. In *The Psychoanalytic Study of Society*, edited by L. B. Boyer and S. Grolnick, vol. 12, pp. xi–xxxix. Hillsdale, NJ: Analytic Press.

Kirmayer, Laurence J. 1987. Abstract/review of *The Culture-Bound Syndromes*, edited by R. C. Simons and C. C. Hughes. *Transcultural Psychiatric Research Review* 24(4): 275–283.

Klarman, Herbert E. 1977. The financing of health care. *Daedalus: Journal of the American Academy of Arts and Sciences* 106: 215–233.

Klein, Melanie. 1946. Notes on some schizoid mechanisms. In *Envy and Gratitude and Other Works*, by M. Klein, pp. 1–24. New York: Basic Books.

Kleinman, Arthur M. 1973. Toward a comparative study of medical systems. *Science, Medicine and Man* 1: 55–65.

———. 1975. Explanatory models in health care relationships. In *Health of the Family*, pp. 159–172. Washington, DC: National Council for International Health.

———. 1978. Clinical relevance of anthropological and cross-cultural research: Concepts and strategies. *American Journal of Psychiatry* 135(4): 427–431.

———. 1980. *Patients and Healers in the Context of Culture: An Exploration of the Borderland Between Anthropology, Medicine, and Psychiatry.* Berkeley: University of California Press.

———. 1983a. The cultural meanings and social uses of illness: A role for medical anthropology and clinically oriented social science in the development of primary care theory and research. *Journal of Family Practice* 16(3): 539–545.

———. 1983b. Editor's note. *Culture, Medicine and Psychiatry* 7(1): 97–99.

Kleinman, Arthur M., Leon Eisenberg, and Byron Good. 1978. Culture, illness, and care: Clinical lessons from anthropologic and cross-cultural research. *Annals of Internal Medicine* 88(2): 251–258.

Kluckhohn, Clyde. 1944. *Navaho Witchcraft*. Boston: Beacon Press.

———. 1951. The study of culture. In *The Policy Sciences*, edited by D. Lerner and H. D. Lasswell, pp. 86–101. Stanford, CA: Stanford University Press.

Kluckhohn, Florence R. 1953. Dominant and variant value orientations. In *Personality in Nature, Society, and Culture*, edited by C. Kluckhohn and H. A. Murray. New York: Knopf.

Kluckhohn, Florence R., and Fred Strodtbeck. 1961. *Variations in Value Orientations.* Evanston, IL: Row Peterson.

Koenigsberg, Richard A. 1975. *Hitler's Ideology: A Study in Psychoanalytic Sociology.* New York: Library of Social Science.

Kohn, Hans. 1960. *Panslavism: Its History and Ideology.* New York: Vintage Books.

Kohut, Heinz. 1971. *The Analysis of the Self.* New York: International Universities Press.

———. 1984. *How Does Analysis Cure?* Chicago: University of Chicago Press.

Kormos, Harry R. 1984. The industrialization of medicine. In *Advances in Medical Social Science*, edited by J. L. Ruffini, vol. 2, pp. 323–339. New York: Gordon and Breach Science Pubs.

Korzybski, Alfred. 1941. *Science and Sanity.* New York: Science Press.

Kovel, Joel. 1971. *White Racism: A Psychohistory.* New York: Vintage/Random House.

Krantzler, Nora J. 1986. Media images of physicians and nurses in the United States. *Social Sciences and Medicine* 22(9): 933–952.

Kren, George, and Leon Rappoport. 1980. *The Holocaust and the Crisis of Human Behavior.* New York: Holmes and Meier.

Kroeber, Alfred L. 1948. *Anthropology.* New York: Harcourt, Brace and World (orig. 1923).

———. 1952. *The Nature of Culture.* Chicago: University of Chicago Press.

Kurtz, Irma. 1987. Health educators—The new puritans. *Journal of Medical Ethics* 13: 40–41, 48.

La Barre, Weston. 1951. Family and symbol. In *Psychoanalysis and Culture: Essays in Honor of Geza Roheim*, edited by G. Wilbur and W. Muensterberger, pp. 156–167. New York: International Universities Press.

———. 1954. *The Human Animal.* Chicago: University of Chicago Press.

———. 1956. Social cynosure and social structure. In *Personal Character and Cultural Milieu*, edited by D. G. Haring, pp. 535–563. Syracuse, NY: Syracuse University Press.

———. 1962. Transference cures in religious cults and social groups. *Journal of Psychoanalysis in Groups* 1(1): 66–75.

———. 1969. *They Shall Take Up Serpents: Psychology of the Southern Snake-Handling Cult.* New York: Schocken (orig. 1962).

———. 1971. Anthropological perspectives on sexuality. In *Sexuality: A Search for Perspective*, edited by D. Grumman and A. M. Barclay, pp. 38–53. New York: Van Nostrand Reinhold.

______. 1972. *The Ghost Dance: The Origins of Religion*. New York: Dell.

______. 1974. Review of *The Mind Game: Witchdoctors and Psychiatrists*, by E. Fuller Torrey. *Social Casework* 55(1): 57–58.

______. 1977. Review of *Cultural Beyond*, by E. Hall. *American Ethnologist* 4: 783–784.

______. 1978. The clinic and the field. In *The Making of Psychological Anthropology*, edited by G. D. Spindler, pp. 258–299. Berkeley: University of California Press.

______. 1980. *Culture in Context: Selected Writings of Weston La Barre*. Durham, NC: Duke University Press.

______. 1984. *Muelos: A Stone Age Superstition About Sexuality*. New York: Columbia University Press.

Lakoff, George, and Mark Johnson. 1980. *Metaphors We Live By*. Chicago: University of Chicago Press.

La Mettrie, Julien Offray de. 1748. *L'Homme Machine*. Leyde, France: E. Luzac.

Laplanche, J., and J.-B. Pontalis. 1973. *The Language of Psycho-Analysis*. New York: Norton.

Lawton, Henry W. 1982. The myth of altruism. *Journal of Psychohistory* 9(3): 265–308.

Lazarus, Ellen S. 1988. Theoretical considerations for the study of the doctor-patient relationship: Implications of a perinatal study. *Medical Anthropology Quarterly* 2(1): 34–58.

Leach, Edmund R. 1954. *Political Systems of Highland Burma*. Boston: Beacon Press.

Lerner, Stephen. 1979. The excessive need to treat: A countertherapeutic force in psychiatric hospital treatment. *Bulletin of the Menninger Clinic* 43: 463–471.

Lifton, Robert Jay. 1984. Medicalized killing in Auschwitz. In *Psychoanalytic Reflections on the Holocaust: Selected Essays*, edited by S. A. Luel and P. Marcus, pp. 11–34. New York: Holocaust Awareness Institute, Center for Judaic Studies, University of Denver, and KTAV Publishing House.

______. 1986. *The Nazi Doctors*. New York: Basic Books.

Light, Donald. 1980. *Becoming Psychiatrists: The Professional Transformation of the Self.* New York: Norton.

Lincoln, Yvonna S., and Egon G. Guba. 1985. *Naturalistic Inquiry*. Beverly Hills, CA: Sage.

Litman, Theodor J. 1974. The family as a basic unit in health and medical care. *Social Science and Medicine* 8: 495–519.

Littlewood, Roland, and Maurice Lipsedge. 1986. The "culture-bound syndromes" of the dominant culture: Culture, psychopathology and biomedicine. In *Transcultural Psychiatry*, edited by J. Cox, pp. 253–273. London: Croom Helm.

Lock, Margaret. 1983. Review of *Medusa's Hair: An Essay on Personal Symbols and Religious Experience*, by G. Obeyesekere. *Transcultural Psychiatric Research Review* 20(4): 266–269.

______. 1986a. Castigations of a selfish housewife: National identity and menopausal rhetoric in Japan. Paper presented at the American Ethnological Society Meetings, Wrightsville Beach, North Carolina.

______. 1986b. Plea for acceptance: School refusal syndrome in Japan. *Social Science and Medicine* 23: 99–112.

______. 1987. Introduction: Health and medical care as cultural and social phenomena. In *Health, Illness, and Medical Care in Japan: Cultural and Social Dimensions*, edited by E. Norbeck and M. Lock, pp. 1–23. Honolulu: University of Hawaii Press.

Lock, Margaret, and Pamela Dunk. 1987. My nerves are broken: The communication of suffering in a Greek-Canadian community. In *Health in Canadian Society: Sociological*

Perspectives, edited by D. Coburn, C. D'Arcy, P. New, and G. Torrence. Toronto: Fitzhenry and Whiteside.

Ludwig, Arnold M., and Ekkehard Othmer. 1977. The medical basis of psychiatry. *American Journal of Psychiatry* 134: 1087–1092.

Mack, John E. 1986a. Review of *The Other Walls: The Politics of the Arab-Israeli Peace Process*, by Harold H. Saunders. *Middle East Journal* 40(4): 743–744.

———. 1986b. Some thoughts on the nuclear age and the psychological roots of anti-Sovietism. *Psychoanalytic Inquiry* 6(2): 267–285.

———, ed. 1986c. Special journal issue on "aggression and its alternatives in the conduct of international relations." *Psychoanalytic Inquiry* 6(2).

———. 1988. Conversations for wholeness: The challenge of corporate self-responsibility. Unpublished manuscript. Quoted with permission.

Mager, Robert F. 1962. *Preparing Instructional Objectives*. Palo Alto, CA: Fearon.

Mahler, Margaret S. 1958. Autism and symbiosis, two extreme disturbances of identity. *International Journal of Psychoanalysis* 39: 77–83.

———. 1968. *On Human Symbiosis and the Vicissitudes of Individuation*. New York: International Universities Press.

Main, Thomas F. 1957. The ailment. *British Journal of Medical Psychology* 30: 129–145.

Maranhão, Tullio. 1984. Family therapy and anthropology. *Culture, Medicine and Psychiatry* 8: 255–279.

Martin, Clarence J. 1981. Address to the Pennsylvania Psychological Association, June 19. *Behavior Today* 12(27): 5–8.

Martin, Emily. 1987. *The Woman in the Body: A Cultural Analysis of Reproduction*. Boston: Beacon Press.

Masterson, James F. 1983. *Countertransference and Psychotherapeutic Technique*. New York: Brunner/Mazel.

———. 1985. *The Real Self*. New York: Brunner/Mazel.

May, William F. 1983. *The Physician's Covenant: Images of the Healer in Medical Ethics*. Philadelphia: Westminster Press.

McGoldrick, Monica, and Randy Gerson. 1985. *Genograms in Family Assessment*. New York: Norton.

McLuhan, Marshall. 1967. *The Mechanical Bride: Folklore of Industrial Man*. Boston: Beacon Press.

Mead, Margaret. 1947. The concept of culture and the psychosomatic approach. *Psychiatry* 10: 57–76.

Mechanic, David. 1968. *Medical Sociology: A Selective View*. New York: Free Press.

Mengel, Mark B. 1985. Collaboration with family therapists: Dealing with physician's family of origin issues. *Working Together* 1: 10–11.

———. 1987. Physician ineffectiveness due to family-of-origin issues. *Family Systems Medicine* 5(2): 176–190.

Menninger, Karl A. 1957. Psychological factors in the choice of medicine as a profession. *Bulletin of the Menninger Clinic* 21: 51.

Miller, Alice. 1981. *The Drama of the Gifted Child*. New York: Basic Books.

Mishler, Elliot G. 1981. *Social Contexts of Health, Illness, and Patient Care*. New York: Cambridge University Press.

Mitscherlich, Alexander, and Margarete Mitscherlich. 1967. *The Inability to Mourn*. New York: Grove Press, 1975.

Mold, James W. 1988. Stroke. Presentation at the Enid Family Medicine Clinic Residency Training Program, Enid, Oklahoma, July 29.

Mold, James W., and Howard F. Stein. 1986. The cascade effect in the clinical care of patients. *New England Journal of Medicine* 314(8): 512–514.

Montville, Joseph V. In press. Psychoanalytic enlightenment and the greening of diplomacy. *Journal of the American Psychoanalytic Association*.

Morantz, Regina M. 1983. Review of *Crusaders for Fitness: The History of American Health Reformers*, by J. C. Wharton. *Science* 219: 381–382.

Morgan, Robert F., ed. 1983. *The Iatrogenics Handbook*. Toronto: IPI Pub.

Morley, Peter C. 1988. From holistic anthropology to holistic health: A personal odyssey. *High Plains Applied Anthropologist* 8(2): 12–28.

Moses, Rafael. 1985. Empathy and dis-empathy in political conflict. *Political Psychology* 6(1): 135–139.

Muensterberger, Warner. 1970. On the biopsychological determinants of social life. In *Man and His Culture*, edited by W. Muensterberger, pp. 81–99. New York: Taplinger.

Mumford, Lewis. 1971. *Technics and Human Development: The Myth of the Machine*. New York: Harcourt Brace Jovanovich.

Munroe, Ruth H., Robert Munroe, and John Whiting. 1981. Male sex-role resolutions. In *Handbook of Cross-Cultural Human Development*, edited by R. Munroe, R. Munroe, and B. Whiting, pp. 611–632. New York: Garland STPM Press.

Munson, Ronald. 1981. Why medicine cannot be a science. *Journal of Medicine and Philosophy* 6: 183–208.

Nedelmann, Carl. 1986. A psychoanalytical view of the nuclear threat—from the angle of the German sense of political inferiority. *Psychoanalytic Inquiry* 6(2): 287–302.

Nelson, Marie Coleman, ed. 1977. *The Narcissistic Condition*. New York: Human Sciences Press.

Nichter, Mark. 1981. Idioms of distress: Alternatives in the expression of psychosocial distress: A case study from South India. *Culture, Medicine and Psychiatry* 5: 379–408.

Nichter, Mark, Gordon Trockman, and Jean Grippen. 1985. Clinical anthropologist as therapy facilitator: Role development and clinician evaluation in a psychiatric training program. *Human Organization* 44(1): 72–81.

Nolen, William A. 1987. Medical zealots. *The American Scholar* 56(1): 45–56.

Nosal, Roger A. 1987. Reviews of *Manipulation, Traction, and Massage*, edited by J. F. Basmajina, and *Chiropractic Spinography: A Manual of Technology and Interpretation*, by R. W. Hildebrandt. *Family Medicine* 19(3): 237.

Nurnberg, George H., and Leon M. Shapiro. 1983. The central organizing fantasy. *The Psychoanalytic Review* 70(4): 493–503.

Ober, K. Patrick. 1987. Uncle Remus and the cascade effect in clinical medicine: Brer Rabbit kicks the Tar-Baby. *American Journal of Medicine* 82: 1009–1013.

Obeyesekere, Gananath. 1981. *Medusa's Hair: An Essay on Personal Symbols and Religious Experience*. Chicago: University of Chicago Press.

Ohnuki-Tierney, Emiko. 1984. *Illness and Culture in Contemporary Japan: An Anthropological View*. Cambridge: Cambridge University Press.

Opler, Marvin. 1957. Schizophrenia and culture. *Scientific American* 197: 103–110.

Parin, Paul. 1988. The ego and the mechanism of adaptation. In *The Psychoanalytic Study of Society*, edited by L. B. Boyer and S. A. Grolnick, vol. 12, pp. 97–130. Hillsdale, NJ: Analytic Press.

Paris, Joel. 1988. Abstract/review of Littlewood and Lipsedge. *Transcultural Psychiatric Research Review* 25(2): 107–109.

Parker, Beulah. 1962. *My Language Is Me: Psychotherapy with a Disturbed Adolescent*. New York: Basic Books.

Parry, Katherine K. 1984. Concepts from medical anthropology for clinicians. *Physical Therapy* 64(6): 929–933.

Parsons, Talcott. 1951. *The Social System*. Glencoe, IL: Free Press.

Pattison, E. Mansell. 1984. The holocaust as sin: Requirements in psychoanalytic theory for human evil and mature morality. In *Psychoanalytic Reflections on the Holocaust: Selected Essays*, edited by S. A. Luel and P. Marcus, pp. 71–91. New York: Holocaust Awareness Institute, Center for Judaic Studies, University of Denver, and Ktav Publishing House.

Paul, Robert A. 1978. Instinctive aggression in man: The Semai case. *Journal of Psychological Anthropology* 1(1): 65–79.

______. 1988. Response to Robarchek and Dentan. *American Anthropologist* 90(2): 418–420.

Payer, Lynn. 1988. *Medicine and Culture: Varieties of Treatment in the United States, England, West Germany, and France*. New York: Henry Holt.

Pendagast, Eileen G., and Charles O. Sherman. 1977. A guide to the genogram family systems training. *The Family* 5(1): 3–14.

Phares, E. Jerry. 1979. *Clinical Psychology*. Homewood, IL: Dorsey Press.

Phillips, Michael R. 1985. Can "clinically applied anthropology" survive in medical care settings? *Medical Anthropology Quarterly* 16(2): 31–36.

Pollitt, Katha. 1982. The politically correct body. *Mother Jones* (May): 66–67.

Powell, Thomas J. 1987. *Self-Help Organizations and Professional Practice*. Silver Springs, MD: National Association of Social Workers.

Prince, Raymond. 1985. The concept of culture-bound syndromes: Anorexia nervosa and brain-fag. *Social Science and Medicine* 21(2): 197–203.

______. 1987. Review of *Holy Anorexia*, by Rudolph Bell. *Journal of Psychoanalytic Anthropology* 10(3): 301–305.

Prince, Raymond, and Francoise Tcheng-Laroche. 1987. Culture-bound syndromes and international disease classifications. *Culture, Medicine and Psychiatry* 11(1): 19; plus comments by R. C. Simons, B. Beiser, M. Lock, R. L. Kapur, and A. Kleinman, pp. 21–52.

Quill, Timothy E. 1983. Partnerships in patient care: A contractual approach. *Annals of Internal Medicine* 98: 228–234.

Reed, J. D. 1981. The fitness craze: America shapes up. *Time* (2 November): 94–106.

Reich, Annie. 1951. On counter-transference. *International Journal of Psychoanalysis* 32: 25–31.

Reiser, Stanley, J. 1978. *Medicine and the Reign of Technology*. New York: Cambridge University Press.

Richards, Audrey Isabel. 1956. *Chisungu: A Girl's Initiation Ceremony Among the Bemba*. London: Faber and Faber.

Ritzer, George. 1987. Beyond "McDoctors": The McDonaldization of American medicine. Unpublished manuscript.

Ritzer, George, and David Walczak. 1986. The changing nature of American medicine. *Journal of American Culture* 9(4): 43–51.

______. 1987. Rationalization and the deprofessionalization of physicians. Unpublished manuscript.

Rochlin, Gregory. 1973. *Man's Aggression: The Defense of the Self*. Boston: Gambit.

Rodnick, Jonathan E. 1987. Family medicine: A retrospective view. *STFM Research News* 2(5): 3, 5.

Roemer, Milton I. 1986. *An Introduction to the U.S. Health Care System*. New York: Springer.

Róheim, Geza. 1943. *The Origin and Function of Culture*. Nervous and Mental Disease Monographs, no. 69. New York: Nervous and Mental Disease Pubs.

Rosenstock, Irwin M. 1960. What research in motivation suggests for public health. *American Journal of Public Health* 50: 295–302.

Rubenstein, Richard. 1978. *The Cunning of History*. New York: Harper & Row.

Rubinstein, Roberta A., and Ronald T. Brown. 1984. An evaluation of the validity of the diagnostic category of attention deficit disorder. *American Journal of Orthopsychiatry* 54(3): 398–414.

Ryan, William. 1971. *Blaming the Victim*. New York: Vintage Books.

Rycroft, Charles. 1968. *Anxiety and Neurosis*. Baltimore: Penguin.

Sammons, James H. 1988. Letter to AMA members, October 28. (Letter courtesy of James W. Mold, M.D.)

Sander, Fred M. 1979. *Individual and Family Therapy: Toward an Integration*. New York: Jason Aronson.

Sandler, Joseph, and Anne-Marie Sandler. 1978. On the development of object relationships and affects. *International Journal of Psycho-Analysis* 59: 285–296.

Saunders, Harold H. 1985. *The Other Walls: The Politics of the Arab-Israeli Peace Process*. Washington, DC: American Enterprise Institute for Policy Research.

Savitt, Todd. 1982. Graham crackers and corn flakes. Annual History of Medicine Lecture, University of Oklahoma Health Sciences Center, Oklahoma City, April 15.

Scheingold, Lee. 1988. Balint work in England: Lessons for American family medicine. *Journal of Family Practice* 26(3): 315–320.

Scheper-Hughes, Nancy, and Margaret M. Lock. 1987. The mindful body: A prolegomenon to future work in medical anthropology. *Medical Anthropology Quarterly* 1(1): 6–41.

Scheper-Hughes, Nancy, and Howard Stein. 1987. Child-abuse and the unconscious in American popular culture. In *Child Survival: Anthropological Perspectives on the Treatment and Maltreatment of Children*, edited by N. Scheper-Hughes, pp. 339–358. Boston: D. Reidel.

Schilder, Paul. 1950. *The Image and Appearance of the Human Body*. New York: International Universities Press (orig. 1923).

Schmidt, Casper G. 1984. The group-fantasy origins of AIDS. *Journal of Psychohistory* 12(1): 37–78.

Schwartzman, Helen B., Anita W. Kniefel, Linda Barbera-Stein, and Eliana Gaviria. 1984. Children, families and mental health service organizations: Cultures in conflict. *Human Organization* 43(4): 297–306.

Schwartzman, John. 1975. The addict, abstinence, and the family. *American Journal of Psychiatry* 132(2): 154–157.

———. 1982. Personal communication.

———. 1986. The natural history of a drug treatment system. *Family Systems Medicine* 4(4): 344–357.

Schwartzman, John, and Peter Bokos. 1979. Methadone maintenance: The addict's family recreated. *International Journal of Family Therapy* 1(4): 338–355.

Schwenk, Thomas L. 1982. Family practice and the behavioral sciences: The need for technology. *Family Medicine* 14(5): 17–20.

Searles, Harold F. 1960. *The Nonhuman Environment in Normal Development and in Schizophrenia*. New York: International Universities Press.

———. 1965. *Collected Papers on Schizophrenia and Related Subjects*. New York: International Universities Press.

———. 1975. The patient as therapist to his analyst. In *Tactics and Techniques in Psychoanalytic Therapy: Countertransference*, edited by P. L. Giovacchini, vol. 2, pp. 95–151. New York: Jason Aronson.

Segal, Hanna. 1955. A psycho-analytical approach to aesthetics. In *New Directions in Psycho-Analysis*, edited by M. Klein, P. Heimann, and R. Money-Kyrle, pp. 384–405. New York: Basic Books.

Shapiro, Warren. 1987. The theoretical importance of pseudo-procreative symbolism. Paper presented at the Symposium on Pseudo-Procreative Symbolism, Eighty-sixth Annual Meeting of the American Anthropological Association. Chicago, Illinois, November 18-22.

———. 1988. Ritual kinship, ritual incorporation and the denial of death. *Man*(N.S.) 23: 275–297.

———. 1989. Thanatophobic man. *Anthropology Today* 5(2): 11–14 [Royal Anthropological Institute, London].

Sharpe, Ella Freeman. 1948. An examination of metaphor. In *The Psychoanalytic Reader*, edited by R. Fliess, pp. 273–286. New York: International Universities Press (orig. 1940).

Shatzman, Rochelle. 1983. Comment on Lawton's "The Myth of Altruism." *Journal of Psychohistory* 10(3): 381–387.

Shelley, Mary Wollstonecraft. 1817. *Frankenstein: Or the Modern Prometheus*. New York: Pocket Books, 1974.

Shweder Richard A., and Edmund J. Bourne. 1984. Does the concept of the person vary cross-culturally? In *Culture Theory: Essays on Mind, Self and Emotion*, edited by R. Shweder and R. LeVine, pp. 158–199. New York: Cambridge University Press.

Simons, Ronald C., and Charles C. Hughes, eds. 1985. *The Culture-Bound Syndromes: Folk Illnesses of Psychiatric and Anthropological Interest*. Boston: D. Reidel.

Smith, Nicholas A. 1981. Review of *Energy, Vulnerability, and War, Alternatives for America*, by Wilson Clark, and Jake Page. *Science* 81: 99–101.

Smith, Robert C. 1984. Teaching interviewing skills to medical students: The issue of "countertransference." *Journal of Medical Education* 59: 582–588.

———. 1986. Unrecognized responses and feelings of residents and fellows during interviews of patients. *Journal of Medical Education* 61: 982–984.

Smith, Robert C., and Howard F. Stein. 1987. A topographical model of clinical decision-making and interviewing: A heuristic for family medicine teaching. *Family Medicine* 19(5): 361–363.

Snarey, John, and Linda Son. 1986. Sex-identity development among kibbutz-born males: A test of the Whiting hypothesis. *Ethos* 14: 99–119.

———. 1987. Sex-identity development and the function of male initiation rites: Commentary on overview article "Homosexuality in Tribal Societies," by R. Endleman. *Transcultural Psychiatric Research Review* 24(1): 72–75.

Snider, Gayle, and Howard F. Stein. 1987. An approach to community assessment in medical practice. *Family Medicine* 19(3): 213–219.

Social Science and Medicine. 1985. Issue 21(2) devoted to symposium on "culture-bound syndromes."

Sontag, Susan. 1978. *Illness as Metaphor*. New York: Vintage/Random House.

Spicer, Edward H. 1971. Persistent cultural systems. *Science* 174: 795–800.

Spiegel, John. 1971. *Transactions: The Interplay Between Individual, Family, and Society*, edited by J. Papajohn. New York: Science House.

Spiro, Melford E. 1965. Religious systems as culturally constituted defense mechanism. In *Context and Meaning in Cultural Anthropology*, edited by M. E. Spiro, pp. 100–113. New York: Free Press.

———. 1979a. *Gender and Culture: Kibbutz Women Revisited*. Durham, NC: Duke University Press.

———. 1979b. Whatever happened to the id? *American Anthropologist* 81(1): 5–13.

______. 1982a. *Buddhism and Society: A Great Tradition and its Burmese Vicissitudes*, 2nd ed. Berkeley: University of California Press.

______. 1982b. Preface to the second edition. *In Buddhism and Society: A Great Tradition and its Burmese Vicissitudes*, by M. E. Spiro, 2nd ed., pp. xi–xix. Berkeley: University of California Press.

______. 1986. Cultural relativism and the future of anthropology. *Cultural Anthropology* 1(3): 259–286.

Spradley, James P. 1970. *You Owe Yourself a Drunk*. Boston: Little, Brown.

Stamm, Ira. 1987. Countertransference in hospital treatment: Basic concepts and paradigms. Paper series, no. 2. Topeka, KS: Menninger Foundation.

Starr, Paul. 1982. *The Social Transformation of American Medicine*. New York: Basic Books.

Stein, Howard F. 1974a. Freedom and interdependence: American culture and the Adlerian ideal. *Journal of Individual Psychology* 30: 145–158.

______. 1974b. Where seldom is heard a discouraging word: American nostalgia. *Columbia Forum* 3(3): 20–23.

______. 1979a. Review essay on *Illness as Metaphor*, by S. Sontag. *Journal of Psychological Anthropology* 3(1): 33–38.

______. 1979b. The salience of ethno-psychology for medical education and practice. *Social Science and Medicine* 13B: 199–210.

______. 1980a. Bowen "family systems theory"—The problem of cultural persistence, and the differentiation of self in one's culture. *The Family* 8(1): 3–12.

______. 1980b. Culture and ethnicity as group-fantasies: A psychohistoric paradigm of group identity. *Journal of Psychohistory* 8(1): 21–51.

______. 1980c. *An Ethno-Historic Study of Slovak-American Identity*. New York: Arno Press/New York Times Press.

______. 1980d. Wars and rumors of wars: A psychohistorical study of a medical culture. *Journal of Psychohistory* 7(4): 379–401.

______. 1981a. Commentary on article, "When Rational Men Fall Sick: An Inquiry into Some Assumptions Made by Medical Anthropologists," by Allan Young. *Culture, Medicine, and Psychiatry* 5(4): 363–370.

______. 1981b. Family medicine as a meta-specialty and the dangers of overdefinition. *Family Medicine* 13(3): 3–7.

______. 1982a. Adversary symbiosis and complementary group dissociation: An analysis of the U.S./U.S.S.R. conflict. *International Journal of Intercultural Relations* 6: 55–83.

______. 1982b. The annual cycle and the cultural nexus of health care behavior among Oklahoma wheat farming families. *Culture, Medicine, and Psychiatry* 6(1): 81–99.

______. 1982c. Autism and architecture—A tale of inner landscapes. *Continuing Education for the Family Physician* 16(6): 15–19.

______. 1982d. Ethanol and its discontents: Paradoxes of inebriation and sobriety in American culture. *Journal of Psychoanalytic Anthropology* 5(4): 355–377.

______. 1982e. The ethnographic mode of teaching clinical behavioral science. In *Clinically Applied Anthropology: Anthropologists in Health Science Settings*, edited by N. Chrisman and T. Maretzki, pp. 61–82. Boston: D. Reidel.

______. 1982f. "Health" and "wellness" as euphemism: The cultural context of insidious draconian health policy. *Continuing Education for the Family Physician* 16(3): 33–44.

______. 1982g. Neo-Darwinism and survival through fitness. *Journal of Psychohistory* 10(2): 163–187.

______. 1982h. Physician-patient transaction through the analysis of countertransference: A study in role relationship and unconscious meaning. *Medical Anthropology* 6(3): 165–182.

______. 1982i. Toward a life of dialogue: Therapeutic communication and the meaning of medicine. *Continuing Education for the Family Physician* 16(4): 29–45.
______. 1982j. Wellness as illusion. *Delaware Medical Journal* 54(11): 637–641.
______. 1983a. The case study method as a means of teaching significant context in family medicine. *Family Medicine* 15(5): 163–167.
______. 1983b. The influence of counter-transference upon the clinical relationship and decision-making. *Continuing Education for the Family Physician* 18(7): 625–630.
______. 1983c. Investing psyche and capital: Farming and its hidden meanings—Review essay on *Of Time and the Enterprise: North American Family Farm Management in a Context of Resource Marginality*, by John W. Bennett. *Journal of Psychoanalytic Anthropology* 6(1): 91–98.
______. 1983d. Psychoanalytic anthropology and the meaning of meaning. In *Sociogenesis of Language and Human Conduct*, edited by B. Bain, pp. 393–414. New York: Plenum.
______. 1984. A note on patron-client theory. *Ethos* 12(1): 30–36.
______. 1985a. Alcoholism as metaphor in American culture: Ritual desecration as social integration. *Ethos* 13(3): 195–235.
______. 1985b. Comment on article, "The American game of 'smear the queer' and the homosexual component of male competitive sport and warfare," by Alan Dundes. *Journal of Psychoanalytic Anthropology* 8(3): 131–134.
______. 1985c. The culture of the patient as red herring in clinical decision making. *Medical Anthropology Quarterly* 17(1): 2–5.
______. 1985d. In pursuit of maturity in the clinical relationship—Review essay on *The Silent World of Doctor and Patient*, by J. Katz. *Family Systems Medicine* 3: 486–491.
______. 1985e. Portrait of a young physician. *The American Scholar* 54(4): 485–499.
______. 1985f. *The Psychoanthropology of American Culture.* New York: Psychohistory Press.
______. 1985g. *The Psychodynamics of Medical Practice: Unconscious Factors in Patient Care.* Berkeley: University of California Press.
______. 1985h. Psychological complementarity in Soviet-American relations. *Political Psychology* 6(2): 249–261.
______. 1985i. Wars and rumors of wars: A psychohistorical study of a medical culture. In *The Psychoanthropology of American Culture*, by H. F. Stein, pp. 107–127. New York: Psychohistory Press.
______. 1986a. "The bomb drops in 1 1/2 hours": A medical case conference as pedagogical ritual and the compulsion to repeat. *Journal of Psychoanalytic Anthropology* 9(1): 55–66.
______. 1986b. The influence of psycho-geography upon the conduct of international relations: Clinical and meta-psychological considerations. *Psychoanalytic Inquiry* 6(2): 193–222.
______. 1986c. "Sick people" and "trolls": A contribution to the understanding of the dynamics of physician explanatory models. *Culture, Medicine and Psychiatry* 10(3): 221–229.
______. 1987a. The annual cycle and the cultural nexus of health care behavior among Oklahoma wheat farming families. In *From Metaphor to Meaning: Papers in Psychoanalytic Anthropology*, by H. F. Stein and M. Apprey, pp. 156–177. Charlottesville: University Press of Virginia.
______. 1987b. *Developmental Time, Cultural Space: Studies in Psychogeography.* Norman: University of Oklahoma Press.
______. 1987c. Farmer and cowboy: The duality of the midwestern male ethos—A study in ethnicity, regionalism, and national identity. In *From Metaphor to Meaning: Papers*

in Psychoanalytic Anthropology, by H. F. Stein, and M. Apprey, pp. 178–227. Charlottesville: University Press of Virginia.

———. 1987d. Polarities in the identity of family medicine: A psychocultural analysis. In *Family Medicine: The Maturing of a Discipline*, edited by W. Doherty, C. E. Christianson, and M. B. Sussman, pp. 211–233. New York: Haworth Press.

———. 1988. Family diseases and family history. *Family Medicine* 21(1): 13–15.

Stein, Howard F., and Maurice Apprey. 1985. *Context and Dynamics in Clinical Knowledge*. Charlottesville: University Press of Virginia.

———. 1987. *From Metaphor to Meaning: Papers in Psychoanalytic Anthropology*. Charlottesville: University Press of Virginia.

———. 1990. *Clinical Stories and Their Translations*. Charlottesville: University Press of Virginia.

Stein, Howard F., and Daniel P. Fox. 1985. Work as family: Occupational relationships and social transference. In *Context and Dynamics in Clinical Knowledge*, by H. F. Stein, and M. Apprey, pp. 182–197. Charlottesville: University Press of Virginia.

Stein, Howard F., and Robert F. Hill. 1977. *The Ethnic Imperative: Examining the New White Ethnic Movement*. University Park: Pennsylvania State University Press.

———. 1984. American medicine and the enchanted machine. *Continuing Education for the Family Physician* 19(8): 428–430.

———. 1986. We buy what we are: The commercial use of American cultural metaphors in medicine and business. *High Plains Applied Anthropologist* 6(1): 18–20.

Stein, Howard F., and Soughik Kayzakian-Rowe. 1978. Hypertension, biofeedback, and the myth of the machine: A psychoanalytic-cultural study. *Psychoanalysis and Contemporary Thought* 1(1): 119–156.

Stein, Howard F., and James W. Mold. 1988. Stress, anxiety, and cascades in clinical decision-making. *Stress Medicine* 4(1): 41–48.

Stein, Howard F., and James Michael Pontious. 1985. Family and beyond: The larger context of non-compliance. *Family Systems Medicine* 3(2): 179–189.

Stephens, G. Gayle. 1984a. Five aspects of the healer. *Continuing Education for the Family Physician* 19(12): 663–666.

———. 1984b. The medical supermarket: Futuristic or decadent? *Continuing Education for the Family Physician* 19(5): 243–245.

———. 1984c. The medical supermarket: Futuristic or decadent? Part II. *Continuing Education for the Family Physician* 19(11): 600–610.

———. 1984d. Personal communication, March 20.

———. 1985. Why can't we avoid the horror of dying? Presentation for Alabama Gerontological Society Geriatric Intensive, Birmingham, February 22.

———. 1988a. At the graduation of family practice residents: Seeing over one's shoulder, and out of the corner of one's eye. Unpublished manuscript presented in Bellevill, Illinois, and Birmingham, Alabama.

———. 1988b. Confessions of a post-Flexnerian physician. In *The Task of Medicine: Dialogue at Wickenburg*, by Kerr L. White, pp. 172–189. Menlo Park, CA: Henry J. Kaiser Family Foundation.

Stierlin, Helm. 1972. Family dynamics and separation patterns of potential schizophrenics. In *Proceedings of the Fourth International Symposium on Psychotherapy of Schizophrenia*, edited by D. Rubinstein and Y. O. Alanen, pp. 169–179. Amsterdam: Excerpta Medica.

———. 1973. The adolescent as delegate of his parents. *Australian and New Zealand Journal of Psychiatry* 7: 249–256.

———. 1974. *Separating Parents and Adolescents: A Perspective on Running Away, Schizophrenia, and Waywardness*. New York: Times Books.

______. 1976. *Adolf Hitler: A Family Perspective.* New York: Psychohistory Press.
Stoller, Robert J. 1985. *Observing the Erotic Imagination.* New Haven, CT: Yale University Press.
Strupp, Hans H., and Allen E. Bergin. 1969. Some empirical and conceptual bases for coordinated research in psychotherapy: A critical review of issues, trends, and evidence. *International Journal of Psychiatry* 7: 18–90.
Szasz, Thomas S., and Marc H. Hollender. 1975. A contribution to the philosophy of medicine: The basic models of the doctor-patient relationship. In *Medical Behavioral Science,* edited by T. Millon, pp.432–440. Philadelphia: W. B. Saunders.
Tähkä, Veikko. 1984. *The Patient-Doctor Relationship.* Boston: ADIS Health Science Press.
Tassel, Janet. 1985. Gunther Schuller: Composer, conductor and musical conscience. *Ovation* 6(10): 23–26.
Tausk, Viktor. 1948. On the origin of the "influencing machine" in schizophrenia (orig. 1919). In *The Psychoanalytic Reader: An Anthology of Essential Papers with Critical Introductions,* edited by R. Fliess, pp. 31–64. New York: International Universities Press.
Taylor, Frederick Winslow. 1911. *The Principles of Scientific Management.* New York: Harper.
Thomas, Lewis. 1983. *Late Night Thoughts on Listening to Mahler's Ninth Symphony.* New York: Viking Press.
______. 1984. Cancer risk: Less than we fear. *Reader's Digest* 124: 142–143.
Trautman, Joanne, and Carol Pollard. 1975. *Literature and Medicine.* Philadelphia: Society for Health and Human Values.
Trostle, James A., W. Allen Hauser, and Ida S. Susser. 1983. The logic of noncompliance: Management of epilepsy from the patient's point of view. *Culture, Medicine and Psychiatry* 7: 35–56.
Turkle, Sherry. 1984. *The Second Self: Computers and the Human Spirit.* Greenville, NC: S. and S. Publishers.
Turner, Victor. 1967. *The Forest of Symbols.* Ithaca, NY: Cornell University Press.
______. 1969. *The Ritual Process: Structure and Anti-Structure.* Chicago: Aldine.
Tuzin, Donald F. 1977. Reflections of being in Arapesh water symbolism. *Ethos* 5(2): 195–223.
______. 1980. *The Voice of the Tambaran: Truth and Illusion in Ilahita Arapesh Religion.* Berkeley: University of California Press.
U.S. Government. 1979. *Healthy People: The Surgeon General's Report on Health Promotion and Disease Prevention; and Background Papers,* 2 vols. Washington, DC: U.S. Dept. of Health, Education, and Welfare/Public Health Service.
U.S. News & World Report. 1982. "America's Fitness Binge," May 3.
Uzzell, Douglas. 1974. Susto revisited: Illness as strategic role. *American Ethnologist* 1(2): 369–378.
Van Gennep, Arnold. 1908. *The Rites of Passage.* Chicago: University of Chicago Press, 1960.
Vogel, Albert V. 1981. Placebo and the physician-patient relationship. *Colloquy* (October): 4–8.
Volkan, Vamık D. 1976. *Primitive Internalized Object Relations.* New York: International Universities Press.
______. 1979. *Cyprus—War and Adaptation: A Psychoanalytic History of Two Ethnic Groups in Conflict.* Charlottesville: University Press of Virginia.
______. 1984. Psychological formulations developed at the conferences on the Middle East. Unpublished manuscript. Quoted with permission.

———. 1986. Nuclear weapons and the need to have enemies: A psychoanalytic perspective. Presented at the Symposium, "Psychoanalytic Explorations of the Nuclear Threat: Aggression, Projection and Identity," sponsored by the Boston Psychoanalytic Society and Institute, Boston, Massachusetts, March 22.

———. 1987. Psychological concepts useful in the building of political foundations between nations: Track II diplomacy. *Journal of the American Psychoanalytic Association* 35(4): 903–935.

———. 1988. *The Need to Have Enemies and Allies: From Clinical Practice to International Relations*. New York: Jason Aronson.

Volkan, Vamık D., and David R. Hawkins. 1971. A field-work case in the teaching of clinical psychiatry. *Psychiatry in Medicine* 2: 160–176.

———. 1972. The learning group. *American Journal of Psychiatry* 128: 1121–1126.

von Mering, Otto. 1961. Healing experience and disease causation. In *Family Centered Social Work in Illness and Disability: A Preventive Approach*, pp. 51–67. Silver Spring, MD: National Association of Social Workers.

———. 1970. Medicine and psychiatry. In *Anthropology and the Behavioral and Health Sciences*, edited by O. von Mering and L. Kasdan, pp. 272–306. Pittsburgh: University of Pittsburgh Press.

Wallace, Anthony F.C. 1961. *Culture and Personality*. New York: Random House.

———. 1966. *Religion: An Anthropological View*. New York: Random House.

Wallerstein, Robert S. 1986. The transformation of thought that the nuclear age requires: Can we achieve it? *Psychoanalytic Inquiry* 6(2): 303–312.

Watzlawick, Paul, Janet H. Beavin, and Don D. Jackson. 1967. *Pragmatics of Human Communication*. New York: Norton.

Watzlawick, Paul, John Weakland, and Richard Fisch. 1974. *Change: Principles of Problem Formation and Problem Resolution*. New York: Norton.

Waxler, Nancy E. 1981. The social labeling perspective on illness. In *The Relevance of Social Science for Medicine*, edited by L. Eisenberg, and A. Kleinman, pp. 283–306. Boston: D. Reidel.

Weidman, Hazel H., and Janice A. Egeland. 1973. A behavioral science perspective in the comparative approach to the delivery of health care. *Social Science and Medicine* 7: 845–860.

Weisman, Avery D., and Robert K. Kastenbaum. 1968. *The Psychological Autopsy*. New York: Human Sciences Press.

Weppner, Robert S. 1973. An anthropological view of the street addict's world. *Human Organization* 32(2): 111–121.

Wharton, James C. 1982. *Crusaders for Fitness: The History of American Health Reformers*. Princeton, NJ: Princeton University Press.

White, Leslie A., ed. 1949. *The Science of Culture*. New York: Farrar Straus and Cudahy.

Whitehead, Alfred North. 1925. *Science and the Modern World*. New York: Macmillan.

———. 1926. *Religions in the Making*. New York: Macmillan, 1965.

Whiting, John W. M. 1960. Resource mediation and learning by identification. In *Personality Development in Children*, edited by I. Iscoe and M. Stevenson, pp. 112–126. Austin: University of Texas Press.

Whiting, John W. M., R. Kluckhohn, and A. Anthony. 1958. The function of male initiation ceremonies at puberty. In *Readings in Social Psychology*, edited by E. Maccoby, T. Newcomb, and E. Hartley, pp. 359–370. New York: Wiley.

Wilkinson, Rupert. 1984. *American Tough: The Tough-Guy Tradition and American Character*. Westport, CT: Greenwood Press.

Worsley, Peter. 1982. Non-Western medical systems. *Annual Review of Anthropology* 11: 315–348.

Wright, Ann L. 1987. Thorns in the flesh: "Problem patients" and the struggle for control. Presentation at the Eighty-sixth Annual Meeting of the American Anthropological Association, Chicago, Illinois, November 19.

Wylie, Philip. 1979. *A Generation of Vipers*. Marietta, GA: Larlin, (orig. 1979).

Wynne, Lymon C. 1965. Some indications and contraindications for exploratory family therapy. In *Intensive Family Therapy: Theoretical and Practical Aspects by 15 Authors*, edited by I. Boszormenyi-Nagy, and J. L. Framo, pp. 289–322. Hagerstown, MD: Harper & Row.

Yap, Pow Meng. 1969. The culture-bound reactive syndromes. In *Mental Health Research in Asia and the Pacific*, edited by W. Caudill and T. Y. Lin, pp. 33–53. Honolulu: East-West Center.

Yates, Alayne, Kevin Leehey, and Catherine M. Shisslak. 1983. Running—An analogue of anorexia? *New England Journal of Medicine* 308(5): 251–255.

Young, Allan. 1976. Internalizing and externalizing medical belief systems: An Ethiopian example. *Social Science and Medicine* 10(3/4): 147–156.

Zborowski, Mark. 1969. *People in Pain*. San Francisco: Jossey-Bass.

Zola, Irving Kenneth. 1972. Studying the decision to see a doctor. In *Advances in Psychosomatic Medicine* 8: 216–236.

INDEX